MW00843691

ADHD in Preschool Children

ADHD in Preschool Children

ASSESSMENT AND TREATMENT

EDITORS

JASWINDER K. GHUMAN, M.D.

Associate Professor of Psychiatry & Pediatrics
Director, Infant and Preschool Program
The University of Arizona College of Medicine

HARINDER S. GHUMAN, M.D.

Professor of Psychiatry & Pediatrics
Director, Child & Adolescent Psychiatry
The University of Arizona College of Medicine

FOREWORD BY

LAURENCE L. GREENHILL, M.D.

Ruane Professor of Clinical Psychiatry, Columbia University
Director, Research Unit of Pediatric
Psychopharmacology–Psychosocial Intervention
New York State Psychiatric Institute
AACAP President 2009–2011

OXFORD
UNIVERSITY PRESS

OXFORD
UNIVERSITY PRESS

Oxford University Press is a department of the University of
Oxford. It furthers the University's objective of excellence in research,
scholarship, and education by publishing worldwide.

Oxford   New York
Auckland   Cape Town   Dar es Salaam   Hong Kong   Karachi
Kuala Lumpur   Madrid   Melbourne   Mexico City   Nairobi
New Delhi   Shanghai   Taipei   Toronto

With offices in
Argentina   Austria   Brazil   Chile   Czech Republic   France   Greece
Guatemala   Hungary   Italy   Japan   Poland   Portugal   Singapore
South Korea   Switzerland   Thailand   Turkey   Ukraine   Vietnam

Oxford is a registered trademark of Oxford University Press
in the UK and certain other countries.

Published in the United States of America by
Oxford University Press
198 Madison Avenue, New York, NY 10016

© Oxford University Press 2014

All rights reserved. No part of this publication may be reproduced, stored in
a retrieval system, or transmitted, in any form or by any means, without the prior
permission in writing of Oxford University Press, or as expressly permitted by law,
by license, or under terms agreed with the appropriate reproduction rights organization.
Inquiries concerning reproduction outside the scope of the above should be sent to the
Rights Department, Oxford University Press, at the address above.

You must not circulate this work in any other form
and you must impose this same condition on any acquirer.

Library of Congress Cataloging-in-Publication Data
ADHD in preschool children : assessment and treatment / editors, Jaswinder K. Ghuman,
Harinder S. Ghuman.
    p. ; cm.
Includes bibliographical references.
ISBN 978–0–19–994892–5 (alk paper)
I. Ghuman, Jaswinder K., editor of compilation.   II. Ghuman, Harinder S., editor of compilation.
[DNLM: 1. Attention Deficit Disorder with Hyperactivity—diagnosis.   2. Attention Deficit Disorder
with Hyperactivity—therapy.   3. Child, Preschool. WS 350.8.A8]
RJ506.H9
618.92′8589—dc23   2013026894

9 8 7 6 5 4 3 2 1
Printed in the United States of America
on acid-free paper

This book is dedicated to all the children and their parents and the clinicians who deal with mental health issues in preschool children. The clinicians include trainees who are in the process of learning as well as the experienced mental health professionals who are open to learning.

To the memory of our parents for their love, care, and encouragement.

To our children, Avniel and Sapna, for their love and support, and our grandchildren, Karuna and Anisha, for bringing much happiness and excitement in our lives.

Contents

Section 1.   OVERVIEW AND ASSESSMENT OF ATTENTION-DEFICIT/HYPERACTIVITY DISORDER IN PRESCHOOL CHILDREN

Section 2.   TREATMENT INTERVENTIONS

Foreword

I am not clear why, but I find that I resist edited books about attention-deficit/ hyperactivity disorder (ADHD). Jaswinder Ghuman is the great exception, and deservedly so. My initial impulse, when confronted with a book, is to see it as a long study, requiring time not set aside in a hectic life. Yet this extraordinary book commanded my attention. The more I read, the more I learned and understood about preschoolers with ADHD. This extraordinary book more than justified the time I spent enjoying its contents.

Much of my pleasure in reading this volume came from my early involvement in the new field of preschool ADHD back in 1998, some 15 years ago. At that time, I had accompanied James Swanson, Ph.D., Professor of Psychiatry and Pediatrics at the University of California at Irvine, and Benedetto Vitiello, Director of NIMH's Child and Adolescent Treatment and Preventive Intervention Research Branch, to meet with Paul Leber, M.D., then the Director, Division of Neuropharmacological Drug Products, U.S. Food and Drug Administration. Paul Leber had a powerful reputation for brilliance, eloquence, and, at times, a difficulty suffering fools quietly. Once seated in the FDA's small but comfortable conference room, I timidly asked if Dr. Leber would listen to our recommendation for the FDA to review an anomaly in their indications for treating young children with ADHD. The lower limit of age for FDA-approved ADHD treatment with methylphenidate was 6, but it was age 3 for dextroamphetamine. Yet the published controlled data for methylphenidate for 3- to 5-year-olds with ADHD included 240 children from seven publications, whereas there was then only a single case report showing its safe use in a 3-year-old with ADHD. Dr. Leber agreed that the disparity was interesting but noted the FDA could review methylphenidate's age indication criterion only if its "innovator" (initially Ciba-Geigy, then Novartis) would agree to write a letter to the agency requesting re-review. Otherwise, Dr. Leber said, we would have to generate the data for FDA review through a multisite clinical trial.

Later, when Novartis replied that it was not interested in a review, Dr. Swanson and I, and four other investigators, submitted a grant application for a multisite study to test methylphenidate's efficacy and safety in preschoolers with ADHD. The review of this application was given extra urgency when Julie Zito's landmark study (Zito et al., 2000) was published. It revealed that the prescribing of methylphenidate to children with ADHD under age 6 had increased markedly from 1991 through 1996. Approval followed by 2000, and Dr. Jaswinder Ghuman found herself working on the NIMH Preschool ADHD Treatments Study (PATS) at its Johns Hopkins site under Dr. Mark

Riddle, principal investigator in Baltimore. The PATS study is described in Chapters 1, 3, 7, and 8 of this book.

That same year, I persuaded the Research Committee of the American Academy of Child and Adolescent Psychiatry (AACAP) to devote the topic of their Research Forum at the association's annual meeting to discussing what might be the most ethical and most fruitful scientific strategies for psychopharmacologic studies in preschoolers. Guidelines for pharmacologic studies in school-age children had just been developed and were in use, but there was no such roadmap for guiding preschoolers and their parents through the rigors of a clinical trial. One of my fondest memories was the quick agreement from the most talented researchers I then knew to attend this forum and participate in its daylong deliberations. AACAP volunteered, without being asked, to employ a court stenographer to take down the proceedings verbatim. This was a wise decision, because the attendance at the New York-based 2000 Research Forum exceeded 150, mostly child and adolescent psychiatry and psychology researchers. Decisions reached that day were published in the *Journal of the American Academy of Child and Adolescent Psychiatry* (Greenhill et al., 2003) and led to the NIMH's recommendations for study design of the PATS study as well as for its Data and Safety Monitoring Board. Other recommendations were implemented by forming a subcommittee of AACAP's Research Committee, called the Pediatric Psychopharmacology Initiative, which is the one committee of the association's that permits membership from the pharmaceutical industry and from FDA. It is still in existence and is thriving.

It is now more than 10 years later, and the rapid progress in the field of preschool ADHD studies is most evident in the richness and diversity of the book you now hold in your hands.

Laurence Greenhill, M.D., July 2013

References

Greenhill, L. L., Jensen, P. S., Abikoff, H., Blumer, J. L., Deveaugh-Geiss, J., Fisher, C., Hoagwood, K., Kratochvil, C. J., Lahey, B. B., Laughren, T., Leckman, J., Petti, T. A., Pope, K., Shaffer, D., Vitiello, B., & Zeanah, C. (2003). Developing strategies for psychopharmacological studies in preschool children. *Journal of the American Academy of Child & Adolescent Psychiatry, 42*(4), 406–414.

Zito, J. M., Safer, D. J., dosReis, S., Gardner, J. F., Boles, M., & Lynch, F. (2000). Trends in the prescribing of psychotrophic medications for preschool children. *Journal of the American Medical Association, 283*(8), 1025–1030.

Acknowledgments

We wish to acknowledge all our teachers and mentors who have provided us with the foundation in our education and work with children and inspired and encouraged us at different stages in our professional lives. We especially wish to acknowledge and thank our teachers and mentors, Drs. James Harris, Susan Folstein, Michael Aman, and Mark Riddle for JKG, and Drs. John Romano, E. James Anthony, Roy Mendelsohn, Richard Sarles, and Donald Saidel for HSG. We want to thank our colleagues, staff and trainees at the University of Arizona, Department of Psychiatry for their ongoing support to us in our daily work.

In this effort, we owe much to our esteemed contributors and express our deep appreciation and gratitude for their hard work and availability to write and revise and share their expertise. We also appreciate Dr. Eugene Arnold's guidance and input for the chapter on complementary and alternative treatments. We owe a special debt of gratitude to our publishers at the Oxford University Press for patience and support with this project. David D'Addona, Associate Editor, Psychiatry, Oxford University Press, Meredith Keller, Editorial Assistant, Oxford University Press, Prasad Tangudu, Project Manager, Newgen Knowledge Works Pvt Ltd., and Wendy Walker have provided us with great deal of encouragement and direction in moving this project along.

We are most grateful to our friends and family, especially our children, Avniel and Sapna, and grandchildren, Karuna and Anisha, for their love and affection.

Contributors

Regina Bussing, M.D., M.S.H.S.
Professor of Psychiatry
Division of Child and Adolescent
　Psychiatry
Department of Psychiatry
University of Florida, Gainesville, FL

Harinder S. Ghuman, M.D.
Professor of Psychiatry and Pediatrics
Director, Child and Adolescent
　Psychiatry
Department of Psychiatry
University of Arizona College of
　Medicine, Tucson, AZ

Jaswinder K. Ghuman, M.D.
Associate Professor of Psychiatry and
　Pediatrics
Director, Infant and Preschool Clinic
Department of Psychiatry
University of Arizona College of
　Medicine, Tucson, AZ

Elizabeth Hurt, Ph.D.
Postdoctoral Researcher
Nisonger Center
The Ohio State University,
　Columbus, OH

Nicholas Lofthouse, Ph.D.
Clinical Assistant Professor of
　Psychiatry
Child and Adolescent Psychiatry
Department of Psychiatry
The Ohio State University College of
　Medicine, Columbus, OH

E. Mark Mahone, Ph.D., ABPP
Director of Neuropsychology, Kennedy
　Krieger Institute
Professor of Psychiatry and Behavioral
　Sciences
Johns Hopkins University School of
　Medicine, Baltimore, MD

William N. Marshall, Jr., M.D.
Professor of Clinical Pediatrics,
　Department of Pediatrics
University of Arizona College of
　Medicine, Tucson, AZ

Desiree W. Murray, Ph.D.
Associate Professor
Social Science Research Institute
Department of Psychiatry/
　Medical Center
Duke University, Durham, NC

Alison E. Pritchard, Ph.D., ABPP
Program Director, Neuropsychology
    Research Lab
Kennedy Krieger Institute
Instructor in Psychiatry
Johns Hopkins University School of
    Medicine, Baltimore, MD

Jamila Reid, Ph.D.
Clinical Psychologist
University of Washington
Seattle, WA

Sydney A. Rice, M.D.
Associate Professor of Pediatrics
Department of Pediatrics
University of Arizona College of
    Medicine, Tucson, AZ

Mark Stein, Ph.D., ABPP
Professor of Psychiatry and Pediatrics
Institute of Juvenile Research
University of Illinois, Chicago, IL

Carolyn Webster- Stratton, M.P. H., Ph.D.
Professor Emeritus, University of
    Washington
Founding Director, the
    Parenting Clinic
University of Washington School of
    Nursing, Seattle, WA

Margaret D. Weiss, M.D., Ph.D., FRCP
Clinical Professor of Psychiatry
University of British Columbia
West Vancouver, British
    Columbia, Canada

Introduction

Attention-deficit/hyperactivity disorder (ADHD) in preschool children is a common, chronic, and impairing disorder. Preschoolers with untreated ADHD are at risk for persistent impairment through the school years and beyond, resulting in considerable stress for the entire family and a staggering socioeconomic burden to schools and society at large. In the clinical practice of child and adolescent psychiatry, psychology, and primary healthcare, ADHD is one of the most commonly diagnosed and treated mental health disorders. Despite extensive research on various aspects of diagnosis and treatment interventions in ADHD, there is much controversy regarding the validity of ADHD diagnosis, especially in young children, underdiagnosis and undertreatment versus overdiagnosis and overtreatment, and the efficacy and safety of treatment interventions, especially pharmacologic interventions in preschool children.

Preschoolers are increasingly being referred for evaluation and treatment of ADHD symptoms. There is a limited pool of experienced clinicians with expertise in working with young children with behavior problems. Our objective in writing this book is to provide information to clinicians regarding essentials of assessment and treatment interventions in preschool children with ADHD.

This book is intended to provide a guide to more experienced child and adolescent mental health and primary healthcare practitioners, as well as trainees in child and adolescent psychiatry, psychology, pediatrics, social work, mental health, and nursing who evaluate and treat preschool children with ADHD. Due to both the increased emphasis and controversy regarding mental health issues, especially ADHD in preschool children, we believe this book will be helpful to both national and international mental health professionals working with very young children and their families.

Overview

The impetus to provide early diagnosis and treatment to very young children with ADHD has largely been driven by increased understanding of concerns regarding the deleterious short- and long-term effects of untreated ADHD and emerging consensus regarding the efficacy of early interventions. Assessing and treating preschool children with ADHD is complicated by the normal developmental variation during early years and the impact of environmental factors and comorbid disorders. This book is intended to provide updated information to our readers regarding assessment, diagnosis, differential diagnosis and comorbid disorders, and treatment interventions in a clinical context as it pertains to preschool children. To this end, the book is divided in two sections. The first section provides an overview and assessment of ADHD in preschool children.

In Chapter 1, J. and H. Ghuman provide a brief history of the concept of modern-day ADHD terminology and nomenclature and possible underlying causes and interventions noted in the medical literature as it evolved over the last two to three centuries. Although the majority of the past literature is focused on older children, there are accounts of behavior problems in preschool children that are very similar to the present-day descriptions of ADHD. Past symptom focus varied in emphasis on either overactivity/hyperactivity or inattention being the core feature of ADHD. It is only recently that both inattention and hyperactivity symptoms were included as part of one disorder. However there continues to be a debate whether attention-deficit disorder (ADD) and ADHD are two separate and distinct disorders. Next, recent epidemiologic information on the prevalence of ADHD in preschool children is provided, followed by a summary of the etiology of ADHD, including genetics, pathophysiology, and environmental factors. Most of the information in the literature on ADHD etiology is derived from studies conducted in older children, adolescents and adults. A comprehensive discussion of developmental issues and temperamental influences is presented along with diagnostic challenges in evaluating preschool children with ADHD. A case example highlights the importance of giving careful consideration to behavioral, interactional, and relational contexts while assessing preschool children for ADHD. The chapter concludes with a description of the DSM-5 diagnostic criteria for ADHD along with the changes relevant to preschoolers.

Chapter 2, also by J. and H. Ghuman, addresses the evaluation process and essentials of clinical assessment of ADHD in preschoolers. An in-depth discussion of various factors and challenges that may influence data collection, history-taking, and clinical observations is presented. The American Academy of Child and Adolescent Psychiatry and the American Academy of Pediatrics practice guidelines for the assessment of ADHD in preschool children are reviewed. Specifics of the evaluation process are addressed, including information on scheduling, evaluation setting, preparing the preschooler for the assessment process, history-taking, child interview, and observation of parent–child interaction. The authors provide examples of the relevant interview topics and questions to aid in eliciting responses from preschoolers regarding ADHD and comorbid disorders symptoms. Child observation and mental status examination processes are discussed. The authors emphasize the importance of obtaining information from multiple sources, informants, settings, and contexts. A table is included with examples of complaints of caregivers of preschoolers regarding specific DSM-5 ADHD criteria. The chapter concludes with a discussion of integration of data, diagnostic and treatment plan formulation, and recommendations to parents.

Neuropsychological assessment measures can aid in clarifying the diagnosis and delineating the severity of symptoms and specific cognitive components that are affected in a preschooler. Chapter 3, by Mahone and Pritchard, addresses neuropsychological assessment of ADHD in preschool children and provides valuable insights into executive functioning deficits in preschoolers with ADHD. The authors highlight the limited availability of standardized instruments for children in this age range. Rating scales have become an essential component in the diagnostic process and monitoring of treatment outcome in preschool children with ADHD. The chapter provides a comprehensive and thoughtful review of performance-based measures, rating scales, and structured interviews that can be used with preschool children and their families. The authors conclude the chapter with a discussion of issues related to the future of neuro-psychological assessment in preschoolers in light of diagnostic changes in DSM-5.

Preschool children with ADHD are at considerable risk for comorbid disorders. There are also a number of medical and psychiatric disorders that may mimic ADHD symptoms in preschoolers. In Chapter 4, Rice and Marshall provide a primary health-care perspective in evaluating and treating preschool children with ADHD and describe pertinent issues related to early diagnosis and clinical presentation of behavior disorders including ADHD in preschoolers. A careful review of what takes place in a primary healthcare provider's office and essentials of medical assessment are presented. Rice and Marshall provide a thoughtful discussion of the need for adequate time to assess the child and the caregiver and the impact of the relationship and communication between the primary healthcare provider and the caregiver. Medical conditions and psychiatric disorders that can be comorbid with ADHD or mimic the symptoms of ADHD are reviewed, along with a discussion of how a clinician can clarify the diagnosis or diagnoses.

Section 2 of the book addresses specific treatment interventions, including psychosocial and behavioral, pharmacologic, and complementary and alternative treatments, in preschool children with ADHD. There is strong empirical support for psychosocial interventions, which are considered first-line treatments in preschoolers with ADHD, especially due to concerns about the safety and efficacy of psychopharmacologic interventions at such a young and vulnerable age. Chapters 5 and 6 describe psychosocial and behavioral interventions for preschool children with ADHD. In Chapter 5, Bussing and Murray provide an overview of psychosocial and behavioral interventions for pre-schoolers with ADHD, including background and rationale, theoretical underpinnings, and common elements of parent management training (PMT). Recent studies on evidence for PMT's efficacy are reviewed. Interventions addressing disruptive behavior in young children, combination treatments of parent and classroom interventions, and behavioral interventions directly targeting children without concurrent parent training are discussed. Bussing and Murray describe three well-established evidence-based PMT programs that have been used for preschoolers with ADHD: Parent–Child Interaction Therapy (PCIT), Incredible Years (IY) Parent Program, and Positive Parenting of Preschoolers (Triple P). A thorough discussion for one of the empirically supported parenting programs, PCIT, is provided, along with an excellent case report describing the practical application of PCIT in a clinical setting.

Using the Incredible Years interventions for young children with ADHD is the topic of Chapter 6, by Webster-Stratton and Reid. The IY treatment programs have over 25 years of research base. The authors review research on the effectiveness of these treatment programs for children with behavior problems, including preschoolers with ADHD. They offer a comprehensive discussion on how the IY Parent Program can be tailored to preschoolers with ADHD. Webster-Stratton and Reid outline ways a therapist can work with parents to improve parents' skills in coaching their children to sustain attention in play activities and strengthen emotion regulation skills, and the importance of providing immediate feedback and consequences. In addition, there is a discussion on problem solving with children and on promoting positive communication between parents and teachers. Webster-Stratton and Reid provide practical and detailed information on how to modify the children's small group training series, Dina Dinosaur's social skills, emotion, and problem-solving small group therapy, to preschoolers with ADHD. They emphasize the need for shorter circle-time lessons and more movement by including more songs, more physical activities, and more hands-on group activities to meet the developmental needs, attention span, and activity level of preschoolers with ADHD.

The next two chapters, by J. and H. Ghuman, describe psychopharmacologic interventions for preschool children with ADHD. In Chapter 7, they review prescribing trends, practice guidelines, and the role of the FDA and the impact of the Modernization Act in promoting meaningful pharmacologic research in preschool children. There is a thorough discussion of controversies, dilemmas, and challenges in prescribing medications to preschoolers. A comprehensive review and discussion of studies of various stimulant and nonstimulant pharmacologic agents used in the treatment of ADHD in preschool children is presented, along with details of dosing, efficacy, and treatment-emergent adverse events. The NIMH-funded Preschool ADHD Treatment Study (PATS) is the largest trial and is considered the landmark study for pharmacologic treatment of ADHD in preschool children, the findings of this study are described in detail. This chapter also provides helpful information on pharmacologic treatment issues in preschoolers with developmental disorders and symptoms of ADHD, and preschoolers who experience pill-swallowing difficulties.

Chapter 8 describes clinical practice for prescribing medication in preschool children with ADHD and includes a discussion of the need for medical assessment, including physical examination, laboratory workup, and an electrocardiogram. Assessment of the family's ability to safely administer and store medication is emphasized. In addition, the authors provide detailed information regarding psychoeducation of parents about the use of medication and the process for informed consent. A review of ADHD medications includes stimulants, with emphasis on relevant formulations for preschoolers, atomoxetine and alpha-2 adrenergic agonists. The authors offer a thorough discussion of medication titration and monitoring of response and adverse effects. The increased sensitivity of preschoolers to ADHD medications in comparison to older children is emphasized, and strategies to manage various adverse effects and the pros and cons of drug holidays are described. Clinical strategies for dealing with comorbid disorders that are associated with ADHD are discussed.

Caregivers often look into and may prefer complementary and alternative treatments (CATs) for their preschoolers due to concerns of adverse effects with traditional ADHD medications. Moreover, dietary and other alternative interventions are more applicable in younger children due to better parental control of children's diet and activities—yet remain controversial. In Chapter 9, Lofthouse and Hurt provide a comprehensive review of ingestible and noningestible CATs for preschoolers with ADHD. For each of the CATs, authors describe the intervention, rationale, and research evidence for its use. In addition, they apply "Sensible, Easy, Cheap, and Safe" criteria to make recommendations for use in preschoolers. The authors discuss clinical recommendations to consider when prescribing CATs to preschoolers with ADHD.

Preschool children with ADHD often experience sleep problems, which can be exacerbated due to the adverse effects of the psychopharmacologic agents used for treatment of ADHD. In Chapter 10, Stein and Weiss provide a careful and thoughtful review of sleep problems in preschoolers with ADHD. They discuss various studies pertinent to sleep problems in preschool children in general and preschoolers with ADHD. The clinical presentation of various sleep problems in preschool children is described, along with possible etiology. Guidance to primary health and mental health practitioners is provided regarding how to assess and treat preschool children with sleep problems and ADHD. Detailed information on how to monitor sleep problems and how to manage circadian issues and stimulant-induced sleep problems is presented.

Conclusion

The chapters in this volume make a strong case for careful evaluation and treatment of ADHD in preschool children. Not identifying and treating ADHD in the early years can have serious negative academic, social, and vocational consequences. Misdiagnosis and inappropriate treatment are also fraught with risk to the child's physical and emotional health and can lead to the wasting of resources, as well as mistrust of mental health professionals by parents and society. More empirical research is necessary to promote understanding of the prevalence, etiology, presentation, assessment, and treatment of ADHD in preschool children.

OVERVIEW AND ASSESSMENT OF ATTENTION-DEFICIT/HYPERACTIVITY DISORDER IN PRESCHOOL CHILDREN

1

ADHD in Preschool Children

Overview and Diagnostic Considerations

JASWINDER K. GHUMAN AND

HARINDER S. GHUMAN

Recent research efforts have focused on the etiology, treatment, and long-term outcomes of attention-deficit/hyperactivity disorder (ADHD) and extending the study of ADHD to younger children, adolescents, and adults. There has been an increased interest in studying various aspects of ADHD in preschool children, including symptomatology, diagnosis, and treatment interventions, which are emphasized throughout the book. In the first section of this chapter we provide an overview of the history, epidemiology, and etiologic considerations in ADHD. In the second part, we focus on diagnostic considerations and discuss developmental issues, diagnostic controversies, and diagnostic criteria for ADHD in preschool children.

Overview

DEFINITION AND HISTORICAL BACKGROUND

ADHD is one of the most studied, diagnosed, and treated child and adolescent psychiatric disorders. There has been a great deal of controversy regarding its diagnosis, etiology, and treatment. Over the years, as psychiatry has tried to refine the nomenclature and criteria for diagnosis, different terms have emerged in describing this disorder that encompasses a core symptom complex of overactivity, impulsivity, and inattention. Some of the past terms have included "hyperkinetic disease," "minimal brain dysfunction," "minimal brain damage," "hyperactive impulse disorder," "hyperactive child syndrome," and "hyperactive child."

Although the modern history of this disorder has been attributed to the writings of Sir George Frederick Still (1902) and Alfred Tredgold (1908), there are case reports describing children with symptoms of hyperactivity, impulsivity, and inattention as far back as the middle of the nineteenth century (Clouston, 1899; Hoffman, 1845; Maudsley, 1867). Several reviews on the history of ADHD have been published, including a recent one by Lange and colleagues (Lange, Reichl, Lange, Tucha, & Tucha, 2010). Recently, Barkley and Peters (2012) reported on the discovery of a chapter in a 1775 medical textbook by the German physician Melchior Adam Weikard on "Lack of Attention, 'Attentio Volubilis.'" This chapter describes patient characteristics ("Unwary, careless, flighty and bacchanal," "every humming fly, every shadow, every sound, the memory of old stories will draw him off task"), causes ("when children are taught a hundred things at the same time, when they are not given enough time, or when they do not get into the habit of examining things"), and treatment ("the inattentive person is to be separated from the noise or any other objects; he is to be kept in solitary, in the dark, when he is too active"). Scottish physician Alexander Crichton wrote a medical textbook on mental disorders in 1798, *An Inquiry Into The Nature and Origin of Mental Derangement*, and one of the chapters, "On Attention and its Diseases," provided a very detailed description of attention problems ("The incapacity of attending with a necessary degree of constancy to any object almost always arises from an unnatural or morbid sensibility of the nerves, by which means this faculty is incessantly withdrawn from one impression to another"), discussion of possible etiology ("It may be either born with a person or it may be the effect of accidental diseases"), treatment (" these children needed special education"), and prognosis ("and what is very fortunate, it is generally diminished with age").

In 1899, Clouston reported a series of conditions in children including "simple hyperexcitability" affecting children from age 3 years to puberty, manifested by overactivity and restlessness, and attributed this condition to an explosive condition of the nerve cells in the higher cortex. In 1902, Sir George Still, a pediatrician who is famous for his description of chronic rheumatoid arthritis in children (Still's disease), described 20 children who showed hyperactivity and an abnormal incapacity for sustained attention and displayed mischievous, destructive, and violent behavior. He reported that this behavior was evident in early school years and was seen more frequently in males. Still proposed that these behaviors were the result of some morbid physical condition that was either inherited or the result of peri- or post-natal injury to the brain. Tredgold (1908) postulated that brain damage, including birth injury or mild anoxia, could result in behavior or learning problems. He reported that a number of these children showed physical anomalies including abnormal head shape and size, soft neurologic signs, abnormalities of the palate, and poor coordination. He further proposed that criminal behavior by these children was the result of organic abnormality in the higher levels of the brain, where the sense of morality was located. There are case reports describing personality changes, emotional instability, cognitive deficits, learning difficulties, sleep reversal, poor motor control, and tics in affected children who survived the epidemic encephalitis lethargica that spread around the world from 1917 to 1928. Bender (1942) proposed the "postencephalitic behavior disorder" to be "best understood as an organic driveness of brain stem origin." In the 1930s, Kramer and Polnow described "hyperkinetic disease" commencing in the third and fourth year of life with marked restlessness and distractibility and speech problems. They distinguished it from other conditions with similar symptoms, such as postencephalitic behavior disorder.

Charles Bradley's discovery, in 1937, of the beneficial effects of Benzedrine on children's hyperactive behavior and school performance was a landmark in the history of ADHD treatment and etiologic postulation. From early on in the history of ADHD, there has been recognition of multiple etiologic factors, including biological and environmental factors, underlying the ADHD symptom complex. However, diagnostic nomenclature and treatment have often been influenced by clinicians and researchers who emphasize either biology or environment as the primary etiology underlying ADHD. Brain damage was seen as the primary etiology for ADHD from the 1930s to 1950s (Strauss & Werner, 1943), hence the term "minimal brain damage." The emphasis on ADHD etiology was later attributed to functional disturbance in the brain rather than anatomic damage, and the criticism that brain damage should not be inferred from behavior alone (Bax & MacKeith, 1963) led to a change in the terminology to "minimal brain dysfunction." Pharmacologic treatment was not widely used until the 1960s due to the prominent influence of psychoanalytical and behavioral theorists who emphasized poor parenting as the causative factor for ADHD.

In the late 1950s and 1960s, hyperactivity was emphasized as the core symptom and the terms "hyperkinetic behavior syndrome" and "hyperactive impulse disorder" were introduced (Laufer & Denhoff, 1957). Chess (1960) described 36 hyperactive children in her practice and proposed that this disorder was due to "physiological hyperactivity." This spurred a number of studies in the ensuing decade on the psychophysiology of hyperactivity. This is also reflected in the inclusion of the "Hyperkinetic Reaction of Childhood" in the second edition of the *Diagnostic and Statistical Manual of Mental Disorders* (DSM) (American Psychiatric Association [APA], 1968).

Another landmark in the history of ADHD was a shift in emphasis from hyperactivity to a deficit in the ability to sustain attention, as proposed by Douglas (1972). This shift in emphasis was reflected in the DSM-III (APA, 1980) by changing the nomenclature to "Attention-Deficit Disorder." Two subtypes were described, one with hyperactivity and one without. The condition was later conceptualized as a single entity with inattentive, hyperactive, and impulsive symptoms and was renamed as "Attention-Deficit/Hyperactivity Disorder (ADHD)" in the DSM-III-Revised (APA, 1987). Children without hyperactivity were considered to have "undifferentiated attention deficit disorder." In the DSM-IV, three ADHD subtypes were included, predominately inattentive type, predominately hyperactive-impulsive type, and combined type (APA, 1994).

The debate continues to the present day in an effort to define and refine the nomenclature. Diamond (2005) recently postulated that attention deficit disorder (ADD) and ADHD are two separate disorders that have different cognitive and behavioral profiles, comorbidities, responses to medication, and underlying neurobiologies and are not simply two subtypes of ADHD. Barkley (2003) has theorized that poor inhibition and deficient executive functioning (self-regulation) are central to the disorder.

EPIDEMIOLOGY

Studies of prevalence of ADHD in preschool children are limited in number. Varied prevalence rates of ADHD in preschool children are reported depending on whether checklists (binary vs. threshold cutoff, parent report/teacher report/both), diagnostic methods, or impairment criteria are used. Lavigne and colleagues (1996) reported on prevalence rates and correlates of psychiatric disorders in 510 children, aged 2 through 5 years, recruited from primary care clinics during their visit to the Chicago-area pediatricians. Using parent report and clinical consensus, the prevalence rate of ADHD was reported at 2% and was almost always comorbid with other disorders, especially oppositional defiant disorder (ODD).

Pineda and colleagues (1999) used a checklist to estimate the prevalence of ADHD in a general preschool population of 181 children (4 to 5 years of age) in Colombia, South America. The authors devised a scale based on the 18 DSM-IV ADHD symptoms and asked parents to rate the preschooler's behavior on a scale of 0 (never) to 3 (almost always). An overall prevalence rate of ADHD symptoms was reported at 18.2%; they were found to be more frequent in children with low socioeconomic status. The same authors recently conducted a prevalence study in a general preschool population of 104 children (4 to 5 years of age) using a semistructured diagnostic interview and several rating scales completed by parents and teachers (Pineda et al., 2003), and the prevalence rate of ADHD was found to be 7.7%.

Bhatia and colleagues (1991) conducted clinical and psychological assessments in children attending a pediatric outpatient clinic in a children's hospital in India. The prevalence rate of ADHD was 5.2% in children aged 3 to 4 years and 10% in children aged 5 to 6 years. Boys were diagnosed with ADHD more often than girls, with a male:female ratio of 5.6:1 in 3- to 4-year-olds and 7.8:1 in 5- to 6-year-olds.

Egger, Kondo, and Angold (2006) used a semistructured parent interview, Preschool Age Psychiatric Assessment (PAPA), and reported a 3.3% overall prevalence rate of ADHD in 307 preschoolers (age range 2 to 5 years) attending a pediatric clinic in the United States. Hyperactive/impulsive subtype was reported in 1.8% and combined type in 1.5%. Boys were two times more likely to meet criteria for ADHD than girls. Combined-type ADHD was more common in boys than girls, with a ratio of about 10:1.

Willoughby and colleagues (2012) conducted a prospective longitudinal parent survey to ascertain patterns of developmental changes in ADHD symptomatology in a representative sample of 1,155 children from 3 to 5 years of age living in two major areas of the United States with high poverty rates. Caregivers completed the ADHD Rating Scale (DuPaul, Power, Anastopoulos, & Reid, 1998) for their child's current ADHD behaviors at the 3-, 4-, and 5-year assessments. Caregiver ratings indicated that 8.4% of the children had persistently high levels of hyperactivity symptoms and 3.5% had increasing levels of hyperactivity symptoms from age 3 to 5 years. Stable low levels of hyperactivity symptoms were reported in 71.7% of the children, and moderate levels of hyperactivity symptoms that decreased over time were reported in 16.4% of the children. There was a significant difference in the mean number of ADHD symptoms in children in the low-stable trajectory compared to the children in the persistently high hyperactivity trajectory. At the 3-, 4-, and 5-year assessments, the respective mean numbers of ADHD (both hyperactive-impulsive and inattentive) symptoms were 12.2, 12.8, and 12.1 in the persistently elevated trajectory group and 1.8, 1.8, and 1.5 in the low-stable trajectory group. Comparable reductions were observed over time in both the hyperactive-impulsive and inattentive symptoms (Willoughby, Pek, & Greenberg, 2012).

In a community prevalence study of psychiatric disorders in preschool children born in 2003 or 2004 in Trondheim, Norway, 2,475 children aged 4 years were screened using the Strengths and Difficulties Questionnaire (SDQ) given to parents (Wichstrom et al., 2012). A screen-stratified random subsample of 995 parents also participated in a structured diagnostic interview, the PAPA. The prevalence rate for ADHD was 1.9%

(hyperactive/impulsive 1.6%, inattentive 0.2%, and combined 0.3%). Boys had ADHD more often than girls.

A recent prevalence study of ADHD symptoms was conducted in 1,403 three- to six-year-olds attending kindergarten in Tehran, Iran. A 19-item observer rating questionnaire was generated to assess ADHD symptoms, the validity of the questionnaire was established by "expert's opinion," and the score related to ADHD symptoms was based on five questions. The questionnaire was completed by both teachers and parents. Parent ratings identified 362 children (25.8%) and teacher ratings identified 239 (17%) children as having ADHD symptoms (Meysamie et al., 2011).

ETIOLOGIC CONSIDERATIONS

Genetics. ADHD often runs in families, with siblings and parents of affected children having a two- to eight-fold increase in risk for ADHD. Twin, family, and adoption studies have reported variable heritability estimates for ADHD ranging from 60% to 90% depending on the specific behavioral rating scale used. Molecular genetic studies into the etiology of ADHD are more recent and ongoing. Genome-wide association studies use single nucleotide polymorphisms (SNPs) to determine and compare allele frequencies in populations with and without a particular medical condition. Many different comparisons are made during this type of analysis, so large numbers of subjects and controls are needed to achieve statistical significance. To date, no individual SNP with the requisite statistical significance has been confirmed to be associated with ADHD. However, the use of SNPs to identify DNA duplications or deletions, referred to in the aggregate as copy number variants (CNVs), has revealed evidence of ADHD-associated CNVs, with many of the genes being involved in neurodevelopment (Elia et al., 2010; Glessner, Connolly, & Hakonarson, 2012; Stergiakouli et al., 2012; Yang et al., 2013). The available data are consistent with the hypothesis that ADHD symptoms and clinical course result from the interactions of several genes with environmental factors. According to this polygenic model, consideration of environmental factors (see below) and the mechanisms by which they trigger, maximize, or minimize psychopathology could lead to new prevention and therapeutic strategies.

Candidate gene studies have primarily focused on the dopaminergic and noradrenergic systems implicated in ADHD pathogenesis, bolstered in part by behavioral studies in mouse models with mutations in one of the genes (Russell, 2007). A number of studies have focused on the dopamine transporter gene DAT1 (*SLC6A3*) at chromosome 5p15.3, a region that, on the basis of affected sibling pairs in two independent samples, contains an ADHD risk gene (Ogdie et al., 2006), dopamine receptor genes, particularly the D4 receptor (DRD4) but also the D2, D3, and D5 receptors, and dopamine synthesis genes, including the dopamine beta-hydroxylase and tyrosine hydroxylase gene. Findings have been mixed. Results for the noradrenergic alpha-2a receptor gene and the serotonin transporter gene in ADHD have been less consistent. On the other hand, recent meta-analyses of candidate gene studies strengthened the connection between ADHD and polymorphisms in genes encoding DAT1, dopamine receptors DRD4, DRD5, 5HTT, HTR1B, and SNAP25 (Gizer et al., 2009; Wu et al., 2012).

Pathophysiology. *Neuroimaging studies.* Neuroimaging studies have focused on prefrontal cortices (important for complex and focused behavior), the basal ganglia/striatum (important for response control), the cerebellum (involved in information processing and motor control), and the corpus callosum (involved in integrating information). Neuroimaging studies show relatively smaller right prefrontal cortex volume; reduced dorsolateral prefrontal cortex volume; reduced volume of caudate and pallidum; decreased right cerebellar volume with reduced size of vermis, especially the posterior-inferior lobules; corpus callosum with smaller rostrum; and abnormalities of the posterior regions linked to temporal and parietal cortices in the splenium (Castellanos et al., 2002; Giedd et al., 2001; Seidman et al., 2005). As a group, children with ADHD show a 5% reduction in total brain volume and a 12% reduction in volume of key frontal and subcortical structures (Nigg & Nikolas, 2008). Castellanos and colleagues (2002) reported that these volumetric reductions are present early in life, are not progressive, and are unrelated to stimulant medication treatment. This suggests inherited or early acquired alterations in the brain structures as opposed to a progressive developmental process or delay.

Shaw and colleagues (2007) conducted a longitudinal magnetic resonance imaging (MRI) study and mapped out growth trajectories in cortical thickness from 824 MRI scans, obtained prospectively from 223 children with ADHD and 223 typically developing controls; the mean interval between scans was 2.8 years. They reported a 3- to 5-year delay in reaching peak cortical thickness (median age of 7.5 years in typically developing children and 10.5 years in the ADHD group) in most of the cerebral regions in the ADHD group; the delay in prefrontal regions was most noticeable.

In children with ADHD, functional MRI (fMRI) studies have shown hypoactivity in the dorsal anterior cingulate cortex, which is involved in attention, cognition, and decision making. There are altered activation patterns in the striatum, including the left caudate nucleus (Durston et al., 2003). Dickstein and colleagues (2006) reported on a meta-analysis of 16 fMRI studies of ADHD showing consistent brain activation deficits in all regions of the prefrontal cortex as well as other brain regions, suggesting abnormal functioning in the frontostriatal and frontoparietal circuitry in ADHD. In a recent meta-analysis of 55 fMRI studies of ADHD in children (39 studies) and adults (16 studies), Cortese and colleagues (2012) reported that the frontoparietal (lateral frontal pole, dorsal anterior cingulate, dorsolateral anterior prefrontal cortex, lateral cerebellum, anterior insula, and inferior parietal lobe) and the ventral attention networks (temporoparietal junction, supramarginal gyrus, frontal operculum, and anterior insula) were hypoactivated in children with ADHD relative to comparison subjects. The frontoparietal network helps goal-directed executive processes and decision-making processes by integrating external information with internal representations, whereas the ventral attention network supports attentional reorienting to salient and behaviorally relevant external stimuli (Corbetta et al. 2008). Cortese and colleagues (2012) also reported ADHD-related hyperactivation in the somatomotor and visual systems, supporting the hypothesis that persons with ADHD compensate for impaired prefrontal and anterior cingulate cortex function by overreliance on brain regions associated with visual, spatial, or motoric processing (Fassbender & Schweitzer, 2006).

Disruption of cortical asymmetry has been implicated in the pathogenesis of various neurodevelopmental disorders, including ADHD. Shaw and colleagues (2009) reported on the development of cortical asymmetry, comparing longitudinal findings from MRI scans in 358 typically developing and 218 ADHD children and adolescents. They found that in right-handed typically developing children and adolescents, the *left* orbitofrontal and inferior frontal gyrus and the *right* medial occipital region (medial aspect of superior parietal lobule and motor cortex and medial occipitotemporal junction) were relatively thicker early on in life. However, by late adolescence the asymmetry reversed, and the *right* orbitofrontal region and inferior frontal gyrus and the *left* occipital cortical regions were relatively thicker, similar to the adult pattern of asymmetry. Thus in childhood, the anterior region was thicker on the left, and by late adolescence the anterior region was thicker on the right. The opposite was true for the posterior region: it was thicker on the right in early childhood but by late adolescence it was thicker on the left.

Shaw and colleagues (2009) further reported that the right-handed ADHD group also showed a gain in relative cortical thickness with age in the *left* posterior temporo-occipital region, as seen in the typically developing group. However, the ADHD group did not show increasing relative *right* hemisphere thickness with age in the frontal cortex, as seen in the typically developing group. They concluded that loss of the prefrontal component of this evolving asymmetry in ADHD is compatible with disruption of prefrontal function in this disorder. However, since about two thirds of the ADHD participants were treated with psychostimulants during the study (information on nonpharmacologic interventions was not provided), it is difficult to tease out the impact of intervention on the changing pattern of asymmetry in ADHD. Gilliam and colleagues (2011) reported a higher rate of growth in the anterior-most region of the corpus callosum in right-handed ADHD youths compared to their typically developing peers.

Most of the neuroimaging studies have been conducted in children over 6 years of age, since MRI scanning without sedation is challenging in preschoolers. Recently, Mahone and colleagues (2011) examined cortical and basal ganglion volumes in preschoolers between the age of 4 and 5 years with ADHD (n = 13; 8 boys) and without ADHD (n = 13; 5 boys). Magnetization prepared rapid gradient recalled echo (MPRAGE) images were used for volumetric assessment. Preschool children required special behavioral training and participated in one or two practice scans with a mock scanner, contingent praise, and reward to prepare them for an unsedated MRI scan. There was no significant difference in the cortical volume, surface area, or thickness; however, the authors reported significantly reduced caudate volumes bilaterally in ADHD preschoolers compared to controls, and the left caudate volume was a significant predictor of hyperactive/impulsive symptom severity. These findings of early anomalous caudate development (more than cortical development) suggest developmental differences in children presenting with early onset of ADHD symptoms.

Magnetoencephalography (MEG) findings. MEG is a noninvasive tool that records the magnetic fields generated by intracellular electrical current flow and offers an excellent temporal resolution of milliseconds with reasonable (~1 cm) spatial resolution (Ghuman, McDaniel, & Martin, 2011; Hämäläinen, Hari, Ilmoniemi, Knuutila, & Lounasmaa, 1993). In a MEG study of children with ADHD, magnetic activity of the brain was recorded during performance of a modified version of the Wisconsin Card Sort test. Results indicated lower activation of the prefrontal dorsolateral cortex than the anterior cingulate cortex of the left hemisphere during the first 400 milliseconds after reception of a negative feedback (Capilla et al., 2004). Prefrontal regions are essential for executive functioning (Capilla-Gonzalez et al., 2004), and anterior cingulate cortex is involved in the allotment of attentional resources (Bush et al., 2000). Mulas and colleagues (2006) used MEG to measure event-related brain activity during a simplified version of the Wisconsin Card Sort Test in 12-year-olds with ADHD and controls. A lower degree of activation in the medial temporal lobe and anterior cingulate cortex was reported in children with ADHD, supporting frontal dysfunction in ADHD. In contrast, early activity in the left inferior parietal lobe and posterior superior temporal gyrus was reported in children with ADHD; these regions were not activated in control children. Mulas and colleagues (2006) postulated that in addition to the frontal dysfunction, deficits in higher-level functions may be secondary to disruptions in earlier limbic processes.

Fernandez and colleagues (2009) obtained MEG recordings during resting conditions in 14 boys with ADHD and 14 control boys (age 8 to 12 years). Based on the brain complexity models of Lempel-Ziv, complexity scores in the anterior regions of the brain were significantly higher in controls compared to boys with ADHD. The difference in the complexity scores between controls and ADHD subjects increased as function of age. The model used in this study correctly classified ADHD and control subjects with 93% sensitivity and 79% specificity; it was strongly correlated with increasing age and reached 100% specificity in children over 9 years of age (Fernandez et al., 2009).

Environmental factors. A number of environmental factors have been considered as risk factors for or directly causing ADHD. These factors include diet, pre- and post-natal insult/injury to the developing brain, and parent-, home-, and school-centered stressors. Certain foods, including caffeine and sugar, dietary insufficiencies, and allergic reactions or intolerance to food additives (colors, flavors, and preservatives) may contribute to ADHD. Maternal smoking and drinking (Mick et al., 2002), lead exposure (Chiodo et al., 2004), and low birth weight (<2,500 g) (Breslau & Chilcoat, 2000) have been identified as risk factors for ADHD.

Low social class, maternal psychopathology, family conflict, a chaotic home and/ or school environment, and cultural issues may contribute to the risk for ADHD, especially in the formative preschool years when the child is in the process of developing self-control, language, and reciprocal socialization in a transactional manner. In a recent prospective cohort study, children of parents reporting both intimate partner violence and parental depression in the first 3 years of a child's life were four times more likely to have a diagnosis of ADHD between the ages of 3 and 6 years (Bauer et al., 2013). Another recent pair-matched case-control study, conducted in Beijing in 5- to 18-year-olds with ADHD, showed that the ADHD participants were 11 times more likely to suffer from emotional abuse compared to normal controls. There was also strong association between ADHD and being a single child. As China has a one-child policy, the authors of this study wondered whether parents of a single child were more likely to seek medical attention for assessment and treatment (Carroll et al., 2012).

The quality of the parent–child relationship can influence whether an at-risk child will follow the developmental pathway that leads to or away from developing ADHD. In a prospective longitudinal study of development of inattention and hyperactivity, the quality of caregiving (parental intrusiveness and overstimulation) in early childhood predicted distractibility and hyperactivity in kindergarteners more strongly than early biological or temperament factors (Jacobvitz & Sroufe, 1987). The quality of caregiving and contextual factors (mother's relationship status and emotional support) significantly predicted hyperactivity in middle childhood (Carlson, 1995). Contextual variables (changing support for caregivers and changing primary caregiver relationship status) in the early preschool period modified the child's expression of attentional and hyperactivity problems at a later age (Carlson, 1995; Sroufe, 1997).

Biometrics. Objective testing for ADHD would clarify the diagnostic process and improve diagnostic validity. Evaluation of several biomarkers to identify ADHD is ongoing, including the use of eye-movement patterns. A recent study showed that eye movements while watching videos differentiated ADHD children from those with fetal alcohol spectrum disorder (Tseng et al., 2013). The authors propose that examining eye-movement patterns can provide a potential screening tool that is objective, automated, low in cost, and time-effective, especially in young children, who may have difficulty with traditional evaluation tests.

Diagnostic Considerations

ADHD frequently begins between the age of 2 and 4 years (Connor, 2002; Egger, Kondo, & Angold, 2006; Wilens et al., 2002), and is associated with significant impairment in terms of emotional distress for the preschool child and the caregivers, expulsion from daycare or early education settings, difficulty finding childcare, and demands on the caregiver's time. Preschoolers with ADHD have comorbid mental health and chronic health problems, are prone to accidents, and have other safety concerns (Ghuman & Ghuman, 2012; Ghuman et al., 2001, 2007, 2008, 2009, 2011) and are frequent users of the healthcare system (Rappley et al., 2002). Early onset of ADHD may be associated with greater cognitive and language deficits, higher rates of psychiatric comorbidity, greater psychosocial and academic impairment, and persistence of behavior problems to school-age years (McGee, Williams, & Feehan, 1992; Willoughby, Curran, Costello, & Angold, 2000).

Follow-up of the original Preschool ADHD Treatment Study (PATS) sample reported significant ongoing impairment over 6 years. At the 6-year follow-up assessment, 89% of the study participants met the diagnostic criteria for ADHD, with a 30% higher risk of an ADHD diagnosis if the preschooler had associated comorbid ODD and/or conduct disorder at recruitment (Riddle et al., 2013).

Lahey and colleagues (2004) conducted four annual assessments for ADHD and functional impairment in 4- to 6-year-old children and reported that of the preschool children who met the DSM-IV criteria for ADHD at recruitment, 75% to 85% continued to meet the criteria for ADHD (either the same or another subtype) and displayed marked functional impairment over 3 years across parent, teacher, and interviewer reports. About one third of the children who were impaired in only one setting at the time of recruitment met ADHD diagnostic criteria during at least two subsequent annual assessments.

Richman, Stevenson, and Graham (1982) reported that 62% of the children who exhibited problems with hyperactivity, concentration, discipline, and tantrums at 3 years continued to have persistent problems at 8 years. Pierce, Ewing, and Campbell (1999) reported that 50% of the children who had exhibited ADHD symptoms at 3 years received a diagnosis of ADHD at 6 years and 48% had externalizing disorder at 9 years and at 13 years. The children with ADHD who also had coexisting peer problems and aggressive-antisocial behaviors were more likely to have persistent problems at a later age (Campbell, 1987). In a New Zealand population study of children who showed "pervasive hyperactivity" at age 3, McGee, Williams, and Silva (1987) reported continued problems with poor cognitive skills, lower levels of reading ability, disruptive and inattentive behaviors at home and at school, and higher rates of DSM-III disorder at age 15.

To mitigate current impairment and problems at later ages, it is important to diagnose and intervene early in preschool children with ADHD. However, given the rapidly changing development and the natural exuberance of young children, making the diagnosis of ADHD in preschool children is controversial and extremely challenging. In this section, we will consider developmental issues, diagnostic controversies, and the applicability of the DSM-5 criteria for ADHD in preschool children.

DEVELOPMENTAL ISSUES

When evaluating preschool children for ADHD, it is important to take note of the rapid developmental changes in the central nervous system (CNS) regions implicated in ADHD as well as the vast individual variation in the rate of development among preschoolers. Synaptic density in the prefrontal cortex increases steadily from birth to late childhood and is followed by synaptic elimination and rewiring of connectivity at the neural level (Crandall et al., 2007; Nasrallah et al., 1986). There is a dramatic increase in the local cerebral metabolic rate of glucose utilization between birth and 4 years that coincides with the period of synaptic proliferation in cerebral cortex (Glantz, Gilmore, Hamer, Lieberman, & Jarskog, 2007; Lou, Henriksen, & Bruhn, 1984). The rapid maturation in the brain's attentional systems and associated catecholamine neurotransmitters in prefrontal, striatal, and associated subcortical systems in infancy and preschool years results in a rapidly changing and variable nature of attention skills at this age. Significant developmental progress in effortful control and redirection of attention occurs across the preschool period. By the second year, children begin to be able to inhibit stimulus-driven motor response, and by 45 months effortful control becomes more stable, with further improvements through age 7 years (Kochanska & Knaack, 2003; Rothbart, Ellis, Rueda, & Posner, 2003; Rothbart, Sheese, Rueda, & Posner, 2011). The vast individual differences in regulation of attention, cognition, emotion and stimulus-driven motor response during early years become stable by the end of early childhood.

Temperamental influences. The influence of temperament in the development and expression of ADHD in preschool children is also important to consider. Reactive and regulatory temperamental processes begin to influence the development of attention and behavior early in life. Reactive processes in response to reward- or punishment-salient stimuli can alter the direction of attention in infants as early as 6 to 8 months of age (Rothbart & Ahadi, 1994). The regulatory domain can influence the allocation of attention and consequently the regulation of the reactive responses in the toddler years. For example, infants have been observed to turn attention deliberately away from upsetting information to soothe themselves (Rothbart & Ahadi, 1994). Certain toddler temperamental traits like difficulties with inhibitory control, hostile and aggressive behavior, anger, and difficult temperaments have been shown to predict ADHD symptom scores in kindergarten and first grade (Shaw, Owens, Giovannelli, & Winslow, 2001). It has been proposed that behavioral disinhibition may represent a temperamental precursor to ADHD.

DIAGNOSTIC CONTROVERSIES

The diagnosis of ADHD in preschool children has been the focus of intense debate and continues to be controversial. First, concerns have been raised whether it is even appropriate to consider the diagnosis of ADHD in preschool children; some worry that the normal, developmentally expected behavior of preschool children may be wrongly labeled as ADHD and lead to overdiagnosis. It has also been questioned whether ADHD symptoms in preschool children may represent the extreme end of normal development or extremes of temperament. Proponents of the continuum view of ADHD consider ADHD behaviors as a trait that differs from normality only by degree and contend that viewing ADHD as a discrete condition (Jensen, 2000) pathologizes normal childhood behavior. While some studies using ADHD symptom checklists with binary "yes and no" responses have reported ADHD prevalence rates as high as 18.3% in preschool children (Pineda et al., 1999), studies using appropriate diagnostic measures have reported lower prevalence rates (4.2%), similar to the prevalence rates in older children (Briggs-Gowan, Horwitz, Schwab-Stone, Leventhal, & Leaf, 2000; Earls, 1982; Egger et al., 2006; Keenan, Shaw, Walsh, Delliquadri, & Giovannelli, 1997; Lavigne et al., 1996).

Second, there are political objections to potentially stigmatizing labels in preschool children (Campbell, 2002; Diller, 2002). Political opponents have suggested that "The ADHD diagnosis contains no 'symptoms' that specifically pertain to any emotional suffering in the child. The focus [of ADHD diagnosis] is entirely on child-like behaviors that can at times cause inconvenience or frustration in adults" (Breggin, 1999a, p. 26; 1999b).

Third, differences in the caregiver's perception of children's behavior, especially in the context of the caregiver's mental health and relationship status, also add to the diagnostic controversy. Stressed mothers tend to perceive their children's behavior as more negative (Berg-Nielsen, Solheim, Belsky, & Wichstrom, 2012; Crnic, Gaze, & Hoffman, 2005). Depressed mothers may often overreport externalizing child behavior problems in their offspring compared to nondepressed caregivers (Gartstein, Bridgett, Dishion, & Kaufman, 2009). Mothers' levels of current depressive symptomatology were associated with maternal ratings of their child as more hyperactive, inattentive, and generally more disruptive compared with teacher ratings (Gartstein et al., 2009). Disproportionate rates of false positives in predicting future psychopathology were reported based on depressed mothers' ratings of the child's behavior compared with nondepressed mothers and youth self-report (Najman et al., 2000).

Similarly, caregivers' involvement in abusive relationships have been shown to affect their perceptions of child behaviors (Milner, 2003). Abusive parents are hyperreactive to the misbehavior of their children, become more easily annoyed (Bauer & Twentyman, 1985), and may inaccurately identify more difficulties in their children that are not corroborated by direct observation (Reid, Kavanagh, & Baldwin, 1987). Compared to non-abusive parents, abusive parents reported higher levels of externalizing behavior problems (Lau, Valeri, McCarty, & Weisz, 2006), thus adding to the criticism of ADHD diagnosis being a reflection of adult intolerance of typical child behaviors. Finally, concerns have also been raised about overreporting of externalizing problems for minority children (Reid, Casat, Norton, Anastopoulos, & Temple, 2001).

Hence, it is important to consider behavioral, interactional, and relational contexts in order to differentiate ADHD mimics from ADHD when evaluating preschool children referred for ADHD, as highlighted by the following case example.

MM was a 3½-year-old boy referred by his primary healthcare provider for an ADHD evaluation due to complaints of not sitting still, disrupting and interrupting his current foster and prospective adoptive mother when she was doing something that did not include MM, and impulsively hitting, pushing, and grabbing when he wanted something from her or from other children living in the foster home. The foster/prospective adoptive mother gave history that MM was "very well behaved" whenever she left him in the care of non-family caregivers. MM was removed from his biological mother's custody at age 3 for neglect and physical abuse and placed in a shelter for 30 days. Subsequently, he was placed with an older relative who was in her mid-sixties and was also caring for other children of varying ages living with her. Within 4 weeks, the "elderly relative" asked that MM be removed from her home as she complained that MM was very active and did not want to comply with her well-organized routine that she expected all the children to follow. MM was placed with the current foster mother, who had planned to adopt him. MM had been living with her for 4 months at the time of the evaluation.

During the evaluation, it was observed that MM's current foster/prospective adoptive mother was very slow in her speech and movements and had low energy, and her affect was very constricted. She did not initiate any interaction with MM or tend to his needs during the first, second, or third evaluation session. MM was observed to climb on her back, climb in and out of her lap, and put his juice cup to her lips. He did not engage in any focused play, placing one toy after another in his foster/prospective adoptive mother's lap, pulling on her, and insisting that she play with him or give him something to eat. Both the foster/prospective adoptive mother and the Child Protective Service (CPS) case worker pointed to MM's behaviors and complained that MM was hyperactive, interrupting the adult conversation and disruptive to the evaluation process. When MM was seen separately from his current foster/prospective adoptive mother, he was observed to be more subdued and had a blunted affect. He sat quietly and did not engage in any play activity.

Our evaluation concluded that MM's intrusions, impulsiveness, repetitively "annoying" demands, and overactivity in the presence of his caregiver were most likely stemming from his feelings of anxiety over attachment figures and his unsuccessful attempts to engage his current foster/prospective adoptive mother. His seemingly "intrusive, impulsive, and overactive" behaviors were limited to his interactions with his foster/prospective adoptive mother and were not pervasive in other situations or contexts. Furthermore, there was an obvious mismatch between the foster/prospective adoptive mother's psychomotor retardation and MM's level of energy and activity level. Based on these observations, MM was not given a diagnosis of ADHD. Recommendations were made for caregiver–child dyadic interaction therapy and developmental guidance, individual play therapy for MM, and a psychiatric evaluation for the foster/prospective adoptive mother.

This case example illustrates the importance of taking into account all the diagnostic issues (e.g., contextual influences bolstered by differences in behavioral expression in different settings and lack of pervasiveness of his "ADHD" symptoms) for a more accurate biopsychosocial diagnostic formulation and treatment plan and to avoid overdiagnosis of ADHD.

ADHD DIAGNOSTIC CRITERIA

Research has supported the categorical validity of the DSM-IV diagnostic criteria in younger children (Lahey et al., 1998). The DSM-IV diagnostic criteria have also demonstrated predictive validity, such that young children do appear to maintain their diagnoses and behavioral and academic problems over time (Lahey et al., 2004; McGee, Partridge, Williams, & Silva, 1991).

Similar to the DSM-IV-TR diagnostic criteria (APA, 2000), the DSM-5 symptoms for ADHD are divided into two domains based on hyperactive/impulsive or inattentive behaviors. The DSM-5 ADHD diagnostic criteria for hyperactive/impulsive presentation include six hyperactive symptoms (fidgety, does not stay in his/her seat, running and climbing excessively, difficulty playing quietly, often talking excessively, and "on the go") and three impulsive symptoms (blurting out answers, difficulty waiting turn, and often interrupting others). The inattentive symptoms cluster includes nine inattention symptoms (difficulty sustaining attention, not giving close attention to details, not following through with instructions, often seems not to be listening, difficulty organizing, dislikes tasks that require sustained mental effort, often loses things, forgetful in daily activities, and is often easily distracted). The DSM-5 diagnostic criteria for ADHD require six hyperactive/impulsive symptoms for predominantly hyperactive/impulsive presentation, six inattentive symptoms for predominantly inattentive presentation, or six hyperactive/impulsive and six inattentive symptoms for combined presentation. The symptoms should be persistent (present for a minimum of 6 months) and developmentally inappropriate for the child's age. Several symptoms must be present in two or more settings (at home, school, with friends or relatives, or in other activities) and lead to impairment (for example, interfere or reduce the quality of social and academic/educational functioning or developmentally appropriate learning). Several symptoms must have been present before 12 years of age (APA, 2013).

The DSM-IV-TR ADHD subtypes in preschool and older children have been reported to be highly unstable over time. In a longitudinal study, Lahey and Willcutt (2011) recruited 4- to 6-year-old children and conducted repeated assessments over years 2 to 9. Even though the ADHD diagnosis was highly stable over time, the subtypes shifted from year to year. Accordingly, in DSM-5, the ADHD subtypes are no longer designated at the initial evaluation as a stable diagnosis; instead, predominantly hyperactive/impulsive, inattentive, or combined presentation is specified at each clinical encounter.

Additional changes to the ADHD diagnostic criteria in the DSM-5 that are relevant to preschool ADHD include requiring several ADHD symptoms to be present in two or more settings and removing pervasive developmental disorder from the exclusionary criteria. ADHD is now included under neurodevelopmental disorders (APA, 2013) to reflect brain developmental correlates with ADHD. The remaining changes (reduction of symptom threshold for ADHD in adults, changing age of onset, and elaboration of examples of symptoms for inattentive and hyperactivity/impulsivity symptoms) are mostly geared to adolescents and adults. None of the changes in DSM-5 specifically addresses diagnostic issues in preschool children. Even though descriptions were added to elaborate and exemplify some of the ADHD criteria, no specific examples were included for preschool children. It is disappointing that an opportunity was lost with the recently released DSM-5 to provide guidance related to difficulties associated with differentiating developmentally appropriate inattentive, hyperactive, and impulsive behaviors from clinically significant ADHD symptoms in preschool children.

Summary

Information regarding the epidemiology, etiology, and validity of an ADHD diagnosis in preschoolers is limited. Diagnosis of ADHD in preschool children remains controversial and presents many challenges to the clinician. At the same time, clinicians are increasingly being asked to evaluate children for ADHD at younger and younger ages. Future studies delineating normative development and differentiating it from clinically significant behaviors implicated in ADHD are sorely needed.

Disclosures

Jaswinder K. Ghuman, M.D., has received past funding from the NIMH for a K-23 career development grant, the Arizona Institute for Mental Health Research, and from Bristol-Myers Squibb for a clinical trial in autistic disorder. She received funding from the Health Resources and Services Administration–Maternal and Child Health (HRSA-MCH) for a training grant for the University of Arizona Leadership Education in Neurodevelopmental Disabilities Training Program (AZLEND).

Harinder S. Ghuman, M.D., has no conflicts of interest.

References

APA. (1968). *Diagnostic and statistical manual of mental disorders* (DSM-II). Washington, DC: American Psychiatric Association.

APA. (1980). *Diagnostic and statistical manual of mental disorders* (DSM-III). Washington, DC: American Psychiatric Association.

APA. (1987). *Diagnostic and statistical manual of mental disorders-Revised* (DSM-III-Revised). Washington, DC: American Psychiatric Association.

APA. (1994). *Diagnostic and statistical manual of mental disorders* (DSM-IV). Washington, DC: American Psychiatric Association.

APA. (2000). *Diagnostic and statistical manual of mental disorders, text revision* (DSM-IV-TR). Washington, DC: American Psychiatric Association.

APA. (2013). *Desk reference to the diagnostic criteria from the diagnostic and statistical manual of mental disorders-5* (DSM-5). Washington, DC: American Psychiatric Association.

Barkley, R. A. (2003). Issues in the diagnosis of attention-deficit/hyperactivity disorder in children. *Brain Development, 25*(2), 77–83.

Barkley, R. A., & Peters, H. (2012). The earliest references to ADHD in the medical literature? Melchior Adam Weikard's description in 1775 of "Attention deficit" (mangel der Aumerksamkeit, Attentio volubilis). *Journal of Attention Disorder* (online).

Bauer, N. S., Gilbert, A. L., Carroll, A. E., & Downs, S. M. (2013). Associations of early exposure to intimate partner violence and parental depression with subsequent mental health outcomes. *JAMA Pediatrics, 4*, 1–7.

Bauer, W. D., & Twentyman, C. T. (1985). Abusing, neglectful, and comparison mothers' responses to child-related and non-child-related stressors. *Journal of Consulting & Clinical Psychology, 53*(3), 335–343.

Bax, M. C. O., & Mackeith, R. C. (1963). Minimal brain damage—a concept discarded. In R. C. Mackeith & M. C. O. Bax (Eds.), *Minimal cerebral dysfunction.* Little Club Clinics in Developmental Medicine, No. 10. London: Heinemann

Bender, L. (1942). Postencephalatic behavior disorders in children. In N. B. Neal (Ed.), *Encephalitis: A clinical study* (pp. 361–385). New York, NY: Grunne and Stratton.

Berg-Nielsen, T. S., Solheim, E., Belsky, J., & Wichstrom, L. (2012). Preschoolers' psychosocial problems: in the eyes of the beholder? Adding teacher characteristics as determinants of discrepant parent-teacher reports. *Child Psychiatry & Human Development, 43*(3), 393–413.

Bhatia, M. S., Nigam, V. R., Bohra, N., et al. (1991). Attention deficit disorder with hyperactivity among pediatric outpatients. *Journal of Child Psychology and Psychiatry, 32*, 297–306.

Bradley, C. (1937). The behavior of children receiving Benzedrine. *American Journal of Psychiatry, 94*, 577–585.

Breggin, P. R. (1999a). Psychostimulants in the treatment of children diagnosed with ADHD: Risks and mechanism of action. *International Journal of Risk & Safety in Medicine, 3*–35.

Breggin, P. R. (1999b). Treatment of attention-deficit/hyperactivity disorder. *Journal of the American Medical Association, 281*(16), 1490–1491.

Breslau, N., & Chilcoat, H. D. (2000). Psychiatric sequelae of low birth weight at 11 years of age. *Biological Psychiatry, 47*, 1005–1011.

Briggs-Gowan, M. J., Horwitz, S. M., Schwab-Stone, M. E., Leventhal, J. M., & Leaf, P. J. (2000). Mental health in pediatric settings: distribution of disorders and factors related to service use. *Journal of the American Academy of Child & Adolescent Psychiatry, 39*(7), 841–849.

Bush, G., Luu, P., & Posner, M. I. (2000). Cognitive and emotional influences in anterior cingulate cortex. *Trends in Cognitive Science, 4*, 215–222.

Campbell, S. B. (1987). Parent-referred problem three-year-olds: developmental changes in symptoms. *Journal of Child Psychology & Psychiatry, 28*(6), 835–845.

Campbell, S. B. (2002). *Behavior problems in preschool children: Clinical and developmental issues* (2nd ed.). New York: Guilford Press.

Capilla, A., Etchepareborda, M. C., Fernandez-Gonzalez, S., Mulas, F., Campo, P., Maestu, F., et al. (2004). Sustrato neurofunctional de la rigidez cognitive en al trastorno por deficit de atencion con hiperactividad: resutados preliminaries. *Revista de Neurologia, 38* (Suppl. 1), S145–S148.

Capilla-Gonzalez, A., Fernandez-Gonzalez, S., Campo, P., Maestu, F., Fernandez-Lucas, A., Mulas, F., et al. (2004). La magnetoencefalografia en los tratornos cognitive del lobulo frontal. *Revista de Neurologia, 39*(2), 183–188.

Carlson, E. A., Jacobvitz, D., & Sroufe, L. A. (1995). A developmental investigation of inattentiveness and hyperactivity. *Child Development, 66*(1), 37–54.

Carroll, X., Yi, H., Liang, Y., Pang, K., et al. (2012). Family–environmental factors associated with attention deficit hyperactivity disorder in Chinese children: a case-control study. *PLoS, 7*(11), e50543.

Castellanos, F. X., Lee, P. P., Sharp, W., Jeffries, N. O., Greenstein, D. K., Clasen, L. S., et al. (2002). Developmental trajectories of brain volume abnormalities in children and adolescents with attention-deficit/hyperactivity disorder. *Journal of the American Medical Association, 288*, 1740–1748.

Chess, S. (1960). Diagnosis and treatment of the hyperactive child. *New York State Journal of Medicine, 63*, 575–585.

Chiodo, L. M., Jacobson, S. W., & Jacobson, J. L. (2004). Neurodevelopmental effects of postnatal lead exposure at very low levels. *Neurotoxicology and Teratology, 26*, 259–264.

Clouston, T. S. (1899). Stages of over-excitability, hypersensitiveness, and mental explosiveness in children and their treatment by the bromides. *Scottish Medical and Surgical Journal, IV*(6), 481–490.

Connor, D. F. (2002). Preschool attention deficit hyperactivity disorder: a review of prevalence, diagnosis, neurobiology, and stimulant treatment. *Journal of Developmental & Behavioral Pediatrics, 23*(1 Suppl), S1–S9.

Corbetta, M., Patel, G., & Shulman, G. L. (2008). The reorienting system of the human brain: from environment to theory of mind. *Neuron, 58*, 306–324.

Cortese, S., Kelly, C., Chabernaud, C., Proal, E., Martino, A. D., Milham, M. P., & Castellanos, F. X. (2012). Toward systems neuroscience of ADHD: a meta-analysis of 55 fMRI studies. *American Journal of Psychiatry, 169*(10), 1038–1055.

Crandall, J. E., McCarthy, D. M., Araki, K. Y., Sims, J. R., Ren, J. Q., & Bhide, P. G. (2007). Dopamine receptor activation modulates GABA neuron migration from the basal forebrain to the cerebral cortex. *Journal of Neuroscience, 27*(14), 3813–3822.

Crichton, A. (1798). *An inquiry into the nature and origin of mental derangement: Comprehending a concise system of physiology and pathology of the human mind and a history of the passions and their effects.* London, England: T. Cadell Hr. & W. Davies. (reprinted by AMS Press: New York, 1976).

Crnic, K. A., Gaze, C., & Hoffman, C. (2005). Cumulative parenting stress across the preschool period: relations to maternal parenting and child behavior at age 5. *Infant & Child Development, 14*, 117–132.

Diamond, A. (2005). Attention-deficit disorder (attention-deficit/hyperactivity disorder without hyperactivity): a neurobiologically and behaviorally distinct disorder from attention-deficit/ hyperactivity disorder (with hyperactivity). *Developmental Psychopathology, 17*(3), 807–825.

Dickstein, S. G., Bannon, K., Castellanos, F. X., & Milham, M. P. (2006). The neural correlates of attention deficit hyperactivity disorder: An ALE meta-analysis. *Journal of Child Psychology and Psychiatry, 47*, 1051–1062.

Diller, L. H. (2002). Lessons from three year olds. *Journal of Developmental & Behavioral Pediatrics, 23*(1 Suppl), S10–S12.

Douglas, V. I. (1972). Stop, look and listen: the problem of sustained attention and impulse control in hyperactive and normal children. *Canadian Journal of Behavioral Science, 4*, 259–282.

DuPaul, G. J., Power, T. J., Anastopoulos, A. D., & Reid, R. (1998). *ADHD Rating Scale-IV.* New York: Guilford Press.

Durston, S., Tottenham, N. T., Thomas, K. M., Davidson, M. C., Eisgsti, I. M., Yang, Y., et al. (2003). Differential patterns of striatal activation in young children with or without ADHD. *Biological Psychiatry, 53*, 871–878.

Earls, F. (1982). Application of DSM-III in an epidemiological study of preschool children. *American Journal of Psychiatry, 139*(2), 242–243.

Egger, H. L., Kondo, D., & Angold, A. (2006). The epidemiology and diagnostic issues in preschool attention-deficit/ hyperactivity disorder: A review. *Infants & Young Children, 19*(2), 109–122.

Elia, J., Gai, X., Xie, H. M., et al. (2010). Rare structural variants found in attention-deficit hyperactivity disorder are preferentially associated with neurodevelopmental genes. *Molecular Psychiatry, 15*(6), 637–646.

Fassbender, C., & Schweitzer, J. B. (2006). Is there evidence for neural compensation in attention deficit hyperactivity disorder? A review of the functional neuroimaging system. *Clinical Psychology Review, 26*, 445–465.

Fernandez, A., Quintero, J., Hornero, R., et al. (2009). Complexity analysis of spontaneous brain activity in attention-deficit/hyperactivity disorder: diagnostic implications. *Biological Psychiatry, 65*, 571–577.

Gartstein, M. A., Bridgett, D. J., Dishion, T. J., & Kaufman, N. K. (2009). Depressed mood and maternal report of child behavior problems: another look at the depression-distortion hypothesis. *Journal of Applied Developmental Psychology, 30*(2), 149–160.

Ghuman, A. S., McDaniel, J. R., & Martin, A. (2011). A wavelet-based method for measuring the oscillatory dynamics of resting-state functional connectivity in MEG. *Neuroimage, 56*(1), 69–77.

Ghuman, J. K., Aman, M. G., Ghuman, H. S., Reichenbacher, T., Gelenberg, A., Wright, R., et al. (2009). Prospective, naturalistic, pilot study of open-label atomoxetine treatment in preschool children with attention-deficit/hyperactivity disorder. *Journal of Child &Adolescent Psychopharmacology, 19*(2), 155–166.

Ghuman, J. K., Arnold, L. E., & Anthony, B. J. (2008). Psychopharmacological and other treatments in preschool children with attention-deficit/hyperactivity disorder: current evidence and practice. *Journal of Child & Adolescent Psychopharmacology, 18*(5), 413–447.

Ghuman, J. K., Byreddy, S., & Ghuman, H. S. (2011). Methylphenidate transdermal system in preschool children with attention-deficit/hyperactivity disorder. *Journal of Child & Adolescent Psychopharmacology, 21*(5), 495–498.

Ghuman, J. K., & Ghuman, H. S. (2012). Pharmacologic intervention for attention-deficit hyperactivity disorder in preschoolers: is it justified? *Paediatric Drugs, 15*(1), 1–8.

Ghuman, J. K., Ginsburg, G. S., Subramaniam, G., Ghuman, H. S., Kau, A. S., & Riddle, M. A. (2001). Psychostimulants in preschool children with attention-deficit/hyperactivity disorder: clinical evidence from a developmental disorders institution. *Journal of the American Academy of Child & Adolescent Psychiatry, 40*(5), 516–524.

Ghuman, J. K., Riddle, M. A., Vitiello, B., Greenhill, L. L., Chuang, S. Z., Wigal, S. B., et al. (2007). Comorbidity moderates response to methylphenidate in the Preschoolers with Attention-Deficit/Hyperactivity Disorder Treatment Study (PATS). *Journal of Child & Adolescent Psychopharmacology, 17*(5), 563–580.

Giedd, J. N., Blumenthal, J., Molloy, E., & Castellanos, F. X. (2001). Brain imaging of attention deficit/hyperactivity disorder. *Annals of the New York Academy of Science, 931*, 33–49.

Gilliam M., Stockman M., Malek M., Sharp W., Greenstein D., Lalonde F., et al. (2011). Developmental trajectories of the corpus callosum in attention-deficit/hyperactivity disorder. *Biol Psychiatry, 69*(9), 839–846.

Gizer, I. R., Ficks, C., & Waldman, I.D. (2009). Candidate gene studies of ADHD: a meta-analytic review. *Human Genetics, 126*, 51–90.

Glantz, L. A., Gilmore, J. H., Hamer, R. M., Lieberman, J. A., & Jarskog, L. F. (2007). Synaptophysin and postsynaptic density protein 95 in the human prefrontal cortex from mid-gestation into early adulthood. *Neuroscience, 149*(3), 582–591.

Glessner, J. T., Connolly, J. J., & Hakonarson, H. (2012). Rare genomic deletions and duplications and their role in neurodevelopmental disorders. *Current Topics in Behavioral Neurosciences, 12*, 345–360.

Hämäläinen, M., Hari, R., Ilmoniemi, R., Knuutila, J., & Lounasmaa, O. (1993). Magnetoencephalography—theory, instrumentation, and applications to noninvasive studies of the working human brain. *Reviews of Modern Physics, 65*, 1–93.

Hoffman, H. (1845). *Der Struwwelpeter.* Frankfurt: Literarische Anstalt.

Jacobvitz, D., & Sroufe, L. A. (1987). The early caregiver-child relationship and attention-deficit disorder with hyperactivity in kindergarten: a prospective study. *Child Development, 6*, 1496–1504.

Jensen, P. S. (2000). Commentary: the NIH ADHD Consensus Statement: win, lose, or draw? *Journal of the American Academy of Child & Adolescent Psychiatry, 39*(2), 194–197.

Keenan, K., Shaw, D. S., Walsh, B., Delliquadri, E., & Giovannelli, J. (1997). DSM-III-R disorders in preschool children from low-income families. *Journal of the American Academy of Child & Adolescent Psychiatry, 36*(5), 620–627.

Kochanska, G., & Knaack, A. (2003). Effortful control as a personality characteristic of young children: antecedents, correlates, and consequences. *Journal of Personality, 71*(6), 1087–1112.

Kramer, F. & Pollnow, H. (1930). Hyperkinetische Zustandsbilder im Kindesalter. *Zentralblatt für die gesamte Neurologie und Psychiatrie, 57*, 844–845.

Laufer, M. W., & Denhoff, E. (1957). Hyperkinetic behavior syndrome in children. *Journal of Pediatrics, 50*, 463–474.

Lahey, B. B., Pelham, W. E., Loney, J., Kipp, H., Ehrhardt, A., Lee, S. S., et al. (2004). Three-year predictive validity of DSM-IV attention deficit hyperactivity disorder in children diagnosed at 4-6 years of age. *American Journal of Psychiatry, 161*(11), 2014–2020.

Lahey, B. B., Pelham, W. E., Stein, M. A., Loney, J., Trapani, C., Nugent, K., et al. (1998). Validity of DSM-IV attention-deficit/hyperactivity disorder for younger children. *Journal of the American Academy of Child & Adolescent Psychiatry, 37*(7), 695–702.

Lahey, B. B., & Willcutt, E. G. (2011). Predictive validity of a continuous alternative to nominal subtypes of attention-deficit/hyperactivity disorder for DSM-V. *Journal of Clinical Child & Adolescent Psychology, 39*(6), 761–775.

Lange, K. W., Reichl, S., Lange, K. M., Tucha, L., & Tucha, O. (2010). The history of attention deficit hyperactivity disorder. *Attention Deficit Hyperactivity Disorder, 2*(4), 241–255.

Lau, A. S., Valeri, S. M., McCarty, C. A., & Weisz, J. R. (2006). Abusive parents' reports of child behavior problems: relationship to observed parent-child interactions. *Child Abuse & Neglect, 30*(6), 639–655.

Lavigne, J. V., Gibbons, R. D., Christoffel, K. K., Arend, R., Rosenbaum, D., Binns, H., et al. (1996). Prevalence rates and correlates of psychiatric disorders among preschool children. *Journal of the American Academy of Child & Adolesc Psychiatry, 35*(2), 204–214.

Lou, H. C., Henriksen, L., & Bruhn, P. (1984). Focal cerebral hypoperfusion in children with dysphasia and/or attention deficit disorder. *Archives of Neurology, 41*(8), 825–829.

Mahone, E. M., Crocetti, D., Ranta, M. E., et al. (2011). A preliminary neuroimaging study of preschool children with ADHD. *The Clinical Neuropsychologist, 25*(6), 1009–1028.

Maudsley (1867). *The physiology and pathology of mind*. London: Macmillan.

McGee, R., Partridge, F., Williams, S., & Silva, P. A. (1991). A twelve-year follow-up of preschool hyperactive children. *Journal of the American Academy of Child & Adolescent Psychiatry, 30*(2), 224–232.

McGee, R., Williams, S., & Feehan, M. (1992). Attention deficit disorder and age of onset of problem behaviors. *Journal of Abnormal Child Psychology, 20*(5), 487–502.

McGee, R., Williams, S., & Silva, P. A. (1987). A comparison of girls and boys with teacher-identified problems of attention. *Journal of the American Academy of Child & Adolescent Psychiatry, 26*(5), 711–717.

Milner, J. S. (2003). Social information processing in high-risk and physically abusive parents. *Child Abuse & Neglect, 27*(1), 7–20.

Meysamie, A., Fard, M. D., & Mohammadi, M. (2011). Prevalence of attention-deficit/hyperactivity disorder symptoms in preschool-aged Iranian children. *Iran Journal of Pediatrics, 21*(4), 467–472.

Mick, E., Biederman, J., Faraone, S. V., et al. (2002). Case-control study of attention-deficit hyperactivity disorder and maternal smoking, alcohol use, and drug use during pregnancy. *Journal of the American Academy of Child and Adolescent Psychiatry, 41*, 378–385.

Mulas, F., Capilla, A., Fernandez, S., et al. (2006). Shifting-related brain magnetic activity in attention-deficit/hyperactivity disorder. *Biological Psychiatry, 59*, 373–379.

Najman, J. M., Williams, G. M., Nikles, J., Spence, S., Bor, W., O'Callaghan, M., et al. (2000). Mothers' mental illness and child behavior problems: cause-effect association or observation bias? *Journal of the American Academy of Child & Adolescent Psychiatry, 39*(5), 592–602.

Nasrallah, H. A., Loney, J., Olson, S. C., McCalley-Whitters, M., Kramer, J., & Jacoby, C. G. (1986). Cortical atrophy in young adults with a history of hyperactivity in childhood. *Psychiatry Research, 17*(3), 241–246.

Nigg, J., & Nikolas, M. (2008). Attention-deficit/hyperactivity disorder. In T. P. Beauchaine & S. P. Hinshaw (Eds.), *Child and adolescent psychopathology* (pp. 301–34). Hoboken, NJ: John Wiley & Sons, Inc.

Ogdie, M. N., Bakker, S. C., Fischer, S. E., et al. (2006). Pooled genome-wide linkage data on 424 ADHD ASPs suggest genetic heterogeneity and a common risk locus at 5p13. *Molecular Psychiatry, 11,* 5–8.

Pierce, E. W., Ewing, L. J., & Campbell, S. B. (1999). Diagnostic status and symptomatic behavior of hard-to-manage preschool children in middle childhood and early adolescence. *Journal of Clinical Child Psychology, 28*(1), 44–57.

Pineda, D., Ardila, A., Rosselli, M., Arias, B. E., Henao, G. C., Gomez, L. F., et al. (1999). Prevalence of attention-deficit/hyperactivity disorder symptoms in 4- to 17-year-old children in the general population. *Journal of Abnormal Child Psychology, 27*(6), 455–462.

Pineda, D. A., Lopera, F., Palacio, J.D., Ramirez, D., & Henao G. C. (2003). Prevalence estimations of attention-deficit/hyperactivity disorder: Differential diagnosis and comorbidities in a colombian sample. *Internation Journal of Neuroscience, 113*(1), 49–71.

Rappley, M. D., Eneli, I. U., Mullan, P. B., Alvarez, F. J., Wang, J., Luo, Z., et al. (2002). Patterns of psychotropic medication use in very young children with attention-deficit hyperactivity disorder. *Journal of Developmental & Behavioral Pediatrics, 23*(1), 23–30.

Reid, R., Casat, C.D., Norton, H. J., Anastopoulos, A.D., & Temple, E.P. (2001). Using behavior rating scales for ADHD across ethnic groups: The IOWA Conners. *Journal of Emotional and Behavioral Disorders, 9*, 210–218.

Reid, J. B., Kavanagh, K., & Baldwin, D. V. (1987). Abusive parents' perceptions of child problem behaviors: an example of parental bias. *Journal of Abnormal Child Psychology, 15*(3), 457–466.

Richman, N., Stevenson, J., & Graham, P. J. (1982). *Pre-school to school: a behavioural study*: London: Academic Press.

Riddle, M. A., Yershova, K., Lazzaretto, D., Paykina, N., Yenokyan, G., Greenhill, L., et al. (2013). The Preschool Attention-Deficit/Hyperactivity Disorder Treatment Study (PATS) 6-year follow-up. *Journal of the American Academy of Child & Adolescent Psychiatry, 52*(3), 264–278, e262.

Rothbart, M. K., & Ahadi, S. A. (1994). Temperament and the development of personality. *Journal of Abnormal Psychology, 103*(1), 55–66.

Rothbart, M. K., Ellis, L. K., Rueda, M. R., & Posner, M. I. (2003). Developing mechanisms of temperamental effortful control. *Journal of Personality, 71*(6), 1113–1143.

Rothbart, M. K., Sheese, B. E., Rueda, M. R., & Posner, M. I. (2011). Developing mechanisms of self-regulation in early life. *Emotion Review, 3*(2), 207–213.

Russell, V. A. (2007). Reprint of "Neurobiology of animal models of attention-deficit hyperactivity disorder." *Journal of Neuroscience Methods, 166*(2), I–XIV.

Seidman, K. J., Biederman, J., Monteaux, M. C., et al. (2005). Impact of gender and age on executive functioning: Do girls and boys with or without attention-deficit hyperactivity disorder differ neuropsychologically in the preteen and teenage years? *Developmental Neuropsychology, 27*, 79–105.

Shaw, P., Eckstrand, K., Sharp, W., et al. (2007). Attention-deficit/hyperactivity disorder is characterized by a delay in cortical maturation. *Proceedings of National Academy of Sciences, USA 104*(49), 19649–19654.

Shaw, D. S., Owens, E. B., Giovannelli, J., & Winslow, E. B. (2001). Infant and toddler pathways leading to early externalizing disorders. *Journal of the American Academy of Child & Adolescent Psychiatry, 40*(1), 36–43.

Shaw, P., Lalonde, F., Lepage, C., et al. (2009). Development of cortical asymmetry in typically developing children and its disruption in attention-deficit/hyperactivity disorder. *Archives of General Psychiatry, 66*(8), 888–896.

Sroufe, L. A. (1997). Psychopathology as an outcome of development. *Developmental Psychopathology, 9*(2), 251–268.

Stergiakouli, E., Hamshere, M., Holmans, P., et al. (2012). Investigating the contribution of common genetic variants to the risk and pathogenesis of ADHD. *American Journal of Psychiatry, 169*(2), 186–194.

Still, G. F. (1902). Some abnormal psychical conditions in children. *Lancet, 1,* 1008–1012, 1077–1082, 1163–1168.

Strauss, A. A., & Werner, H. (1943). Comparative psychopathology of the brain injured child and the brain injured adult. *American Journal of Psychiatry, 99,* 835–838.

Tredgold, C. H. (1908). *Mental deficiency (amentia).* New York: W. Wood.

Tseng, P. H., Cameron, I. G., Pari, G., Reynolds, J. N., Munoz, D. P. & Itti, L. (2013). High-throughput classification of clinical populations from natural viewing eye movements. *Journal of Neurology, 260*(1), 275–284. doi:10.1007/s00415-012-6631-2.

Wichstrom, L., Berg-Nielsen, T. S., Angold, A., et al. (2012). Prevalence of psychiatric disorders in preschoolers. *Journal of Child Psychology & Psychiatry, 53*(6), 695–705.

Wilens, T. E., Biederman, J., Brown, S., Tanguay, S., Monuteaux, M. C., Blake, C., et al. (2002). Psychiatric comorbidity and functioning in clinically referred preschool children and school-age youths with ADHD. *Journal of the American Academy of Child & Adolescent Psychiatry, 41*(3), 262–268.

Willoughby, M. T., Curran, P. J., Costello, E. J., & Angold, A. (2000). Implications of early versus late onset of attention-deficit/hyperactivity disorder symptoms. *Journal of the American Academy of Child & Adolescent Psychiatry, 39*(12), 1512–1519.

Willoughby, M. T., Pek, J., & Greenberg, M. T. (2012). Parent-reported attention deficit/hyperactivity symptomatology in preschool-aged children: factor structure, developmental change, and early risk factors. *Journal of Abnormal Child Psychology, 40*(8), 1301–1312.

Wu, J., Xiao, H., Sun, H., Zou, L, Zhu, L. Q. (2012). Role of dopamine receptors in ADHD: A systematic meta-analysis. *Molecular Neurobiology, 45*(3), 605–620.

Yang, L., Neale, B. M., Liu, L., et al. (2013). Polygenic transmission and complex neurodevelopmental network for attention deficit hyperactivity disorder: Genome-wide association study of both common and rare variants. *American Journal of Medical Genetics B: Neuropsychiatric Genetics.* doi: 10.1002/ajmg.b.32169.

2

Evaluation Process and Essentials
of Clinical Assessment

JASWINDER K. GHUMAN AND

HARINDER S. GHUMAN

Diagnosis of attention-deficit/hyperactivity disorder (ADHD) in preschool children continues to be controversial and challenging despite the accumulating evidence for its diagnostic validity (Lahey et al., 2004, 2006). Concerns have been raised about the lack of sensitivity of the *Diagnostic and Statistical Manual, 4th edition* (DSM-IV) diagnostic criteria to the unique developmental changes that take place during pre-school years. As a result, the American Academy of Child and Adolescent Psychiatry (AACAP) sponsored a task force to develop the Research Diagnostic Criteria Preschool Age (RDC-PA). The task force reviewed empirical studies for reliability and validity of the ADHD diagnosis in preschool children (DuPaul, McGoey, Eckert, & VanBrakle, 2001; Keenan & Wakschlag, 2000; Lahey et al., 1998, 2004, 2006; Speltz, McClellan, DeKlyen, & Jones, 1999; Wilens et al., 2002) and concluded that preschool children can be diagnosed using the ADHD diagnostic criteria as listed in the *Diagnostic and Statistical Manual, 4th edition, Text Revision* (DSM-IV-TR) (AACAP, 2003).

Even though the AACAP task force did not recommend any changes to the DSM-IV-TR ADHD diagnostic criteria for preschoolers, the exemplars for individual ADHD criteria included in the DSM-IV-TR are geared toward school-age children. No guidelines are provided to distinguish between the preschoolers' developmentally appropriate and clinically significant hyperactive, impulsive, and inattentive behaviors (Egger, Kondo, & Angold, 2006). Clinicians must rely on their clinical experience and knowledge about developmental issues in preschool children. The challenges that confront assessment of preschool children presenting with ADHD symptoms (especially given the diagnostic controversies described in Chapter 1) require particular attention.

First, clinicians are faced with the difficult question of determining whether hyperactive, impulsive, and inattentive behaviors in a preschool child merely reflect the wider variation in energy and activity level among preschoolers (Gimpel & Kuhn, 2000) since skills in attention deployment and ability to inhibit unnecessary motor behaviors are still developing in preschoolers (Espy, Kaufmann, McDiarmid, & Glisky, 1999).

Second, young children may not be in school and may have fewer demands placed on them to sit in their seats or attend to a task, making it difficult to assess impairment in the child's functioning. Third, even if some children attend a preschool or a family daycare program, the level of structure of a preschool and daycare program may vary widely and differs from the structure in an elementary school. The daily schedule in a preschool and a daycare program does not routinely include independent seatwork or structured classroom instruction delivered to the entire classroom, a setting that is more problematic for a child with ADHD (Pelham, Chacko, & Wymbs, 2004). Instead, the schedule usually involves frequent free choice of activities, and the structured periods are more interactive (e.g., circle time, story time, craft activities, or snack or meal times). Additionally, the preschool and daycare providers vary widely in their qualifications and training. In contrast to elementary school teachers, there are no required training standards or guidelines for preschool and daycare "teachers." Fourth, it is also important to be aware of any "teacher" bias and cultural beliefs that might either over- or under-identify behavior or mental health problems in preschool children (Pelham et al., 2004). Daycare, preschool, and kindergarten "teachers" vary in their beliefs about maintaining strict or lenient structure and discipline in the classroom. There are daycare, preschool, and kindergarten "teachers" who encourage children to move around and talk to peers, incorporate manual activities, and keep any pre-academic activities short, and view the preschoolers' and kindergartners' high physical activity level as positive. Other "teachers" may prefer a more sedentary classroom and may view the preschoolers' and kindergartners' high physical activity level as problematic (Pellegrini & Horvat, 1995).

A fifth difficulty occurs when the child's ADHD behaviors are present only in certain contexts, such as specific caregiving situations or school activities requiring a particular skill, indicating the need to explore particular relationships or demands of those situations that exacerbate the problems. Alternatively, are there environmental accommodations that may be masking the child's problematic symptoms? Many times, caregivers and "teachers" may provide regulatory strategies, supports, and structure to manage the child's behavior and set limits to minimize the escalation of negative behaviors (Carter, Briggs-Gowan, & Davis, 2004). Hence, it is important for clinicians to enquire about any environmental accommodations, management strategies, supports, structure, and limits caregivers and teachers may be providing to regulate the child's behavior.

Sixth, clinicians have to determine whether ADHD symptoms in the preschool child are a manifestation of an underlying anxiety or mood disturbance or language or cognitive impairment (Blackman, 1999). Often anxious or depressed preschool children may appear unfocussed, restless, and hyperactive, whereas the underlying reason for the restlessness and hyperactivity may be due to the child's feelings of anxiety and nervousness rather than ADHD.

Finally, clinicians need to differentiate whether the behavioral symptoms presented by a preschool child are an expression of other issues. For example, is there a mismatch between caregiver and/or "teacher" expectations and the child's level of energy and curiosity? Parents may have developmentally inappropriate expectations (de Lissovoy, 1973; Thompson, Powell, Patterson, & Ellerbee, 1995) of their child's ability to sit and participate in structured activities (e.g., due to inexperience of first-time parents). There may be a mismatch between the child's and the caregiver's energy levels—for example, physical limitations of parents due to health problems, older parents, or grandparents with primary caregiving or significant childcare responsibilities. Does the caregiver have psychiatric difficulties, like depression or cognitive limitation, that may make it difficult for him or her to manage the preschool child's behavioral challenges? Is the caregiver overly stressed or in an abusive relationship and thus overly sensitive to the preschooler's developmentally expected exuberance and mild misbehaviors? (Bauer & Twentyman, 1985; Berg-Nielsen, Solheim, Belsky, & Wichstrom, 2012).

Behavioral Variability Related to Context

In addition to the assessment challenges described above, it is important to consider the contexts in which the behaviors occur. A preschooler's behavior can differ significantly depending on the relational and the interactional contexts and the situation, setting, and the motivational contexts (Dirks, De Los Reyes, Briggs-Gowan, Cella, & Wakschlag, 2012). For example, young children with ADHD have been shown to display better behavioral control in the presence of the father (Nidiffer, Ciulla, Russo, & Cataldo, 1983) and exhibit fewer symptoms and problematic behaviors when they are with an unfamiliar person or are in an unfamiliar environment or situation (Purper-Ouakil, Lepagnol-Bestel, Grosbellet, Gorwood, & Simonneau, 2010). Many parents have expressed their disbelief as to how well behaved their preschooler was during psychiatric assessment in our clinic as opposed to the child's behavior at home and/or at the daycare center.

Behavioral differences among preschoolers with versus without ADHD may become more evident in group activities than in activities with one-on-one adult attention. Frequently caregivers give us histories that their preschooler does better at home when alone with the caregiver and becomes more disruptive and hyperactive when his or her siblings return from school, when visiting family members, or when attending family activities. These clinical findings are corroborated by lower overall mean rates of disruptive behavior and more efficient task performance on pre-academic tasks in young children with one-on-one attention in individual settings than in group play and group teaching situations (Nidiffer et al., 1983).

Motivational context also affects a child's behavior. Often children with ADHD are less attentive when they are expected to do tasks they do not understand (Pellegrini & Horvat, 1995), for example when attempting new tasks. Children with ADHD are usually more responsive and attentive when they receive immediate attention and positive reinforcement from adults and are involved in a novel and interesting activity. Preschoolers with ADHD were less attentive than non-ADHD controls during a passive circle-time task when they were required to listen to the teacher read a story (Alessandri, 1992). In contrast, preschoolers with ADHD did not differ from non-ADHD controls in the level of attention during circle time when they were required to listen to music and respond periodically by singing, clapping, dancing, or playing instruments when cued by the teacher (Alessandri, 1992).

Complaints of problematic behaviors are reported more often in overly stimulating situations—for example, when ADHD preschoolers accompany caregivers to a store, mall, or restaurant—than in free-play situations (Barkley, 2003). Symptoms and dysfunction are more likely to manifest in situations when preschool children with ADHD are required to sit for prolonged periods of time, for example during church services.

In this chapter, we present the AACAP and the American Academy of Pediatrics (AAP) guidelines for preschool ADHD assessment followed by a detailed description of the clinical evaluation processes, emphasizing the need to obtain information from multiple sources.

AACAP and AAP Guidelines for Preschool ADHD Assessment

Both the AACAP and AAP practice guidelines advocate using the DSM-IV-TR diagnostic criteria for diagnosing ADHD in preschool children. The AACAP practice parameters recommend that screening questions regarding the major symptom domains of ADHD (inattention, impulsivity, and hyperactivity) should be asked during every psychiatric evaluation regardless of the nature of the chief complaint. Full evaluation for ADHD should be performed if indicated and should include a thorough assessment of presenting symptoms and the child's functioning at home and preschool or daycare, comorbid psychiatric disorders, and medical, social, and family histories. Rating scales and questionnaires for ADHD symptoms should be completed by parents and teachers (Pliszka, 2007).

The AAP clinical practice guidelines recommend that an evaluation for ADHD should be initiated for any child ages 4 through 18 years who presents with academic or behavioral problems and symptoms of inattention, hyperactivity, or impulsivity. The primary healthcare clinician should rule out any alternative cause for the presenting problems and include assessment for other conditions that might coexist with ADHD, including emotional or behavioral (e.g., anxiety, depressive, oppositional defiant, and conduct disorders), developmental (e.g., learning and language disorders or other neurodevelopmental disorders), and physical (e.g., tics, sleep apnea) conditions (AAP, 2011).

Evaluation Process

In most clinical settings, the parents' first contact is usually via telephone with scheduling office staff. It is important to educate the scheduling staff regarding the basic details of the evaluation process and structure. Members of the scheduling staff in our Infant and Preschool Psychiatry Clinic inform the parents that the evaluation will take place over multiple sessions, with a 90-minute initial session and 45- to 60-minute follow-up sessions. The scheduling staff obtains information about the reasons for the call, asking details to clarify the specific referral request. If parents have other specific questions or need further clarification, the staff refers the parents to the clinician.

Clinicians contact the parents to discuss their concerns and explain that the first session is usually devoted to obtaining psychiatric history from the parents. Follow-up appointments are scheduled for child interview, assessment of parent–child interaction, and discussion of treatment planning and recommendations. Parents are informed that they will be asked detailed historical and background information, the preschool child will also be seen by herself or himself, and collateral information will be collected from multiple sources both through interview and rating scales and questionnaires. The collateral informants may include the other parent if not present during the initial evaluation session, other important family members with whom the child interacts frequently, and daycare/preschool "teachers." Rating scales and questionnaires are mailed for parents and "teachers" to complete prior to the initial evaluation. Parents are requested to bring the completed forms to the initial evaluation appointment along with any other records the child may have from previous evaluations and/or school evaluations and reports. Parents are assured that the clinic/office is child-friendly with age-appropriate toys, books, drawing paper, washable nontoxic crayons, and child-sized furniture, and we try to make the child as comfortable as possible.

EVALUATION SETTING

Preschoolers may be fearful about going to "the doctor's office." It is important to prepare the office and the playroom to make it inviting. Toys and other play materials can help to engage the child as well as keep the child occupied during the parent interview. At the same time, precautions should be taken for the safety of the preschooler and others who may be present during the evaluation. There should be a limited number of toys so as not to overwhelm and overly distract the child. Appropriate toys include building blocks, a dollhouse, a doll family, toy figurines, a variety of toy animals (e.g., dinosaurs, farm animals), hand puppets, plain paper, and nontoxic and washable crayons and markers. Not recommended are toys that are easily breakable, heavy toys that could hurt if thrown, and toys with small parts, as they may present a choking hazard. It may be best to see the child in a playroom rather than in the office to minimize distractions for the child and the need for vigilance on the part of the evaluator and parents to ensure that the child does not get into papers, computers, drawers, and other materials in the office.

REASONS FOR EVALUATION REQUEST

Frequently preschool children are referred for evaluation for ADHD because of impulsive, disruptive, and aggressive behaviors resulting in problems in peer and social relationships and childcare difficulties. Often, hyperactivity and inattentive behaviors are elicited during the evaluation process and may not have been the specific reason for the referral request. A quick survey of the preschool children seen in our Infant and Preschool Psychiatry Clinic revealed that of the 53 preschoolers who received a diagnosis of ADHD, 64% (n = 34) had presenting complaints related to hyperactivity and/or inattentive symptoms and 36% (n = 19) had presenting complaints related to associated behavior problems (e.g., aggression, problems getting along with peers, and disruptive behavior). Parents often complain that their preschooler does not have many friends, is not invited to peer social events, and is not welcome at family gatherings due to his or her impulsive behavior.

By the time preschoolers present for psychiatric evaluation, many have already been suspended and/or expelled from daycare or early education settings, and their parents have experienced difficulty finding childcare. In a study of preschool children attending a large pediatric clinic, more than 40% of the preschoolers with ADHD had been suspended compared to 0.5% of the preschoolers without ADHD, and almost 16%

of the ADHD preschoolers had been expelled (Egger et al., 2006; Ghuman, Arnold, & Anthony, 2008). Parents often worry about their job security because of added demands on their time (Ghuman et al., 2008). Parents get frequent calls from the child's preschool or daycare center to inform them about the child's disruptive behavior and/ or to ask them to pick up the child early. Parents often express their reluctance to take the preschooler to a store or a restaurant in order to avoid public embarrassment and scrutiny due the child's impulsive, loud, and disruptive behaviors (Egger et al., 2006).

Parents are concerned that their child's overactivity, impulsivity, and inattention may interfere with his or her ability to learn new skills. They often express frustration that their child does not know the alphabet or numbers even though they have been working with him or her. They are concerned that their child does not seem to retain what he or she has just learned. They fear that their child won't be ready for school and may be falling behind peers. They are further worried that their child's co-occurring temper tantrums, aggression, defiance, and noncompliance behaviors will be disruptive to their classroom peers and question whether the preschool "teacher" will be able to manage their child's behavior. One mother told us that she could not "subject the 'teacher'" to her child's difficult-to-manage behaviors.

The following examples highlight some of the ADHD-related presenting complaints and impairments that were the impetus for the preschoolers' referral to our Infant and Preschool Psychiatry Clinic. It is important to note that these behaviors constitute a consistent pattern of repeated occurrences of problematic behaviors across different settings, and that a single such occurrence would not qualify a preschooler for an ADHD diagnosis.

- A mother reported that despite moving all the cleaning supplies to the top cabinets, her 2½-year-old son climbed up on the shelves to get to the cleaning supplies. Eventually she had to put locks on the top cabinets also.
- A mother told us that her 4-year-old son was always "on the go" and would climb up on objects without regard to his safety. She called our clinic for an evaluation after he climbed on top of a soda machine when she took her eyes off of him for few seconds while talking to somebody.
- A 4½-year-old child presented with a history of an accidental fracture at age 4 when he jumped off the table and did not look to see if there was anything in the way.
- A mother reported that her 5-year-old foster child had impulsively shoved a corn kernel in ear; it needed surgical removal.
- Another caregiver told us that she had tried to manage her 4-year-old adopted child's need to be constantly moving by scheduling back-to-back outdoor activities all day long. As a result she was exhausted and unable to pay adequate attention to her other children and her household duties and had started to experience problems in her marital relationship.

PREPARING/INFORMING THE PRESCHOOLER REGARDING THE REASONS AND PROCESS OF ASSESSMENT

It is important to inform and prepare the preschooler regarding the reasons for and process of assessment. We encourage the parents to talk to the preschooler about difficulties during recent events—for example, having to return home early from the store because the child was running in the aisles, time-out at the preschool for running around in the classroom, becoming angry and hitting a classmate/teacher, and similar difficulties related to getting along with siblings, cousins, and/or other family members. Parents can explain to the preschooler that because the child has been having problems at home/preschool, they are going to see a professional, a "talking doctor," who can help. Parents are encouraged to explain to the preschooler that they will talk together with the professional, and the child will also talk to the professional by herself or himself. Preschoolers' fears are usually allayed by preparing them ahead of time and also explaining that there will be a playroom with toys, books, crayons, and drawing paper and that there will be "no needles." Following are examples of the preschoolers' understanding as to why their parents brought them to the clinic.

Recently a 4-year-old preschooler told us that he gets mad when his brother tries to play with his toys. He pushes his brother to get him away from his toys. He gets mad when his mom tells him to stop playing his video game because he "really, really" wants to get to the next level. At school when he pushes another child, the teacher sends him to time-out. He does not want to sit in the time-out chair or for circle time to listen to a story because "it is boring" and because it is "fun to run around." Another 4-year-old told us that she is "too talky" in the classroom and she does not raise her hand because her "hand gets tired" as her teacher "never calls on me," an observation that was not confirmed by her mother, who had observed that the teacher always called on her first.

Diagnostic Process

Psychiatric evaluation for a DSM-5 diagnosis of ADHD includes a comprehensive psychiatric history from the caregiver(s), child interview, observation of child behavior and parent–child interaction, mental status examination of the preschooler, and collateral information regarding the child's symptoms and functioning in settings outside of the home. We routinely interview the parents with the child present as we believe that it is important for the child to hear the parents' concerns about his or her behavior. Additionally, having the child present during the parent interview provides an opportunity to observe casual child behavior, parent–child interaction, and parenting behaviors. At the beginning of the interview, it is important to ask the parents if there are particularly sensitive issues that they do not feel comfortable discussing in the presence of the child. In that case, the parents can be interviewed without the child for part of the psychiatric history.

HISTORY OF PRESENT ILLNESS

Detailed information is obtained from the parents about the history of the present illness, the child's functioning at home, preschool, or daycare (if the child is attending preschool or daycare), and peer and social relationships. The parents are asked to provide detailed information regarding the 18 DSM-5 ADHD symptoms (9 hyperactive and impulsive and 9 inattentive symptoms) with examples and probes to assess the frequency, severity, pervasiveness, and functional impairment from each symptom across preschool, home, and public settings. Parents are asked about the child's behavior during participation in activities and situations that are pertinent to a preschool child's daily life (e.g., circle time, story time, craft activities, or meal, snack, or nap times. See Table 2.1 for examples of typical behavioral descriptions provided by parents pertaining

Table 2.1. **Examples of Complaints of Caregivers of Preschool Children Regarding Specific DSM-5 ADHD Criteria**

DSM-5 Criteria	*Examples of ADHD behaviors/parent complaints in preschool children*
Hyperactive/Impulsive Presentation	
Hyperactivity	
Fidgets with hands or feet or squirms in seat	Always touching something, "teachers" always telling the child to keep hands to self, always has to have something in hand, kicks bottom of the table top when seated at the dinner table, kicks the seat in front of him/her when sitting in the car, slides down the chair, sits under the table, sits on the arm of the chair
Leaves seat in classroom or in other situations in which remaining seated is expected	Does not sit during circle time, meals, or story time at the library, won't even sit to watch television (stands or walks around when watching television) or to eat in a restaurant
Runs about or climbs excessively in situations where it's inappropriate	Always running through the house, always runs to wherever he/she has to go, gets bruises and bumps from running into objects or people, climbs onto the counters, bookshelves, jumps on the furniture, jumps on the bed, slides down the staircase railing, careless accidents, runs through the aisles in the store, runs away from the caregiver when they go to the mall
Is always "on the go" or acts as if "driven by a motor"	Like the "Energizer Bunny," is never still, goes all day and does not stop until he/she falls asleep, may slow down only if he/she is sick
Talks excessively	"Motor mouth," talks non-stop, talks during story time and Sunday school, won't be quiet during naptime
Difficulty playing or engaging in leisure activities quietly	Noisy play, banging toys together, slamming into things, wakes the entire household once gets up in the morning
Impulsivity	
Difficulty waiting in lines or awaiting turn in games or group situations	Always wants to be first, butts in front of the line when waiting for his/her turn to go on the slide or to get a snack from the preschool "teacher", if wants to play with a toy snatches the toy from the other child's hand, starts to clown around or becomes very impatient when caregiver is waiting turn at the cashier line

(continued)

Table 2.1. (**Continued**)

DSM-5 Criteria	Examples of ADHD behaviors/parent complaints in preschool children
Blurts out answers to questions before the questions have been completed	Blurts out answers during story time or circle time, does not raise hand even when reminded repeatedly, starts talking before finding out whether the question was addressed to him/her or to somebody else
Interrupts or intrudes on others	Interrupts when caregiver is on the phone or talking to someone, interrupts sibling when sibling is playing a game even when the caregiver tries to engage him/her in a different but interesting activity
Inattentive Presentation	
Difficulty sustaining attention in tasks or play activities	Goes from one toy or one activity to another, does not finish even a simple puzzle, does not finish listening to a story from a nursery book, starts coloring but leaves it in the middle, does not finish watching a cartoon on TV
Difficulty organizing tasks and daily activities	Comes out of the room half-dressed, starts doing an activity before gathering all the materials, does not put shoes or jacket in their designated spots, puts shirt on backwards
Does not follow through on instructions and fails to finish schoolwork or chores	Starts to take backpack to his/her room but gets distracted and starts to do something else, leaving the backpack on the way
Avoids, expresses reluctance about, or has difficulties engaging in tasks that require mental effort	Complains it is too difficult, "I don't like it," wants caregiver to help or wants the caregiver to do it, refuses to practice writing his/her name or the alphabet
Loses things necessary for tasks or activities	Can't find toys, crayons, shoes or favorite possessions (e.g., stuffed toy)
Does not seem to listen to what is being said	Name has to be called several times before looks up
Easily distracted by extraneous stimuli	Gets distracted if sees a bird fly by the window, brother/sister comes in the room, or hears a noise, gets up to see the bird or follow brother/sister and stops what he is doing
Forgetful in daily activities	Forgets to brush teeth, comb hair, put shoes on when going outside or put backpack away
Fails to give close attention to details or makes careless mistakes in schoolwork, work, or other activities	Scribbles on the paper as wants to get done fast, even though able to write name when gets 1:1 attention, coloring is messy as rushes through and doesn't take care to stay within lines

to the DSM-5 ADHD diagnostic criteria. It is important to ask for sufficient detail about each symptom regarding age of onset and progression trajectory (improving, remaining the same, or worsening). Information regarding any variability in the child's behavioral expression in different contexts (i.e., situations, settings, structure, and environmental demands) in which the child's symptoms are exaggerated or minimized should be explored. Parents should be asked about any specific strategies they have found to be helpful.

It should be determined if the parents' complaints regarding the child's activity level, impulsivity, or inattention are excessive compared to what is expected of the child's developmental age peers. Do the child's behaviors impair his or her ability to make developmental progress or interfere in functioning in the areas of learning new skills, relationships with authority figures, peer relationships, and self-perception and self-image? The impact of the child's ADHD symptoms in terms of stress on the physical environment (e.g., breaking things, destruction of property) as well as peer and caregiver distress, safety concerns, and need for environmental accommodations should be evaluated.

In addition to the parent interview, we ask that parents complete parent rating scales and questionnaires. See Chapter 3 for commonly used rating scales.

REVIEW FOR COMORBID DISORDERS

A detailed history regarding comorbid disorders/coexisting conditions (both behavioral and developmental disorders, such as communication disorders, learning issues) should be obtained, and their contribution, if any, to the child's ADHD symptoms or vice versa should be evaluated. The need for any other assessments to determine the role of communication, cognitive, or other learning disorders in the child's ADHD symptoms should be identified. See Chapter 4 regarding details about disorders that are frequently comorbid with ADHD.

FAMILY AND SOCIAL HISTORY

Family history should be obtained to look for a genetic predisposition for ADHD or other psychiatric disorders in the family. Parents should be asked about learning issues, school behavior problems, depressive and anxiety symptoms, drug abuse, police involvement, and stress or other emotional concerns in themselves and other family members. Social history is obtained regarding the child's living situation, the parents' marital situation and relationship, custody issues/disputes, visitation arrangements and/or conflicts if any, CPS involvement, parents' educational and occupational status, and any financial concerns. Information is also obtained regarding childcare arrangements, daycare/preschool attendance and any behavioral concerns, and peer relations.

Psychosocial factors (family stress, family psychopathology, parent–child relationship, differences in parenting styles of the caregivers, adequacy of the caregiving environment) affecting the child's ADHD symptoms and psychosocial intervention needs should be assessed. The adequacy of, as well as current and past history of changes in, primary caregiver relationship status and social support network and need for respite resources should be explored. As discussed in Chapter 1, the mother's relationship status, emotional support, and the adequacy of the caregiving environment were found to influence and predict the trajectory of progression of ADHD symptoms in at-risk infants and preschoolers (Carlson, Jacobvitz, & Sroufe, 1995; Jacobvitz & Sroufe, 1987).

DEVELOPMENTAL AND MEDICAL HISTORY

Detailed information should be obtained to determine the contribution of developmental, medical, and dietary history to the child's ADHD symptoms. The developmental history should include details regarding the mother's pregnancy with the child, the parents' age at the time of the pregnancy, whether this was a planned/unplanned and/or wanted/unwanted pregnancy, the parents' relationship at that time, emotional support and emotional and/or social stress, and family support during the pregnancy. Details should be obtained about the mother's health status during the pregnancy, any history of fever, infections, or hospitalizations, and any in utero exposure to illicit substances or prescribed medications. Parents should be asked about any complications during delivery or with the child's health status at birth, and whether the child was born at full term or prematurely. Details about early development should include information on the child's birth weight, condition at delivery, Apgar scores, any complications, the child's temperament, and developmental milestones.

The medical history should include any medical conditions, drug allergies, surgery, or hospitalizations in the child. Is the child taking any prescribed medications, supplements, or over-the-counter medications that may predispose to, mimic, or exacerbate ADHD symptoms or may interact with ADHD medications? Permission to obtain medical records from the primary healthcare provider should be obtained. Parents should be asked about any concerns regarding the child's appetite, eating habits, dietary sensitivities, and adequate nutritional intake. Chapter 4 gives further details about obtaining the medical history, medical risk factors, and medical differential diagnoses for ADHD, and Chapter 10 discusses specific etiologies that might support consideration of complementary and alternative treatments.

CHILD INTERVIEW AND OBSERVATION
OF CHILD BEHAVIOR

We usually ask the preschooler about his or her understanding of the problems and issues at the start of the initial psychiatric evaluation appointment before asking the parents for detailed information. Before starting the interview process, it is important to allow time for the child and parents to get acclimated to the clinic/playroom/office setting and to invite the child to play with the toys to help him or her feel comfortable in the new surroundings. Often commenting on the child's play and/or what the child is wearing (e.g., a super-hero shirt) helps to engage the child. Conversations should be kept short and simple, using language appropriate to the child's chronological and developmental age level.

In addition to the conversation with the preschooler during the parent interview, a 25- to 30-minute interview should be scheduled with the child alone. The child interview is usually conducted after the initial psychiatric evaluation appointment so the

child has had an opportunity to become familiar with the clinic/playroom/office setting. Occasionally, a preschooler may experience excessive separation distress and may
refuse to meet alone without support from the parents.

The preschooler should be invited to play with the toys and the clinician should join
the child's play following the child's lead. A combination of approaches is used for the
child interview depending on what seems to work best with a particular child's interactional style. Many preschoolers with ADHD are outgoing and easily engage in conversation and respond to questions while they play. We try to weave interview questions
as naturally as possible as we play with the preschooler and as opportunities arise. For
example, if the child gets frustrated with a certain play activity, we may ask about other
such frustrations the child experiences at preschool and/or at home and how he or she
deals with them.

Following are examples of the interview topics and questions that we may ask a preschooler. Questions may need to be modified and additional/alternative questions may
be asked depending on the child's age, developmental status, presenting concerns, and
the psychiatric history provided by the parents.

Social relationships. Do you have friends? What are their names? Do you like to
play with other kids? Who do you play with? What toys do you like to play with? What
toys and games do you play with your friends? Do the kids like to play with you? Do
you like school? What is your "teacher"s name? Do you get along with your classmates/
brothers/sisters/cousin/other family members?

ADHD symptoms. During circle time, do you sit on the carpet and listen to the
"teacher" read a story? Do you run around when the "teacher" is reading a story? Do you
talk to the other kids when the "teacher" is reading a story? Does your mom/"teacher"
tell you a lot of times to keep your hands to yourself? Does your mom/"teacher" have to
tell you a lot of times to sit in your seat? Do you jump on the sofa even when your mom
tells you not to? Do you take naps at school? Do you get up from your cot and start play-
ing/talking/running around when it is nap time? Does your "teacher" tell you to read a
book/draw a picture/play quietly when the other kids are taking a nap?

Associated and comorbid psychiatric symptoms. Do you sleep okay at night?
Do you like going to bed? Do you come out of your room after your mom/dad tells
you to go to sleep? Do you sleep in your own room/own bed? Do you share your room
with ___? Do you get up at night and go to your parents' room? Do you sleep in your
parents' room? Do you sleep in their bed? Do you have dreams at night? Are they good
dreams or bad dreams? Tell me what dream did you have. Do you have a TV in your
room? Do you watch TV before going to sleep? Do you watch TV when you get up at
night and can't go back to sleep?

Do you get into trouble at school? Do you get into trouble at home? What kind of
things do you get into trouble for? Does your mom/"teacher" send you to time-out? Do
you fight with other children? What was the fight about? Did anybody get hurt? Did
you get hurt?

How do you feel? Do you feel happy? What makes you happy? Do you get sad sometimes? Do you get sad a lot? What makes you feel sad? What do you do when you get
sad? Do you cry sometimes? Do you cry a lot? Do you get angry sometimes? Do you
get angry a lot? What makes you angry? What do you do when you are angry? Do you
worry sometimes? Do you worry a lot? What do you worry about? What do you do

when you get worried? Do you think about your parents when you are at school? Do you worry if they are okay?

Do you get scared at night? Are you scared of the dark? Do you tell your mom you don't want to go to your room by yourself when it is dark? Do you see/hear scary things? Do you hear them at night time/daytime? Do your ears/eyes play tricks on you? Do you hear/see something, but when you turn around nobody was there? Do you hear/see something, but nobody else saw/heard it? Does that scare you?

Child's understanding of/insight into the behavioral problems, reason for behavior, impact of behavior on others, thoughts about the fairness/unfairness of the consequences, and need for changing behavior (e.g., fighting, being punished, sent to time-out or restriction of activities, and whether behavior is problematic for self and/or others). What made you fight? Do you feel it was ___'s (the other child's name) fault? Do you feel ___ made you do it? (For example, a preschooler told us that he hit and snatched the toy from a peer because he wanted to play with the toy, but his peer refused to give it to him.)

How did you feel when ___ (the other child's name) got hurt? Did you think it was your fault when ___ got hurt? Did your behavior get you into trouble? Did your behavior get ___ (the other child) into trouble? Did you go to time-out? Did you think it was unfair/fair that you had to go to time-out? Do you think you can stop/control your behavior? Do you think you can't stop your behavior even when you try your best to be good?

Do you wish you could stop hitting? Do you wish you could get along better with your friends/siblings/cousins/parents? What do you think can help? Do you think if you and your mom and dad came back to talk to us, we can all think of some things that can help? Would you like to earn stickers for sitting in circle time when your "teacher" reads a story? Would you like to earn stickers for playing nicely with your brother/sister/friends? What kind of stickers do you like? Would you like to go to the store with your mom/dad to buy the stickers you like? Would you like to put your stickers on the sticker chart? Would you like to put your sticker chart on the fridge or in your room? Would you like to show your sticker chart to mom/dad/siblings?

CHILD OBSERVATION AND MENTAL STATUS EXAMINATION

The AACAP practice parameters for assessment of infants and toddlers provide a reference tool, the Infant and Toddler Mental Status Exam, that incorporates the traditional mental status examination categories for observation of infants and toddlers (Thomas et al., 1997). Mental status examination of the preschoolers is conducted to assess appearance, including dysmorphic features, sensorium, reaction to new settings and people, relatedness to parents, other caregivers, and the examiner, self-regulation strategies, play exploration, play content and structure, thought content, fears, nightmares, affect and mood, vocalization and speech production, receptive language, age-appropriate vocabulary, clarity and understandability of speech, gross and fine motor function, and cognitive functioning (Thomas et al., 1997). Preschoolers should be observed for activity level, attention span, persistence with completing a play activity versus shifting attention from one activity to another, reaction to transitions, frustration tolerance, aggression, and modulation of aggression. Preschoolers should be asked to identify and copy different shapes, such as Gessel figures (Cattel, 1960; Illingsworth, 1972), draw a person (Levine & Gross, 1968; Sinha, 1970; Tramill, Edwards, & Tramill, 1980), draw their family doing something together, tell a short story about the picture, and write their name. Preschoolers should be asked if they recognize emotions, colors, alphabet letters and numbers, read simple words, count, and understand the concept of "more" and "less." If appropriate, preschoolers may be asked to perform simple addition and subtraction. Preschoolers may need visual cues, props, and concrete examples ("Here are two cars and I am going to give you one more car. How many cars do you have now?").

LIMITATIONS OF THE CHILD INTERVIEW AND CLINIC OBSERVATION OF THE PRESCHOOLER

The child interview and clinic observation can provide valuable information regarding the child's behaviors, the child's understanding and acknowledgment of problems, and the child's motivation to get help and change and cooperate with the recommendations, parents, and therapist. However, many times the information obtained from the child interview and observation may be limited. The reliability of the child interview has been questioned; young children may often be unaware of their symptoms of ADHD (Pliszka, 2007). Moreover, there is no standard structure expected in a preschooler's daily life, making it difficult to determine whether the observed child behaviors in the clinic indicate impairment or mere lack of exposure to structured activities. Additionally, as we discussed earlier, due to the novelty of the clinic setting, new toys, unfamiliar individuals, and the one-on-one nature of the clinical assessment, a child's behavior during a clinic visit may be very different from his or her usual behavior.

Hence, observing children on multiple occasions in different settings, contexts, and natural surroundings (e.g., home, clinic, classroom, and community settings) can provide very valuable information. Assessment by observing the child in the classroom can shed light on the child's classroom behavior, peer interactions, the classroom structure, the "teacher's" interactive and disciplining style, and the "teacher–child" fit. Even though multiple observations in varied settings and contexts can be very time-consuming, every attempt should be made to observe children in their natural surroundings. For example, many community mental health centers routinely employ and/or have the capability to do in-home assessment and therapy services and visit the child's school. On the other hand, in many clinic and private office settings, if such observations prove to be impractical, talking with the teacher can provide collateral information about his or her observations of the child's behavior in the classroom, peer relationships, perceptions of peers about the child, relationship with authority figures, history of suspensions or expulsions, and age-appropriate development of and progress in pre-academic skills. Rating scales completed by a preschool child's parents and other caregivers can also serve as a proxy and provide information about a child's behavior in multiple settings and across multiple contexts.

Obtaining history from multiple informants, sources, and settings provides a comprehensive understanding of the child's presentation and can help to distinguish whether the child's symptoms and the resulting impairment are pervasive, isolated, or specific to a certain activity, setting, situation, or person.

OBSERVATION OF PARENT–CHILD INTERACTION

A 25- to 30-minute appointment should be scheduled for observation of parent–child interaction and parenting behaviors. Parents should be instructed to interact and play with the child as they would at home. The child is observed for engagement or initiation of play with the parent, quality and quantity of verbal exchange, and capacity for affective involvement with the parent. The parents are observed for attunement to the child's cues, vigilance, protectiveness, ability to regulate the child's emotional responses, limit setting, facilitating autonomous play in the child, and parenting behaviors (see Chapters 5 and 6 for a detailed description of parenting behavior observation).

DIAGNOSTIC FORMULATION AND COMPREHENSIVE TREATMENT PLANNING AND RECOMMENDATIONS

Integration of all available data from the clinical history, child observation, parent and teacher rating scales and questionnaires, school reports, and reports from previous evaluations helps to formulate a working diagnosis, rule out mimics and narrow the differential diagnosis, and consider comorbid disorders. The data should be evaluated to determine if any further workup is indicated (e.g., speech, language and hearing, cognitive and educational assessments, classroom observation, consultation with primary healthcare provider for any medical issues and medications the child might be taking). A meeting should be scheduled with the parents to discuss the working diagnosis, differential diagnosis and comorbid disorders, recommendations for further assessment, and treatment recommendations.

In keeping with the biopsychosocial approach for comprehensive treatment planning, any specific psychosocial stressors and intervention needs should be addressed. For example, specific recommendations may need to be made if there are differences in parenting styles of the caregivers, inadequate or no psychosocial support networks, and/ or mental health problems in the parents. The parents' participation in parent behavior management skills intervention (discussed in detail in Chapters 5 and 6) should be routinely recommended. Pharmacologic intervention is recommended only if there is insufficient progress with an adequate trial of parent behavior management skills intervention.

If ADHD symptoms and resulting impairment in functioning are limited to specific contexts, it is important to explore the underlying basis for the behavioral problems in the particular context, and specific recommendations to address the situation should be made (Dirks et al., 2012).

If the child has problems getting along with peers, specific strategies to improve peer relationships should be recommended, for example one-on-one peer play dates. It should be emphasized to the parents that to enhance the chances for a successful experience for both the child and the peer, it is important to take care in selecting the peer, plan specific structured activities that are of interest to both the peer and the child, keep the play date short (30 to 60 minutes), take a snack break at transition times, and provide on-hand guidance, support, and supervision during the play date. Practicing ahead of time how to share and choose alternate activities that might be of interest to the peer can be helpful.

It is also important to discuss the need for structure in the child's daily routine. If the child is not yet attending a preschool, it is often recommended that parents look into enrolling the child in a preschool or Head Start program. The preschool setting provides structure to the child's day and more appropriate peer models, allows the child to get accustomed to structured activities, provides an opportunity for the child to learn from experienced educators and/or childcare professionals, and prepares the child for kindergarten. In addition to learning pre-academic skills, it also provides respite for the parent (AAP, 2011). In some cases, the school staff may determine that they are not able to manage the child's behavior in a regular daycare setting or preschool program and may suggest referral to a special education preschool.

If the child is attending preschool, the impact of the child's school and classroom structure and routine (for example, strict and rigid schedule vs. very loosely structured classroom) on the child's behavior should be discussed. If classroom observation and/ or the parents indicate that there is a mismatch between the child's needs and the classroom structure, the "teacher" style, and/or the "teacher–child" fit, recommendations regarding the child's school placement may need to be considered. Occasionally, changing the child's classroom to a more structured classroom and a "teacher" who is firm and has clear, consistent, and predictable expectations can be helpful. It should be emphasized to the parents that it is important to establish frequent, regular, and positive communication with the child's "teacher."

If there are subthreshold ADHD symptoms or a history of improving symptom trajectory, follow-up assessments at 3- to 6-month intervals are recommended to monitor the preschooler's progress in ADHD symptoms and general functioning.

Sometimes there is evidence or suspicion of parental psychopathology (that may be undiagnosed and/or untreated) and/or inadequate social support. It should be emphasized to the parents that it is important for them to take care of their own mental health and social support needs so they are able to meet the child's needs. If indicated, referral should be made for supportive counseling and/or other mental health services, including psychiatric assessment of the parents.

Summary

Rational approaches to diagnosing preschool children with ADHD include a thorough diagnostic workup to rule out mimics. Assessment should be carried out over multiple visits. The baseline diagnostic workup should include detailed clinical information regarding presenting symptoms and whether they are inappropriate for the child's developmental level. Information should be collected from multiple sources, including parents, preschool "teachers," and/or daycare providers regarding the child's functioning, typical behaviors, and problems in different settings and contexts. An assessment should be made of the caregiver and "teacher" bias and cultural beliefs, and environmental accommodations and supports provided to the child. Specificity of the ADHD diagnosis in preschool children can be enhanced if supported by a history of multiple, persistent, and substantial impairments that occur in multiple contexts and in multiple situations and environments and/or in the community.

Future efforts should focus on improving and developing structured and standardized interviews and observation measures that are practical for clinical purposes. Even more importantly, efforts should be focused on training clinicians, providers, and researchers to work with young preschool-age children and develop expertise to address this area of great need.

Disclosures

Jaswinder K. Ghuman, M.D., has received past funding from the NIMH for a K-23 career development grant, the Arizona Institute for Mental Health Research, and from Bristol-Myers Squibb for a clinical trial in autistic disorder. She received funding from the Health Resources and Services Administration–Maternal and Child Health (HRSA-MCH) for a training grant for the University of Arizona Leadership Education in Neurodevelopmental Disabilities Training Program (AZLEND).

Harinder S. Ghuman, M.D., has no conflicts of interest.

References

AACAP. (2003). Research diagnostic criteria for infants and preschool children: the process and empirical support. *Journal of the American Academy of Child and Adolescent Psychiatry, 42*(12), 1504–1512.

AAP. (2011). ADHD: clinical practice guideline for the diagnosis, evaluation, and treatment of attention-deficit/hyperactivity disorder in children and adolescents. *Pediatrics, 128*(5), 1007–1022.

Alessandri, S. M. (1992). Attention, play, and social behavior in ADHD preschoolers. *Journal of Abnormal Child Psychology, 20*(3), 289–302.

Barkley, R. A. (2003). Issues in the diagnosis of attention-deficit/hyperactivity disorder in children. *Brain Development, 25*(2), 77–83.

Bauer, W. D., & Twentyman, C. T. (1985). Abusing, neglectful, and comparison mothers' responses to child-related and non-child-related stressors. *Journal of Consulting Clinical Psychology, 53*(3), 335–343.

Berg-Nielsen, T. S., Solheim, E., Belsky, J., & Wichstrom, L. (2012). Preschoolers' psychosocial problems: in the eyes of the beholder? Adding teacher characteristics as determinants of discrepant parent-teacher reports. *Child Psychiatry Human Development, 43*(3), 393–413.

Blackman, J. A. (1999). Attention-deficit/hyperactivity disorder in preschoolers. Does it exist and should we treat it? *Pediatric Clinics of North America, 46*(5), 1011–1025.

Carlson, E. A., Jacobvitz, D., & Sroufe, L. A. (1995). A developmental investigation of inattentiveness and hyperactivity. *Child Development, 66*(1), 37–54.

Carter, A. S., Briggs-Gowan, M. J., & Davis, N. O. (2004). Assessment of young children's social-emotional development and psychopathology: recent advances and recommendations for practice. *Journal of Child Psychology & Psychiatry & Allied Disciplines, 45*(1), 109–134.

Cattel, P. (1960). *The measurement of intelligence of infants and young children.* New York: Psychological Corporation.

de Lissovoy, V. (1973). Child care by adolescent parents. *Children Today, 2*(4), 22–25.

Dirks, M. A., De Los Reyes, A., Briggs-Gowan, M., Cella, D., & Wakschlag, L. S. (2012). Annual research review: embracing not erasing contextual variability in children's behavior—theory and utility in the selection and use of methods and informants in developmental psychopathology. *Journal of Child Psychology & Psychiatry, 53*(5), 558–574.

DuPaul, G. J., McGoey, K. E., Eckert, T. L., & VanBrakle, J. (2001). Preschool children with attention-deficit/hyperactivity disorder: impairments in behavioral, social, and school functioning. *Journal of the American Academy of Child and Adolescent Psychiatry, 40*(5), 508–515.

Egger, H. L., Kondo, D., & Angold, A. (2006). The epidemiology and diagnostic issues in preschool attention-deficit/ hyperactivity disorder: A review. *Infants & Young Children, 19*(2), 109–122.

Espy, K. A., Kaufmann, P. M., McDiarmid, M. D., & Glisky, M. L. (1999). Executive functioning in preschool children: performance on A-not-B and other delayed response format tasks. *Brain Cognition, 41*(2), 178–199.

Ghuman, J. K., Arnold, L. E., & Anthony, B. J. (2008). Psychopharmacological and other treatments in preschool children with attention-deficit/hyperactivity disorder: current evidence and practice. *Journal of Child & Adolescent Psychopharmacology, 18*(5), 413–447.

Gimpel, G. A., & Kuhn, B. R. (2000). Maternal report of attention deficit hyperactivity disorder symptoms in preschool children. *Child Care Health Development, 26*(3), 163–176.

Illingsworth, R. (1972). *The development of the infant and young child, normal and abnormal* (5th ed.). Baltimore: Williams & Wilkins.

Jacobvitz, D., & Sroufe, L. A. (1987). The early caregiver-child relationship and attention-deficit disorder with hyperactivity in kindergarten: a prospective study. *Child Development, 6*, 1496–1504.

Keenan, K., & Wakschlag, L. S. (2000). More than the terrible twos: the nature and severity of behavior problems in clinic-referred preschool children. *Journal of Abnormal Child Psychology, 28*(1), 33–46.

Lahey, B. B., Pelham, W. E., Chronis, A., Massetti, G., Kipp, H., Ehrhardt, A., et al. (2006). Predictive validity of ICD-10 hyperkinetic disorder relative to DSM-IV attention-deficit/hyperactivity disorder among younger children. *Journal of Child Psychology & Psychiatry, 47*(5), 472–479.

Lahey, B. B., Pelham, W. E., Loney, J., Kipp, H., Ehrhardt, A., Lee, S. S., et al. (2004). Three-year predictive validity of DSM-IV attention deficit hyperactivity disorder in children diagnosed at 4-6 years of age. *American Journal of Psychiatry, 161*(11), 2014–2020.

Lahey, B. B., Pelham, W. E., Stein, M. A., Loney, J., Trapani, C., Nugent, K., et al. (1998). Validity of DSM-IV attention-deficit/hyperactivity disorder for younger children. *Journal of the American Academy of Child and Adolescent Psychiatry, 37*(7), 695–702.

Levine, H. A., & Gross, M. (1968). Suitability of the Harris revision of the Goodenough Draw-a-Man test for a psychiatric population. *Journal of Clinical Psychology, 24*(3), 350–351.

Nidiffer, F. D., Ciulla, R. P., Russo, D. C., & Cataldo, M. F. (1983). Behavioral variability as a function of noncontingent adult attention, peer availability, and situational demands in three hyperactive boys. *Journal of Experimental Child Psychology, 36*(1), 109–123.

Pelham, W. E., Chacko, A., & Wymbs, B. T. (2004). Diagnostic and assessment issues of attention deficit/hyperactivity disorder in the young child. In Del Carmen-Wiggins, R. (Ed.). *Handbook of infant, toddler, and preschool mental health assessment* (pp 399–420). Oxford University Press, New York, NY.

Pellegrini, A. D., & Horvat, M. (1995). A developmental contextualist critique of attention deficit hyperactivity disorder. *Educational Researcher, 24*(1), 13–19.

Pliszka, S. (2007). Practice parameter for the assessment and treatment of children and adolescents with attention-deficit/hyperactivity disorder. *Journal of the American Academy of Child and Adolescent Psychiatry, 46*(7), 894–921.

Purper-Ouakil, D., Lepagnol-Bestel, A. M., Grosbellet, E., Gorwood, P., & Simonneau, M. (2010) [Neurobiology of attention deficit/hyperactivity disorder]. *Medicine Sciences (Paris), 26*(5), 487–496.

Sinha, M. (1970). A study of the Harris revision of the Goodenough Draw-A-Man Test. *British Journal of Educational Psychology, 40*(2), 221–222.

Speltz, M. L., McClellan, J., DeKlyen, M., & Jones, K. (1999). Preschool boys with oppositional defiant disorder: clinical presentation and diagnostic change. *Journal of the American Academy of Child and Adolescent Psychiatry, 38*(7), 838–845.

Thomas, J. M., Benham, A. L., Gean, M., Luby, J., Minde, K., Turner, S., et al. (1997). Practice parameters for the psychiatric assessment of infants and toddlers (0-36 months). American Academy of Child and Adolescent Psychiatry. *Journal of the American Academy of Child and Adolescent Psychiatry, 36*(10 Suppl), 21S–36S.

Thompson, P. J., Powell, M. J., Patterson, R. J., & Ellerbee, S. M. (1995). Adolescent parenting: Outcomes and maternal perceptions. *Journal of Obstetric, Gynecologic, and Neonatal Nursing, 24,* 713–718.

Tramill, J. L., Edwards, R. P., & Tramill, J. K. (1980). Comparison of the Goodenough-Harris Drawing Test and the WISC-R for children experiencing academic difficulties. *Perceptual Motor Skills, 50*(2), 543–546.

Wilens, T. E., Biederman, J., Brown, S., Monuteaux, M., Prince, J., & Spencer, T. J. (2002). Patterns of psychopathology and dysfunction in clinically referred preschoolers. *Journal of Developmental & Behavioral Pediatrics, 23*(1 Suppl), S31–S36.

3

Neuropsychological Assessment of ADHD in Preschoolers

Performance-Based Measures, Rating Scales,

and Structured Interviews

E. MARK MAHONE AND ALISON E. PRITCHARD

ADHD in Preschoolers: Diagnosis, Measurement, and Risks

Attention-deficit/hyperactivity disorder (ADHD) is increasingly diagnosed and treated in younger children (DeBar et al., 2003). The disorder has become the most commonly diagnosed form of psychopathology in the preschool years (Armstrong & Nettleton, 2004) and the most common symptom pattern observed in children referred for assessment (Gadow, Sprafkin, & Nolan, 2001). There are a number of hypotheses for this recent increase, and it remains unclear if those diagnosed earlier represent early-onset forms of the disorder, or whether the earlier diagnoses simply represent misidentification of developmentally normal behaviors as ADHD (Sonuga-Barke, Koerting, Smith, McCann, & Thompson, 2011).

As discussed in detail in other chapters of this volume, the increased prevalence of ADHD in preschoolers represents a significant public health concern and is associated with a poor long-term prognosis (Horn & Packard, 1985; Greenhill, Posner, Vaughan, & Kratochvil, 2008; Lee et al., 2007; Rappley et al., 1999). Moreover, preschool children with ADHD commonly demonstrate multiple developmental deficits over and above the primary symptoms of ADHD, as well as comorbid conditions (Overgaard, Aase, Torgersen, & Zeiner, 2012; Yochman, 2006). By school age, these children's difficulties represent a significant economic cost to society as a whole (over $42 billion total; Robb et al., 2011). Thus, in addition to being at significant risk for social, familial, and academic difficulties, relative to children without ADHD (American Academy of Pediatrics, 2011b), preschoolers with ADHD represent a considerable long-term cost to society, particularly if their symptoms are poorly managed. Despite these risks, the disorder has been studied less extensively in preschool children than in their school-aged counterparts (DuPaul, McGoey, Eckert, & VanBrakle, 2001). These findings suggest that early identification and prevention efforts are needed to offset the societal costs and to minimize the harmful impact of the disorder (Pelham, Foster, & Robb, 2007; Wilens et al., 2002a).

Assessment and Diagnosis of ADHD in Preschoolers

The diagnosis of ADHD in preschool children is challenging since attention problems are very common among children in this age range, and the core symptoms of ADHD— distractibility and hyperactivity—are commonly seen in preschool children referred for any type of developmental evaluation (Shelton & Barkley, 1993). For example, during the first 5 years of life, as many as 40% of children from a community sample had difficulties with attention as rated by parents and preschool teachers (Palfrey, Levine, Walker, & Sullivan, 1985). The rate of behavioral hyperactivity (even at levels falling short of formal DSM-IV diagnostic criteria) is observed to be as high as 3% to 15% in community samples and 50% or higher among clinical referrals (Christophersen & Mortweet, 2003).

The NIH Consensus Statement on ADHD (National Institutes of Health, 1998) released 15 years ago, concluded that many practitioners do not use structured questionnaires or teacher/school input when making the diagnosis of ADHD and called for the development of reliable and valid assessment procedures for younger children. As a result, the last decade has seen an increased interest in assessment and treatment of preschool-aged children presenting with symptoms of ADHD (e.g., Lahey et al., 2004; Massetti et al., 2007). Development of valid, psychometrically sound assessment methods is particularly important because relying on unstandardized parental verbal reports of isolated symptoms of ADHD in preschoolers may lead to over-identification (Gimpel & Kuhn, 2000). It is also important to note that (as in school-aged children), caregiver ratings and performance-based measures often measure different constructs, and ratings may vary widely between settings (Mahone & Hoffman, 2007). For example, Sims and Lonigan (2012) examined associations between parent and teacher ratings of ADHD and performance on a continuous performance test (CPT) in 65 preschoolers ages 4 and 5 years. They found no significant correlations between parent and teacher behavior ratings of the same symptoms. Parent ratings of *both* inattention and hyperactivity/impulsivity accounted for variance in CPT omission (inattention) errors, but parent ratings of impulsivity did not predict CPT commission (impulsivity) errors (Sims & Lonigan, 2012).

Even with reliable, valid, and developmentally appropriate instruments, the practice of actually assessing preschoolers who present with symptoms of ADHD can be difficult since these children tend to tire quickly, struggle to sustain attention during cognitive assessments, and can fail to comply with non-appealing tasks (Anderson & Reidy, 2012). Further, the practice of administering adult-derived tests or scaled-down versions of child tests to younger children is also suspect, since the tests may be of less interest or relevance to preschoolers; the relative novelty and complexity may be greater;

they may tap different skills or greater cognitive resources; and the available normative data may not allow for differentiation of normal versus atypical performance within a developmental context (Anderson & Reidy, 2012).

Primary Differences in Presentation and Diagnosis of ADHD in Preschool Versus School-Age Children

While preschoolers with ADHD are most often found to have similar patterns of comorbid psychopathology and functional impairment to school-age children with ADHD (Wilens et al., 2002b), there are noteworthy differences in the presentation of core symptoms among preschoolers, particularly with regard to subtypes. The combined subtype, for example, is common in both age groups. In contrast, the hyperactive/impulsive subtype is most common in preschool but not in school-age children (i.e., less than 10%), whereas the inattentive subtype is common in school-age children but not in preschoolers (i.e., less than 10%) (American Academy of Pediatrics, 2011a). Some studies even suggest that the inattentive subtype of ADHD occurs in fewer than 1% of preschoolers in the general population (Egger et al., 2006).

Overall ADHD prevalence estimates differ between age groups as well, with estimates of 2% to 8% in preschool children but around 8% to 12% in school-age children (Akinbami, Liu, Pastor, & Reuban, 2011). One reason for this discrepancy may be that there exist fewer validated behavior rating scales for preschool children, compared with the many that are available for older children. It may also be due to the relative absence of appropriately normed neuropsychological instruments for preschoolers, the relative infrequency of referral of preschoolers for neuropsychological assessment, and the trend of neuropsychological training including less focus on preschoolers (Baron & Anderson, 2012).

Issues of Sex Differences in ADHD

Sexually dimorphic patterns of development further complicate the assessment of ADHD symptoms in preschoolers. By school age, boys are diagnosed with ADHD three to four times as often as girls (Akinbami et al., 2011) but only twice as often in the preschool years (Egger & Angold, 2006; Egger et al., 2006); this may reflect the sexually dimorphic patterns of brain development that are associated with girls "aging out" of some of the core ADHD symptoms by school age. Girls present more commonly with the inattentive ADHD subtype than do boys (Hinshaw, Owens, Sami, & Fargeon, 2006; Weiler, Bellinger, Marmor, Rancier, & Waber, 1999). Additionally, symptoms of ADHD tend to decrease in severity with age in parallel with cerebral maturation (Gaub & Carlson, 1997), such that by elementary school age, the disruptive behavioral symptoms are more pronounced in boys (compared to girls) with ADHD. However, recent large-scale studies of preschool children with ADHD reveal that the *opposite pattern* may be true in the preschool years, with girls showing more relative impairment. For example, in preschool children with moderate to severe ADHD studied as part of the multisite Preschool ADHD Treatment Study (PATS), the behavior of girls with ADHD was reported as more deviant, relative to age-matched peers, than that of boys with ADHD on the Conners Parent and Teacher Rating Scales (Posner et al., 2007). Still, the study of girls with ADHD in the preschool years presents a challenge, as the inattentive symptoms (more commonly observed in girls) are not as evident in the preschool years. In fact, Byrne and colleagues (Byrne, Bawden, Beattie, & DeWolfe, 2000) reported that only 4% of children diagnosed with ADHD in preschool (boys and girls) met the criteria for the inattentive subtype, with the large majority meeting the criteria for the hyperactive/impulsive subtype (68%).

ADHD and Executive Functions in Preschool Children

Executive function (EF) involves a set of cognitive processes used in implementing goal-directed behaviors. EF involves developing *and* implementing an approach to performing a task that is not habitually performed. Included in the EF construct are the ability to inhibit inappropriate responses and resist distraction, sustaining attention and behavior for prolonged periods, and planning progressively complex behaviors (Denckla, 1996). These skills are commonly disrupted in children with ADHD and contribute to the functional impairments observed in the disorder. In children, EF and motor control systems appear to develop in parallel with one another, such that both systems display a similarly protracted developmental trajectory. Development of executive and motor control (both skills often disrupted in individuals with ADHD) is dependent on functional integrity and maturation of related brain regions, suggesting a shared neural circuitry that includes frontostriatal systems and the cerebellum—that is, those regions identified as anomalous in neuroimaging studies of ADHD (Mahone, 2011). In children with ADHD, anomalous basal ganglia development appears to play an important role in the early manifestation of the disorder (Mahone et al., 2011); however, widespread cerebellar (Makie et al., 2007) and cortical delays (Shaw et al., 2007, 2012) are also observed and are associated with the behavioral (cognitive and motor) phenotype in children with ADHD.

The early study of executive control is considered crucial in understanding the needs of school-age children, as executive functions are central to successful acquisition and efficient use of academic skills (Biederman et al., 2004), especially in efforts to overcome learning problems (Denckla, 1996). In preschoolers, EF skills (particularly inhibitory control and working memory) play an important role in the development of socialization and the readiness for academic learning; therefore, assessment of these skills is critical in understanding the risks associated with ADHD in preschoolers. Whereas typically developing preschoolers demonstrate rapid, steady development of EF between the ages of 3 and 7 years, including inhibition and set shifting (Espy, 1997; Espy, Kaufmann, McDiarmid, & Glisky, 1999), abstraction (Jacques & Zelazo, 2001), and mental flexibility (Smidts, Jacobs, & Anderson, 2004), preschool children with ADHD commonly demonstrate deficits in response inhibition and working memory. In particular, inhibition problems in preschoolers with ADHD represent the more prominent deficits (Sonuga-Barke, Dalen, Daley, & Remington, 2002) and appear to predict later executive control problems associated with the disorder (Berlin & Bohlin, 2002; Berlin, Bohlin, & Rydell, 2003) in a manner distinct from oppositional defiant disorder (ODD) (Brocki, Nyberg, Thorell, & Bohlin, 2007) but mediated by peer processes (Snyder, Prichard, Schrepferman, Patrick, & Stoolmiller, 2004). Moreover, executive dysfunction among preschool girls represents a notable risk factor, as emotion regulation and inattention are significant predictors of chronic behavior problems at school age (Hill, Degnan, Calkins, & Keane, 2006). Cognitive inhibition problems (e.g., go/no-go commission errors) among preschoolers significantly predict teacher-reported behavior problems in third grade among girls but not boys with ADHD (Von Stauffenberg & Campbell, 2007). Among preschool boys with ADHD, deficits in motor control and persistence appear more prominent (Mariani & Barkley, 1997). Additionally, early motor delays (especially among boys) have been strongly prognostic with respect to which preschoolers are at risk for ADHD; for instance, ability to hop on one foot was the best predictor of "hyperactivity" at age 7 (Nichols & Chen, 1981). Therefore, assessing executive and motor control as part of the neuropsychological examination of preschool children is critical in understanding the risks for ADHD.

Diagnostic Method Used in PATS

Even though much less is known about diagnosing ADHD in preschool children, the practice of prescribing psychotropic medications for very young children has increased in both the United States and Europe (Connor, 2002; Rappley, Eneli, & Mullan, 2002). Funded by the National Institute of Mental Health (NIMH) in 2000, PATS was a large multisite clinical trial that studied the effects of methylphenidate in preschoolers (ages 3 to 6 years) with ADHD. It represented the largest study to date of carefully diagnosed preschool children with ADHD (Abikoff et al., 2007; Greenhill et al., 2006; Swanson et al., 2006; Vitiello et al., 2007). The diagnostic methods used in the PATS studies (which involved standardized diagnostic interviews, caregiver rating scales, and direct assessment of functional impairment) set a strong standard for improving diagnostic reliability in this age range. Additionally, the studies also clarified the rates, types, and moderating effect of comorbidities unique to preschoolers with ADHD (Ghuman et al., 2007) and influenced the most recent American Academy of Pediatrics guidelines for ADHD by requiring symptoms to be present for 9 months (instead of 6 months) for formal diagnosis (Kollins et al., 2006). A number of specific methods and instruments used in the PATS, including the DISC-IV, Conners Rating Scales, Child Behavior Checklist, and Early Child Inventory rating scales, are described in the following section. Due to space limitations, we do not include other measures used in the PATS studies, particularly those originally developed for school-aged children, such as the Hillside Behavior Rating Scale (Gittleman-Klein & Klein, 1976), Strengths and Weaknesses of ADHD Symptoms and Normal Behaviors (SWAN; Swanson, 1992), Swanson, Nolan & Pelham Rating Scale (SNAP; Swanson, 1992), Swanson, Kotkin, Atkins, M-Flynn, and Pelhan Rating Scale (SKAMP; Swanson, 1992), Attention Network Tasks (Fan, McCandliss, Sommer, Raz, & Posner, 2002), and Tower of Hanoi (Simon, 1975), as well as measures that focus on graphomotor skill (e.g., Visuomotor Precision; Korkman et al., 2007).

Neuropsychological Assessment of ADHD in Preschoolers

Comprehensive neuropsychological assessment of children should include a thorough review of the child's history, planned observations, and formal psychometric testing (Mahone & Slomine, 2008). Three primary methods of psychometric assessment have been used to characterize ADHD in preschool children: performance-based tests, rating scales (parent, teacher, clinician), and structured interviews (Mahone, 2005; Mahone & Schneider, 2012). Neuropsychological assessment of a preschool child with ADHD presents a unique set of challenges to the clinician, in part because the manifested behaviors in young children (distractibility, impersistence, impulsivity) can interfere substantially with test administration. As such, specific strategies have been recommended to minimize the interfering behaviors that can potentially contribute to error variance in the resulting test scores (Mahone & Slomine, 2007). These strategies include:

- Keeping unnecessary objects out of reach;
- Providing clear expectations and rules at the outset of assessment;
- Using short directions and visual presentation of rules (e.g., stop sign);
- Giving the preschooler immediate and frequent feedback about his/her behavior, especially reinforcing positive behaviors;
- Frequently changing and rotating salient reinforcers;
- Simplifying and repeating directions as necessary (within standardized procedures for the tests);
- Slowing rate or presentation of material; and
- Alerting and cueing the preschooler before essential information is presented.

A review of relevant published methods for preschool children is provided below, with indications of which are publically versus commercially available and which are most useful for research versus clinical practice.

Performance-Based Tests

CONTINUOUS PERFORMANCE TESTS

The following automated continuous performance measures tap multiple components of attention and executive function. Most of these CPTs include indices of sustained attention and impulsivity (including errors of omission and commission), as well as response latency and response time variability over the course of the task. Clinically, the CPTs can be used to help in determining which of the measured domains, sustained attention or impulsivity, poses greater difficulty for a given patient.

Auditory Continuous Performance Test for Preschoolers (ACPT-P; Mahone, Pillion, & Hiemenz, 2001). The ACPT-P is a computerized go/no-go research-based measure developed for children ages 36 to 78 months. Two auditory stimuli, a dog bark (target stimulus) and a bell (non-target stimulus), are used, with 15 of each stimulus being presented over the course of 5 minutes at fixed inter-stimulus intervals. Children are required to respond as quickly as possible by pressing the space bar in response to target stimuli and ignoring non-targets. During the task, data are collected on omissions, commissions, response latency, and response time variability.

Initial normative data collected on 87 typically developing preschoolers (ages 3 to 5 years) suggested that performance on the task improved with age from 3 to 4 years but leveled off by age 5 (Mahone et al., 2001). Preliminary evidence of concurrent validity of the ACPT-P was also found in this sample, as performance on the task was significantly associated with parent ratings of behavior on the CPRS-R (both the Hyperactivity Scale and the ADHD Index). More recent work has demonstrated concurrent validity of the measure with regard to ADHD diagnostic status (as generated by a combination of clinical interview and parent ratings) among preschoolers (Mahone, Pillion, Hoffman, Hiemenz, & Denckla, 2005).

Gordon Diagnostic System (GDS; Gordon, McClure, & Post, 1986). The GDS is a self-contained, computerized continuous performance measure comprised of 10 separately administered tasks. It is available commercially. Three of the 10 tasks are appropriate for use with 4- and 5-year-old children. The 6-minute-long *Delay* task requires preschoolers to wait 4 seconds before responding to a stimulus by pressing a large blue button. The duration of the required delay is not explicit; however, if a child responds before 4 seconds have passed, a buzzer sounds to indicate an error. When a child successfully completes the 4-second delay, a light flashes and he or she earns a point. The percentage of correct responses on this task is used as an index of impulsivity. Two similar versions of the 6-minute long *Vigilance* task both use the numbers 1 through 9 as stimuli, with numbers being presented one by one at consistent 2-second intervals on the screen. In the first version of the *Vigilance* task, preschool children are required to press a button when they see the number 1 (target) and ignore all other numbers (non-targets). In the second version of the task, the target number changes to 0, but the rest of the task remains the same. The total correct responses and number of commissions are employed as an index of sustained attention.

Normative data for the GDS, collected on a group of children ages 4 through 16 years, offers evidence of moderate test–retest reliability over the course of a 1-year interval (Gordon & Mettelman, 1987). Both convergent and discriminant validity, with respect to ADHD diagnostic classification, have been demonstrated for the measure among school-aged children (McClure & Gordon, 1984). More recent, though limited, evidence of construct validity within a sample of preschoolers was demonstrated using a slightly modified version of the task showing that preschool-aged boys with ADHD had significantly fewer total correct responses on the *Vigilance* task than their typically developing peers (Mariani & Barkley, 1997).

Kiddie Continuous Performance Test (K-CPT; Conners, 2001). The K-CPT is a commercially available computerized attention measure for children ages 4 and 5. Over the course of 7.5 minutes, children respond to 10 black and white "target" pictures and inhibit response to one "non-target" picture, all of which are familiar objects that appear briefly on the screen. The simple motor response involves clicking a mouse or pressing the space bar as quickly as possible following the presentation of the stimulus. Data collected during the task include number of omissions and commissions, an index of perseveration, as well as hit reaction time, reaction time standard error, and reaction time consistency over the course of the task.

Within the normative sample (454 4- and 5-year-olds), adequate split-half reliability and evidence for discriminant validity are reported (Conners, 2001). Sensitivity and specificity with regard to diagnostic classification are also reported as adequate among this sample. Further evidence of construct validity was reported in 237 children, aged 48 to 67 months (Friedman-Weieneth, Harvey, Youngwith, & Goldstein, 2007; Youngwirth, Harvey, Gates, Hashin, & Friedman-Weieneth, 2007), showing that typically developing children evidenced fewer omissions, lower reaction time standard error, less variability, and more stable performance over time on the K-CPT in comparison to children with hyperactive and oppositional behaviors.

Preschool Continuous Performance Test (P-CPT; Kerns & Rondeau, 1998). The P-CPT is a modified version of the Children's Continuous Performance Test (C-CPT), developed by Kerns and Rondeau in 1998. The P-CPT is used in research and involves administration of only the first of the three C-CPT tasks, which require preschoolers to respond by touching (on a touchscreen) target stimuli (sheep) but not non-target stimuli (other animals). A unique feature of the P-CPT is the fact that the visual stimuli are paired with auditory stimuli (i.e., each animal's picture is accompanied by the sound made by that animal). Two hundred stimuli, including 29 targets, are presented with consistent inter-stimulus intervals over the course of 5 minutes. Performance indices collected during the task include correct hits, omission and commission errors, as well as reaction times.

Muller, Kerns, and Konkin (2012) found that among a sample of 33 typically developing children ages 3 to 5, the P-CPT evidenced moderate test–retest reliability for the correct hits, omissions, and reaction time indices (reliability coefficients of 0.65, 0.63, and 0.77 respectively); however, commission errors were significantly less stable over time (reliability coefficient of 0.44). Limited evidence of construct validity is offered by Baron and colleagues (Baron, Kerns, Muller, Ahronovich, & Litman, 2012), who found that preschoolers with a history of prematurity made significantly more commission and omission errors than those born at term.

Tests of Variables of Attention (TOVA; Greenberg, 1996). The TOVA is a commercially available computerized CPT that uses a go/no-go format with a single target stimulus and a single non-target stimulus; visual and auditory formats are available. The visual format employs a monochromatic rectangle with a smaller rectangle placed either in the upper half (for the target stimulus) or the lower half (for the non-target stimulus), while the auditory format uses two tones of different pitch. The inter-stimulus interval for the TOVA is fixed at 2.0 seconds. The target:non-target ratio varies, with a 1:3.5 ratio in the first half of the test and a 3.5:1 ratio in the second half of the test. A unique feature of the TOVA is its specially designed microswitch response button, which reportedly has a very low error of measurement (±1 msec). The TOVA was designed and originally normed for individuals ages 6 years through adulthood. The original version of the TOVA is 21.8 minutes in length. A preschool version of the TOVA is also available for children ages 4 to 5 years; it is 10.9 minutes in length, with all other parameters identical to the original version. Variables measured by the TOVA include variability of response time (consistency), mean response time, commission rate (reflecting impulsivity), errors of omission (inattention), post-commission response times, multiple and anticipatory responses, and an overall "ADHD score," which is a comparison to an age/gender-specific ADHD group. While the TOVA has been used extensively to assess school-age children and adults with suspected ADHD (Greenberg & Dupuy, 2001), there have been no publications using the preschool version of the TOVA; as such, its validity in this age group has not been established.

Other Reaction Time Tasks. In addition to CPTs, several simple reaction time tasks have been used in research, that require children to simply respond as quickly as possible (usually by pressing the space bar or clicking the mouse) when a stimulus is presented on the screen. Typically, performance is evaluated both in terms of overall average response time and variability in response time over the course of the task. The clinical utility of such measures is questionable, however, as preschoolers with ADHD have been found to perform similarly on reaction time tasks to typically developing preschoolers (Gopin, Berwid, Mark, Mlodnicka, & Halperin, 2012).

ADDITIONAL PERFORMANCE-BASED TESTS OF ATTENTION

The performance-based attention measures described here vary greatly in their format, task demands, and components of attention assessed. We review tasks that measure aspects of both visual and auditory attention, as well as more motor-oriented tasks tapping inhibition and persistence. Information obtained from these measures may offer the clinician a more fine-grained understanding of the patient's attentional difficulties. In particular, these measures can provide information regarding whether visual versus auditory domains are differentially implicated in the patient's presentation and the extent to which selective/focused attention, response inhibition, or working memory is problematic for the patient. All of the following measures except one (Picture Deletion Test for Preschoolers) are subtests of norm-referenced standardized tests, widely used for clinical and research purposes, and commercially available. The Picture Deletion Test for Preschoolers was specifically developed for use in research for assessment of attention in preschool children.

Digit Span Measures. For preschoolers, two similar digit span measures exist, both of which tap the span of auditory attention. *Number Recall* from the Kaufman Assessment Battery for Children, Second Edition (KABC-II; Kaufman & Kaufman, 2004), requires the child to repeat several series of verbally presented numbers that increase in length over the course of the subtest. The subtest evidenced good test–retest reliability among 4- and 5-year-old children (0.87 and 0.79, respectively) in the normative sample (Kaufman & Kaufman, 2004). Evidence of construct validity has been established by Mariani and Barkley (1997), who report that preschool boys with ADHD score significantly lower than controls on the Number Recall subtest.

The *Recall of Digits Forward* subtest of the Differential Ability Scales—Second Edition (Elliot, 2007) also requires the child to repeat several series of verbally presented numbers that increase in length. Within the standardization sample, test–retest reliability coefficients for this task among 2.5- to 6-year-olds range from 0.88 to 0.91 (Elliot, 2007). Limited evidence of construct validity is offered by Baron and colleagues

(2011), who found that preschoolers who were born prematurely (who are therefore at risk for developing ADHD) score significantly lower on this task than preschoolers born at term.

Verbal Span Measures. Several verbal span tasks designed for school-aged children have also been adapted for use with preschoolers. These tasks often require the child to repeat increasingly lengthy series of words verbatim (Muller et al., 2012; Wahlstedt, Thorell, & Bohlin, 2008). Because these tasks have been primarily used for research rather than clinical assessment, they will not receive more thorough review here.

Hand Movements (KABC-II; Kaufman & Kaufman, 2004). The Hand Movements subtest of the KABC-II is a measure of visual-motor sequential processing, visual attention span, and short-term memory administered to children ages 3 to 18 years. This 5-minute task requires the child to reproduce a series of hand movements demonstrated by the examiner. Normative data indicate modest to moderate split-half reliability among 4- and 5-year-olds (0.57 and 0.75, respectively) as well as modest test–retest reliability (0.58 across the 4- to 5-year-old age range; Kaufman & Kaufman, 2004). Mariani and Barkley (1997) demonstrated construct validity for the subtest among preschool boys, finding that preschoolers with ADHD performed worse on the task than those without.

Picture Deletion Test for Preschoolers (PDTP; Corkum, Byrne, & Ellsworth, 1995). The PDTP is a visual cancellation task normed on 60 preschoolers, ages 3 to 5 years. The measure requires that children visually scan a randomized array of 15 target and 45 non-target pictures and mark the targets using a self-inking stamp (thus reducing fine motor demands) as quickly as possible. After ensuring that the child is familiar with the target and non-target stimuli, the preschooler completes four tasks over the course of approximately 10 minutes. Three of the tasks require the child to mark varying target stimuli as quickly as possible, while the fourth assesses simple fine motor speed. Performance indices include completion time, as well as omission and commission errors. A revised version of the PDTP is also available, with changes made to the target stimuli as well as the printed layout of the task (Byrne, DeWolfe, & Bawden, 1998).

Evidence for construct validity of the task was preliminarily established within the normative sample, with performance on two of the four trials of the PDTP being significantly associated with commission and omission error rates on the CPTP (Corkum et al., 1995). Children ages 3 to 6 years diagnosed with ADHD were found to make significantly more commission errors and took longer to complete the task than did typically developing controls of the same age (DeWolfe et al., 1999). Similarly, stimulant-naïve preschoolers with ADHD made significantly more commission errors on the PDTP than matched controls. After stimulant treatment, however, the two groups did not differ in performance (Byrne et al., 1998).

Recognition of Pictures (Elliot, 2007). The DAS-II Recognition of Pictures subtest offers an assessment of selective attention and visual attention span for children ages 2 years 6 months through 5 years. The task requires the child to point to target objects within a field of distractor items after a brief visual introduction to the target objects. Over the course of the task, both the number of target objects and their similarity to the distractor items increase. Estimates of test–retest reliability for this task among preschool-aged children range from 0.77 to 0.85 (Elliot, 2007). Literature regarding the construct validity of the test is currently limited to school-aged children; however, among this group, children with ADHD have demonstrated poorer performance on the task relative to controls (Weisen, 2008).

Statue test (Korkman, Kirk, & Kemp, 2007). The NEuroPSYchological Assessment (NEPSY)-II Statue subtest is a measure of motor persistence and inhibition for use with children ages 3 to 6 years. Given the shared neural substrates between motor and attentional control (Diamond, 2000), the subtest represents a time-efficient method of assessing skills commonly disrupted in young children with ADHD. The child is required to stand still in different postures with eyes closed and to refrain from vocalization for 75 seconds, during which time the examiner engages in several potentially distracting behaviors (e.g., coughing, dropping a pencil). Normative data indicate strong test–retest reliability (0.82) for the NEPSY-II Statue subtest among 3- and 4-year-old children (Korkman, Kirk, & Kemp, 2007). Evidence for construct validity of the measure has been found among preschoolers. Preschoolers with behavior problems and those with ADHD specifically have been found to score lower on the Statue subtest than typically developing controls (Mahone et al., 2005; Youngwirth et al., 2007). Similarly, a dimensional measure of ADHD symptomatology was negatively related to performance on the Statue subtest, both concurrently and predictively, among preschoolers (Brocki et al., 2007).

Rating Scales

The following parent and teacher rating scales are useful in evaluating preschool-aged children with ADHD. All of these ratings are commercially available, with the exception of the ADHD Rating Scale-IV—Preschool Version and the Behavior Rating Inventory for Children, both of which have been made available for public use. All of these measures can aid in the process of evaluating ADHD in preschoolers; however, for monitoring treatment progress, the shorter rating scales that are more focused on ADHD symptomatology, such as the ADHD Rating Scale-IV—Preschool Version, the ADHD Symptom Checklist 4, the Attention Deficit Disorders Evaluation Scale 3, the Behavior Rating Inventory for Children, and the Children's Problems Checklist, may be most useful.

ADHD Rating Scale-IV—Preschool Version (DuPaul, Power, Anastopoulos, & Reid, 1998; McGoey et al., 2007). The ADHD-RS-IV—Preschool Version is an 18-item adaptation of the original ADHD-RS-IV (DuPaul, Paul, Power, Anastopoulos, & Reid, 1998), which is a focused measure of ADHD symptomatology. Items on the original measure reflect the 18 behavioral symptom criteria for ADHD, as conceptualized in the *Diagnostic and Statistical Manual of Mental Disorders,* Fourth Edition (DSM-IV; American Psychiatric Association, 1994), and for the Preschool Version symptom statements were modified to better capture behavior that is developmentally inappropriate for children ages 3 through 5—for example, "Avoids tasks that require sustained mental effort (i.e., puzzles, learning ABCs, writing name)," "Loses things necessary for tasks or activities (mittens, shoes, backpack)". Both parents and teachers may complete the measure that requires them to rate each symptom criterion on a 4-point Likert frequency scale. Both inattention and hyperactive/impulsive subscale scores can be calculated, as can a total scale score.

Within the normative sample, internal consistency of the three scales (two subscales and the total scale) of the measure was high, ranging from 0.92 to 0.95 for teacher ratings and from 0.85 to 0.92 for parent ratings. Similarly, test–retest reliability over a 4-week interval was found to be strong for the three scales, with reliability coefficients ranging from 0.93 to 0.96 for the teacher ratings and 0.80 to 0.87 for the parent ratings. Evidence of construct validity was also found within the normative sample, as the ADHD-RS-IV—Preschool Version (both parent and teacher report) was significantly associated with the Conners Rating Scales-Revised (parent and teacher report forms, respectively) Oppositional, Cognitive Problems/Inattention, Hyperactivity, and ADHD Index scales (DuPaul et al., 1998; McGoey et al., 2007).

ADHD Symptom Checklist-4 (ADHD-SC4; Gadow & Sprafkin, 1997). The ADHD-SC4 is a 50-item parent- and teacher-reported rating of ADHD and ODD symptomatology among children ages 3 to 18. In addition to symptoms of ADHD and ODD, the ADHD-SC4, which is rated on a 4-point Likert frequency scale, offers a brief evaluation of peer aggression, as well as a *Stimulant Side Effects Checklist* that can be used to monitor response to medication. Both symptom count and dimensional symptom severity total scores can be calculated. Sprafkin and colleagues (2002) found evidence of good internal consistency and predictive and discriminant validity of the measure relative to diagnostic classification, as well as concurrent validity in relation to other dimensional measures of ADHD symptomatology (e.g., CBCL, Conners).

Attention Deficit Disorders Evaluation Scale-Third Edition (ADDES-3; McGarney & Arthaud, 2004). The ADDES-3 is a parent- and teacher-report rating scale focused on ADHD symptomatology for use with children ages 4 to 18 years. Both the 46-item Home Version and the 60-item School Version of the measure are rated on a 6-point Likert frequency scale. Within the standardization sample, internal consistency, test–retest reliability, and interrater reliability for the measure were all reported as adequate to strong. Further, evidence of strong construct validity, both with respect to ADHD diagnostic classification and dimensional teacher and parent ratings of behavior (e.g., Conners Rating Scales-Revised, ADD-H Comprehensive Teacher's Rating Scale), were found within this sample (McGarney & Arthaud, 2004).

Behavior Assessment Scale for Children-2 (BASC-2; Reynolds & Kamphaus, 2004). The BASC-2 is a broadband behavior rating scale for children. The preschool version of the measure (for ages 2 to 5 years) is offered in both parent- and teacher-report format and contains several subscales of use in the assessment of children with ADHD, including Hyperactivity, Attention Problems, and Aggression. The parent rating scale preschool version comprises 134 items while the teacher preschool version comprises 100 items, all of which are rated on a 4-point Likert frequency scale. Within the preschool portion of the normative sample, internal consistency fell above 0.72 for the Hyperactivity, Attention Problems, and Aggression subtests on both the parent and teacher versions of the measure. Median test–retest reliability of the measure in this subsample of young children was 0.77 for the parent version and 0.82 for the teacher version. Evidence of construct validity was established in the normative sample in relation to both diagnostic classification and dimensional symptom ratings.

Behavior Rating Inventory for Children (BRIC; Gopin et al., 2010). The BRIC is a brief clinician-rated measure of ADHD symptomatology and associated features for children ages 3 to 4 years. The BRIC comprises five items that are rated on a 5-point

Likert scale and offers sample behaviors for each item to help clinicians accurately anchor low-, middle-, and high-severity problem behaviors. The ADHD Symptom Triad subscale comprises three items, each of which assesses one of the three major types of ADHD symptoms (inattention, hyperactivity, and impulsivity). The Mood/Sociability subscale comprises the other two items, which tap into the impairment in social and emotional domains that is often associated with ADHD.

Gopin and colleagues (2010) found that the ADHD Symptom Triad subscale evidenced adequate test–retest reliability when rated by the same examiner on both occasions (0.78), though interrater (two different clinicians) reliability was lower (0.59) in a sample of 214 preschoolers (55 3-year-olds and 159 4-year-olds). Both test–retest and interrater reliability were poor for the Mood/Sociability Factor (0.55 and 0.50 respectively). Within the same sample, the ADHD Symptom Triad (but not the Mood/Sociability subscale) evidenced construct validity in that it predicted differences between a group of hyperactive/inattentive children and a typically developing group. Additionally, Gopin and colleagues found a moderate association between the ADHD Symptom Triad, the Hyperactivity and Inattention subscales of the BASC-2 Preschool version (both parent and teacher report), and the ADHD Rating Scale-IV. Finally, the ADHD Symptom Triad subscale was found to be associated with activity levels measured via actigraph.

Child Behavior Checklist for Ages 1.5 to 5 (CBCL:1.5-5; Achenbach & Rescorla, 2000). The 100-item CBCL for ages 1.5 to 5 offers both parent and teacher ratings of preschool children's problem behaviors. Both internalizing and externalizing domains are included within the measure, as are subscales specific to particular types of problem behavior. The Attention Problems subscale of the CBCL:1.5-5 is the most relevant in the assessment of ADHD in preschoolers; however, subscales such as Aggressive Behavior and Emotional Reactivity may also be useful. Items on the CBCL:1.5-5 are rated on a 3-point Likert scale ranging from 0 (not true) to 2 (very/often true). Problems scales are also included. Within the normative sample, test–retest reliability was high for the majority of the subscales on both the parent- and teacher-report versions of the CBCL for young children (mean reliability above 0.80). Reliability for the Attention Problems scale of the CBCL:1.5-5 was 0.78 for the parent-rated and 0.84 for the teacher-rated versions (Achenbach & Rescorla, 2000).

The CBCL:1.5-5 is often used as a general behavioral screening for preschoolers (Corkum et al., 1995; DeWolfe et al., 1999; Egger et al., 2006; Posner et al., 2007); however, evidence for construct validity of the Attention Problems subscale has been found. Parent-rated Attention Problems subscale scores were found to be significantly higher among children with untreated ADHD than among their typically developing peers. After treatment, the ADHD group's Attention Problems scores were no different from those of their typically developing peers (Byrne et al., 1998). Further, the CBCL:1.5-5 (particularly the Attention Problems subscale) evidences predictive validity for preschoolers in terms of diagnostic categorization as they move through childhood (Hill et al., 2006).

Children's Problems Checklist (CPC; Healey, Miller, Castelli, Marks, & Halperin, 2008). The publicly available CPC was developed to better characterize whether a preschool child's ADHD-like behaviors are, in fact, impairing and therefore clinically significant. Items assess the difficulties associated with ADHD symptomatology (e.g.,

"Does your child disrupt family life?") rather than the presence of symptoms themselves. Both the 7-item parent-report version and the 6-item teacher-report version are rated on a 4-point Likert scale marking the severity of the impairment in terms of the child's disruptiveness, difficulties with peers and adults, and self-esteem, among others. Healy and colleagues (2008) report adequate internal consistency of the measure (0.70 for parent rating and 0.84 for teacher rating), as well as moderate 6-month test–retest reliability (0.69 and 0.70 for parent and teacher, respectively) in a sample of 394 preschoolers aged 36 through 60 months. Additionally, impairment, as measured by the CPC, was significantly correlated with the ADHD-RS-IV, a measure of symptom severity. Most importantly, Healy and colleagues (2008) report that when (even liberal) cross-situational impairment criteria were applied, a very large proportion of the group of children who met the ADHD-RS-IV symptom threshold criteria on the basis of one rater (parent or teacher) no longer met the threshold for ADHD (both symptoms and impairment as required for a DSM diagnosis of ADHD).

Conners Early Childhood (Conners EC; Conners, 2009). The Conners EC offers a broad-based assessment of both problem and adaptive behaviors for children ages 2 to 6 years and is available as a 190-item parent rating and a 186-item teacher rating form (Conners, 2009). Short forms for both parent (49-item) and teacher (48-item) ratings are also available. Of particular use in the assessment of preschool ADHD is the Inattention/Hyperactivity subscale, which is included on the short form of the measure. Within the standardization sample, reliability coefficients for the Conners EC Parent Behavior Scales were internal consistency 0.86, test–retest 0.87, and interrater 0.72. Reliability was slightly higher for the Conners EC-Teacher Behavior Scales: internal consistency 0.89 and test–retest 0.93. The Conners EC Behavior subscales are highly correlated with similar subscales on the BASC-2 and the CBCL:1.5-5 (Conners, 2009).

Early Child Inventory-4 (ECI-4; Sprafkin & Gadow, 1996). The ECI-4 is a broad-based measure of behavioral and emotional problems for use with children ages 3 to 6 years. The ECI-4 items are founded on the DSM-IV diagnostic criteria, and both a 108-item parent-rated and a 77-item teacher-rated version are available. All items are rated on a 4-point Likert frequency scale; however, the measure can be scored either categorically (by counting the number of symptoms rated as "often" or "very often") or dimensionally (by summing the value indicated for each response). The ADHD Inattentive, ADHD Hyperactive-Impulsive, and ADHD Combined indices of the ECI-4 are of particular interest in the assessment of preschool ADHD, though other diagnostically based indices included in the measure (e.g., ODD, Generalized Anxiety Disorder, Major Depressive Disorder) will undoubtedly be valuable in assisting with differential diagnosis and determination of comorbidities.

Sprafkin and colleagues (ECI-4; Sprafkin et al., 1996) found internal consistency of the ECI-4 to be high (above 0.90) for the ADHD dimension. Sensitivity of the measure relative to ADHD diagnosis was similar for parent (0.66) and teacher reports (0.68) but increased substantially when parent and teacher information was used in combination (0.90). Specificity, though generally poor, also improved when parent- and teacher-provided information was used together (0.41). Sprafkin and colleagues (1996) also demonstrated convergent and discriminant validity of the ECI-4, both in relation to diagnostic classification and with the CBCL and TRF dimensional symptom ratings. The ECI-4 has been used extensively in ADHD research, both nationally and internationally (Jane et al., 2006; Nolan, Gadow, & Sprafkin, 2001; Poblano & Romero, 2006).

Preschool and Kindergarten Behavior Scales-Second Edition (Merrell, 2003). The PKBS-2 is a broad-based behavior rating of both social skills and behavior problems for young children (ages 3 to 6 years). The 76-item measure can be completed by a preschooler's parent or teacher. Rated on a 4-point Likert scale, the Attention Problems/ Overactive subscale of the PKBS-2 is of particular interest in the assessment of preschool ADHD. For this subscale, within the standardization sample presented with the first edition of the PKBS, both internal consistency (0.92) and 3-month test–retest reliability (0.74) were adequate (Merrell, 1996). Carney and Merrell (2005) demonstrated evidence of concurrent and discriminant validity in relation to dimensional ratings and diagnostic classification.

Structured Interviews

Diagnostic Interview Schedule, Young Children (DISC-YC; Lucas, Fisher, & Luby, 1998). The DISC-YC is a computerized structured diagnostic interview adapted from the Diagnostic Interview Schedule for Children-IV (DISC-IV) for use with the parents of preschool-aged children. Parents are asked to respond to DSM-IV symptom-based questions presented in a dichotomous (yes/no) format. When symptoms are endorsed at a clinically significant level, follow-up questions related to age of onset, level of impairment, and history of treatment are administered. Due to the highly structured nature of the instrument, the DISC-YC does not require as much clinical judgment as other diagnostic interviews for children this age (e.g., K-SADS, PAPA). It can therefore be administered by a broader range of trained individuals, even those with limited clinical experience. Fisher and Lucas (2006) found acceptable test–retest reliability for the ADHD module of the DISC-YC. Evidence of convergent validity for the DISC-YC, in comparison with the Child Symptom Inventory (CSI), is presented by Lavigne and colleagues (2009). Additionally, McGrath and colleagues (2004) and Shaffer and colleagues (2000) offer evidence of reliability and construct validity of the DISC-IV among school-aged children.

Kiddie-Schedule for Affective Disorders and Schizophrenia-Present and Lifetime Version (K-SADS-PL; Kaufman et al., 1997). The K-SADS-PL is a semistructured diagnostic interview originally developed for use with the parents of children 6 to 18 years of age. Recently, Birmaher and colleagues (2009) have extended the use of the K-SADS-PL to include preschool children ages 2 through 5. The measure includes a module specific to the diagnosis of ADHD, which, among preschoolers, was found to have good interrater reliability. Strong evidence for convergent and discriminant validity of the K-SADS-PL has been established in 204 preschoolers using the Child Behavior Checklist, Early Childhood Inventory-4, and Preschool Age Psychiatric Assessment (Birmaher et al., 2009).

Preschool Age Psychiatric Assessment (PAPA; Egger & Angold, 2004). The PAPA is a semistructured diagnostic interview for use with parents of children ages 2 to 5 years; it asks them to report on their child's behavior over the past 3 months. An ADHD-specific module is one of the 25 diagnosis- and symptom-oriented modules. An advantage of the PAPA is its inclusion of questions that are not part of DSM-IV diagnostic criteria but reflect, developmentally, symptoms that a preschooler might experience (e.g., having trouble concentrating when doing things with an adult; having trouble getting together all of the items necessary to play a game; trying to avoid doing things that require concentration, like puzzles or writing their own name). Egger and colleagues (2006) report adequate test–retest reliability for the ADHD module of the PAPA (0.74), and Tandon and colleagues (2011) have found good stability of ADHD diagnosis between preschool and school-age years using the measure. Limited evidence of construct validity is presented by Sterba and colleagues (2007).

Summary

In the past 10 years, there has been a striking increase in the number of children diagnosed with ADHD (Akinbami et al., 2011), which may be due (in part) to the willingness of clinicians to diagnose and treat ADHD in younger children. Despite advances in diagnostic methods appropriate for preschool children, there remains a considerable need for development and validation of procedures to reliably measure and characterize the core features of ADHD at earlier ages. Unfortunately, at present, the number of instruments appropriate for assessing neurobehavioral dysfunction associated with ADHD in preschoolers lags well behind the number of instruments available for school-age children. This discrepancy raises some concern, since continued advances in medical care, surgical procedures, and infection control have led to greater survival of preterm infants and an increased need for early identification of children at risk for neurodevelopmental disorders (including ADHD).

Among the three primary types of assessment methods used for characterizing the ADHD phenotype (performance-based measures, rating scales, structured interviews), rating scales for preschool children remain the most expedient and practical assessment method. A number of published rating scales are commercially available, and most have nationally representative standardization samples. One notable benefit of the rating scales is that they directly characterize the relative severity of symptoms, subtype, and comorbidity patterns, which will be important for the dimensional characterization of symptom severity required for the DSM-5. At the same time, the majority of preschool rating scales do not permit direct evaluation of current DSM-IV criteria (i.e., symptom counts). One exception is the ADHD Rating Scale—Preschool Version, which allows for assessment of specific DSM-IV diagnostic criteria and facilitates symptom count. Unfortunately, very little research has been done to validate the preschool version of this instrument. Additionally, it is important to emphasize that assessment of functional impairment from the ADHD symptoms is a requirement for a DSM-IV diagnosis of ADHD. Diagnoses based on simple symptom counts can be misleading as they may result in overidentification.

Structured diagnostic interviews facilitate direct assessment of DSM-IV criteria; however, none of the three structured psychiatric interviews reviewed (K-SADS, PAPA, DISC-YC) are commercially available; this has limited their availability and utility for practicing clinicians. Further, all three require considerable clinician train-ing, and the time required for administration may be impractical in some clinic settings. There are a variety of published performance-based measures designed to assess a wide range of cognitive functions in preschool children. None of these measures, however, assesses functions that are unique and specific to ADHD. Among CPTs (which have become a staple in neuropsychological assessment of ADHD in older children), only the K-CPT is both commercially available in this age range *and* developed specifically for preschool children. Nevertheless, despite being released in 2001, there have been remarkably few published validity studies using the K-CPT, and even fewer specific to preschool ADHD. Therefore, despite the increase in number of assessment instru-ments, there remains a relatively sparse literature demonstrating the utility, reliability, and validity among preschool children presenting with symptoms of ADHD. Because hyperactivity and inattentive behaviors are common during typical preschool child development, they may or may not indicate a disorder requiring treatment. Accurate and reliable identification of disordered attentional control in preschoolers can thus be a challenge.

Given these considerations, it is of critical importance for researchers to develop and refine assessment methods that allow for sensitive and specific diagnostic accu-racy, assessment of reliable change, and predictive validity to facilitate earlier identifi-cation of children at risk for ADHD and associated neurodevelopmental conditions. The costly toll that ADHD takes on individual adjustment, family life, schools, health-care, and social services underscores the importance of understanding its develop-mental course, with the ultimate goal of earlier identification and treatment. ADHD is a significant neurodevelopmental disorder, with behavioral anomalies (e.g., neuro-developmental immaturity, increased state organization difficulties) observed as early as infancy among those at risk (Auerbach et al., 2005). By age 4, children with ADHD show significantly reduced volumes of subcortical brain structures (i.e., caudate nucleus) compared to typically developing children, and these reductions strongly predict the severity of hyperactivity symptoms (Mahone et al., 2011). Early neuro-psychological assessment, using the methods described in this chapter, is important for uncovering these early links between brain and behavioral development in ADHD, which can ultimately contribute to identification of important early biomarkers for the disorder. Future prospective research is needed to identify young children at risk for ADHD to better understand the neurodevelopmental pathways that lead to behavioral dysfunction and ultimately the diagnosis of ADHD, as well as those associated with normalization of behavior over time.

Disclosures

This work was supported by the National Institutes of Health Grants R01 HD068425, P30 HD 24061 (Intellectual and Developmental Disabilities Research Center), the Johns Hopkins Brain Sciences Institute, and the Johns Hopkins University School of Medicine Institute for Clinical and Translational Research, an NIH/NCRR CTSA Program, UL1-RR025005.

References

Abikoff, H. B., Vitiello, B., Riddle, M. A., Cunningham, C., Greenhill, L. L., Swanson, J. M., . . . Wigal, T. (2007). Methylphenidate effects on functional outcomes in the Preschoolers with Attention-Deficit/Hyperactivity Disorder Treatment Study (PATS). *Journal of Child & Adolescent Psychopharmacology, 17*, 581–592.

Achenbach, T. M., & Rescorla, L. A. (2000). *Manual for the ASEBA preschool forms and profiles.* Burlington, VT: University of Vermont, Research Center for Children, Youth, & Families.

Akinbami, L. J., Liu, X., Pastor, P. N., & Reuban, C. A. (2011). *Attention deficit hyperactivity disorder among children aged 5–17 years in the United States, 1998–2009.* NCHS Data Brief, 70. Hyattsville, MD: National Center for Health Statistics.

American Academy of Pediatrics. (2011a). ADHD: Clinical practice guideline for the diagnosis, evaluation, and treatment of attention-deficit/hyperactivity disorder in children and adolescents. *Pediatrics,* www.pediatrics.org/cgi/doi/10.1542/peds.2011-2654.

American Academy of Pediatrics. (2011b). Policy statement: Media use by children younger than 2 years. *Pediatrics, 128,* doi:10.1542/peds.2011-1753

American Psychiatric Association. (1994). *Diagnostic and statistical manual of mental disorders* (4th ed.). Washington, DC: APA

American Psychiatric Association. (2000). *Diagnostic and statistical manual of mental disorders* (4th ed., Text Revision). Washington, DC: APA.

Anderson, P. J., & Reidy, N. (2012). Assessing executive function in preschoolers. *Neuropsychology Review, 22,* 345–360.

Armstrong, M. B., & Nettleton, S. K. (2004). Attention deficit hyperactivity disorder and preschool children. *Seminars in Speech Language, 25,* 225–232.

Auerbach, J. G., Landau, R., Berger, A., Arbelle, S., Faroy, M., & Karplus, M. (2005). Neonatal behavior of infants at familial risk for ADHD. *Infant Behavior and Development, 28,* 220–224.

Baron, I. S., & Anderson, P. J. (2012). Neuropsychological assessment of preschoolers. *Neuropsychology Review, 22,* 311–312.

Baron, I. S., Kerns, K. A., Muller, U., Ahronovich, M. D., & Litman, F. (2012). Executive functions in extremely low birth weight and late preterm preschoolers: Effects on working memory and response inhibition. *Child Neuropsychology, 18,* 586–599.

Berlin, L., & Bohlin, G. (2002). Response inhibition, hyperactivity, and conduct problems among preschool children. *Journal of Clinical Child and Adolescent Psychology, 31,* 242–251.

Berlin, L., Bohlin, G., & Rydell, A. M. (2003). Relations between inhibition, executive functioning, and ADHD symptoms: a longitudinal study from age 5 to 8(1/2) years. *Child Neuropsychology, 9,* 255–266.

Biederman, J., Monuteaux, M. C., Doyle, A. E., Seidman, L. J., Wilens, T. E., Ferrero, F., . . . Faraone, S. V. (2004). Impact of executive function deficits and attention-deficit/hyperactivity disorder (ADHD) on academic outcomes in children. *Journal of Consulting and Clinical Psychology, 72,* 757–766.

Birmaher, B., Ehman, M., Axelson, D. A., Goldstein, B. I., Monk, K., Kalas, C., . . . Brent, D. A. (2009). Schedule for affective disorders and schizophrenia for school-age children (K-SADS-PL) for the assessment for preschool children—A preliminary psychometric study. *Journal of Psychiatric Research, 43,* 680–686.

Brocki, K. C., Nyberg, L., Thorell, L. B., & Bohlin, G. (2007). Early concurrent and longitudinal symptoms of ADHD and ODD: relations to different types of inhibitory control and working memory. *Journal of Child Psychology and Psychiatry, 48,* 1033–1041.

Byrne, J. M., Bawden, H. N., Beattie, T. L., & DeWolfe, N. A. (2000). Preschoolers classified as having attention-deficit hyperactivity disorder (ADHD): DSM-IV symptom endorsement pattern. *Journal of Child Neurology, 15,* 533–538.

Byrne, J. M., DeWolfe, N. A., & Bawden, H. N. (1998). Assessment of attention-deficit hyperactivity disorder in preschoolers. *Child Neuropsychology, 4,* 49–66.

Carney, A. G., & Merrell, K. W. (2005). Teacher ratings of young children with and without ADHD: Construct validity of two child behavior rating scales. *Assessment for Effective Intervention, 30,* 67–75.

Christophersen, E. R., & Mortweet, S. L. (2003). *Treatments that work with children: Empirically supported strategies for managing childhood problems.* Washington, DC: American Psychological Association.

Conners, C. K. (2001). *Conners Kiddie Continuous Performance Test (K-CPT).* North Tonawanda, NY: Multi-Health Systems, Inc.

Conners, C. K. (2009). *Conners Early Childhood.* North Tonawanda, NY: Multi-Health Systems, Inc.

Connor, D. F. (2002). Preschool attention deficit hyperactivity disorder: a review of prevalence, diagnosis, neurobiology, and stimulant treatment. *Journal of Developmental & Behavioral Pediatrics, 23,* S1–S9.

Corkum, V., Byrne, J. M., & Ellsworth, C. (1995). Clinical assessment of sustained attention in preschoolers. *Child Neuropsychology, 1,* 3–18.

DeBar, L. L., Lynch, F., Powell, J., & Gale, J. (2003). Use of psychotropic agents in preschool children: associated symptoms, diagnoses, and health care services in a health maintenance organization. *Archives of Pediatric and Adolescent Medicine, 157,* 150–157.

Denckla, M. B. (1996). Biological correlates of learning and attention: what is relevant to learning disability and attention-deficit hyperactivity disorder? *Developmental and Behavioral Pediatrics, 17,* 1–6.

DeWolfe, N. A., Byrne, J. M., Bawden, H. N. (1999). Early clinical assessment of attention. *The Clinical Neuropsychologist, 13,* 458–473.

Diamond, A. (2000). Close interrelation of motor development and cognitive development and of the cerebellum and prefrontal cortex. *Child Development, 71,* 44–56.

DuPaul, G. J., McGoey, K. E., Eckert, T. L., & VanBrakle, J. (2001). Preschool children with attention-deficit/hyperactivity disorder: impairments in behavioral, social, and school functioning. *Journal of the American Academy of Child & Adolescent Psychiatry, 40,* 508–515.

DuPaul, G. J., Power, T. J., Anastopoulos, A. D., & Reid, R. (1998). *ADHD Rating Scale-IV.* New York: Guilford Press.

Egger, H. L., & Angold, A. (2006). Common emotional and behavioral disorders in preschool children: presentation, nosology, and epidemiology. *Journal of Child Psychology & Psychiatry, 47,* 313–337.

Egger, H. L., Kondo, D., & Angold, A. (2006). The epidemiology and diagnostic issues in preschool attention-deficit/hyperactivity disorder: A review. *Infants and Young Children, 19,* 109–122.

Egger, H., & Angold, A. (2004). The Preschool Age Psychiatric Assessment (PAPA): a structured parent interview for diagnosing psychiatric disorders in preschool children. In R. DelCarmen-Wiggins, Carter A. (Ed.), *Handbook of infant, toddler, and preschool mental health assessment* (pp. 223–246). New York: Oxford University Press.

Elliot, C. D. (2007). *Differential ability scales* (2nd ed.). San Antonio: Harcourt Assessment, Inc.

Espy, K. A. (1997). The Shape School: Assessing executive function in preschool children. *Developmental Neuropsychology, 13,* 495–499.

Espy, K. A., Kaufmann, P. M., McDiarmid, M. D., & Glisky, M. L. (1999). Executive functioning in preschool children: performance on A-not-B and other delayed response format tasks. *Brain Cognition, 41,* 178–199.

Fan, J., McCandliss, B. D., Sommer, T., Raz, A., & Posner, M. I. (2002). Testing the efficiency and independence of attentional networks. *Journal of Cognitive Neuroscience, 14,* 340–347.

Fisher, P., & Lucas, C. (2006). *Diagnostic interview schedule for children (DISC-IV)-young child.* New York: Columbia University.

Friedman-Weieneth, J. L., Harvey, E. A., Youngwith, S. D., & Goldstein, L. H. (2007). The relationship between 3-year-old children's skills and their hyperactivity, inattention, and aggression. *Journal of Educational Psychology, 99,* 671–681.

Gadow, K. D., Sprafkin, J., & Nolan, E. E. (2001). DSM-IV symptoms in community and clinic preschool children. *Journal of the American Academy of Child and Adolescent Psychiatry, 40,* 1383–1392.

Gaub, M., & Carlson, C. L. (1997). Gender differences in ADHD: a meta-analysis and critical review. *Journal of American Academy of Child and Adolescent Psychiatry, 36,* 1036–1045.

Ghuman, J. K., Riddle, M. A., Vitiello, B., Greenhill, L. L., Chuang, S. Z., Wigal, S. B.,...Skrobala, A. M. (2007). Comorbidity moderates response to methylphenidate in the Preschoolers with Attention Deficit/Hyperactivity Disorder Treatment Study (PATS). *Journal of Child and Adolescent Psychopharmacology, 17,* 563–580.

Gimpel, G. A., & Kuhn, B. R. (2000). Maternal report of attention deficit hyperactivity disorder symptoms in preschool children. *Child: Care, Health, and Development, 26,* 163–176.

Gittleman-Klein, R., & Klein, D.F. (1976). Methylphenidate effects in learning disabilities. Psychometric changes. *Archives of General Psychiatry, 33,* 655–664.

Gopin, C., Healey, D., Castelli, K., Marks, D., & Halperin, J. M. (2010). Usefulness of a clinician rating scale in identifying preschool children with ADHD. *Journal of Attention Disorders, 13,* 479–488.

Gopin, C. B., Berwid, O., Mark, D. J., Mlodnicka, A., & Halperin, J. M. (2012). ADHD preschoolers with and without ODD: do they act differently depending on degree of task engagement/reward? *Journal of Attention Disorders* (published online Feb 8 prior to publication).

Gordon, M., & Mettelman, B. B. (1987). *Technical guide to the Gordon Diagnostic System.* Syracuse, NY: Gordon Systems, Inc.

Gordon, M., McClure, F. D., & Post, E. M. (1986). *Interpretive guide to the Gordon diagnostic system.* Syracuse, NY: Gordon Systems.

Greenberg, L. M. (1996). *Tests of Variables of Attention.* Los Alamitos, CA: Universal Attention Disorders.

Greenberg, L. M., & Dupuy, T. R. (2001). Test of Variables of Attention. *Neuropsychology, 15,* 136–144.

Greenhill, L. L., Muniz, R., Ball, R. R., Levine, A., Pestreich, L., & Jiang, H. (2006). Efficacy and safety if dexmethylphenidate extended-release capsules in children with attention-deficit/hyperactivity disorder. *Journal of the American Academy of Child and Adolescent Psychiatry, 45,* 817–823.

Greenhill, L. L., Posner, K., Vaughan, B. S., & Kratochvil, C. J. (2008). Attention deficit hyperactivity disorder in preschool children. *Child and Adolescent Psychiatric Clinics of North America, 17,* 347–366, ix.

Healey, D. M., Miller, C. J., Castelli, K. L., Marks, D. J., & Halperin, J. M. (2008). The impact of impairment criteria on rates of ADHD diagnoses in preschoolers. *Journal of Abnormal Child Psychology, 36,* 771–778.

Hill, A. L., Degnan, K. A., Calkins, S. D., & Keane, S. P. (2006). Profiles of externalizing behavior problems for boys and girls across preschool: the roles of emotion regulation and inattention. *Developmental Psychology, 42,* 913–928.

Hinshaw, S. P., Owens, E. B., Sami, N., & Fargeon, S. (2006). Prospective follow-up of girls with attention deficit/hyperactivity disorder into adolescence: Evidence for continuing cross-domain impairment. *Journal of Consulting and Clinical Psychology, 74,* 489–499.

Horn, W. F., & Packard, T. (1985). Early identification of learning problems: A meta-analysis. *Journal of Educational Psychology, 77,* 597–607.

Jacques, S., & Zelazo, P. D. (2001). The Flexible Item Selection Task (FIST): a measure of executive function in preschoolers. *Developmental Neuropsychology, 20,* 573–591.

Jane, M. C., Canals, J., Ballespi, S., Vinas, F., Esparo, G., & Domenech, E. (2006). Parents and teachers reports of DSM-IV psychopathological symptoms in preschool children. *Social Psychiatry Psychiatric Epidemiology 41,* 386–393.

Kaufman, A. S., & Kaufman, N. L. (2004). *Kaufman Assessment Battery for Children-II.* Circle Pines, MN: American Guidance Service.

Kaufman, J., Birmaher, B., Brent, D., Rao, U., Flynn, C., Moreci, P.,...Ryan, N. (1997). Schedule for Affective Disorders and Schizophrenia for School-Age Children-Present and Lifetime Version (K-SADS-PL): initial reliability and validity data. *Journal of the American Academy of Child & Adolescent Psychiatry, 36,* 980–988.

Kerns, K., & Rondeau, L. (1998). Development of a continuous performance test for preschool children. *Journal of Attention Disorders, 2*, 229–238.

Kollins, S., Greenhill, L., Swanson, J., Wigal, S., Abikoff, H., McCracken, J.,...Bauzo, A. (2006). Rationale, design, and methods of the Preschool ADHD Treatment Study (PATS). *Journal of American Academy of Child and Adolescent Psychiatry, 45*, 1275–1283.

Korkman, M., Kirk, U., & Kemp, S. (2007). *NEPSY: Second Edition.* San Antonio, TX: Pearson.

Lahey, B. B., Pelham, W. E., Loney, J., Kipp, H., Ehrhardt, A., Lee, S. S.,...Massetti, G. (2004). Three-year predictive validity of DSM-IV attention deficit hyperactivity disorder in children diagnosed at 4-6 years. *American Journal of Psychiatry, 161*, 2014–2020.

Lahey, B. B., Pelham, W. E., Stein, M. A., Loney, J., Trapani, C., Nugent, K.,...Baumann, B. (1998). Validity of DSM-IV attention deficit/hyperactivity disorder for younger children. *Journal of the American Academy of Child & Adolescent Psychiatry, 37*, 695–702.

Lavigne, J. V., Lebailly, S. A., Hopkins, J., Gouze, K. R., Binns, H. J. (2009). The prevalence of ADHD, ODD, depression, and anxiety in a community sample of 4-year-olds. *Journal of Clinical Child and Adolescent Psychology, 38*, 315–328.

Lee, S. S., Lahey, B. B., Owens, E. B., & Hinshaw, S. P. (2007). Few preschool boys and girls with ADHD are well-adjusted during adolescence. *Journal of Abnormal Child Psychology, 36*, 373–383.

Lucas, C. P., Fisher, P., & Luby, J. L. (1998). *Young Child DISC-IV Research Draft: Diagnostic Interview Schedule for Children.* New York, NY: Columbia University, Division of Children Psychiatry, Joy and William Ruane Center to Identify and Treat Mood Disorders.

Mahone, E. M. (2005). Measurement of attention and related functions in the preschool child. *Mental Retardation and Developmental Disabilities Research Reviews, 11*, 216–225.

Mahone, E. M. (2011). ADHD: Volumetry, motor, and oculomotor functions. In C. Stanford & R. Tannock (Eds.), *Behavioral neuroscience of attention deficit hyperactivity disorder and its treatment. Current Topics in Behavioral Neurosciences, 9* (pp. 17–47). DOI 10.1007/7854_2011_146. Berlin/Heidelberg: Springer-Verlag.

Mahone, E. M., Crocetti, D., Ranta, M. E., Gaddis, A., Cataldo, M., Slifer, K. J., Denckla, M. B., & Mostofsky, S. H. (2011). A preliminary neuroimaging study of preschool children with ADHD. *The Clinical Neuropsychologist, 25*, 1009–1028.

Mahone, E. M., & Hoffman, J. C. (2007). Behavior ratings of executive function among preschoolers with ADHD. *The Clinical Neuropsychologist, 21*, 569–586.

Mahone, E. M., Pillion, J. P., & Hiemenz, J. R. (2001). Initial development of an auditory continuous performance test for preschoolers. *Journal of Attention Disorders, 5*, 93–106.

Mahone, E. M., Pillion, J. P., Hoffman, J., Hiemenz, J. R., & Denckla, M. B. (2005). Construct validity of the auditory continuous performance test for preschoolers. *Developmental Neuropsychology, 27*, 11–33.

Mahone, E. M., & Schneider, H. E. (2012). Assessment of attention in preschoolers. *Neuropsychology Review, 22*, 361–383.

Mahone, E. M., & Slomine, B. S. (2007). Managing dysexecutive disorders. In S. Hunter & J. Donders (Eds.), *Pediatric neuropsychological intervention* (pp. 287–313). Cambridge, UK: Cambridge University Press.

Mahone, E. M., & Slomine, B. S. (2008). Neurodevelopmental disorders. In J. Morgan & J. Ricker (Eds.), *Textbook of clinical neuropsychology* (pp. 105–127). New York: Taylor and Francis.

Makie, S., Shaw, P., Lenroot, R., Pierson, R., Greenstein, D. K., Nugent, T.F. 3rd, Sharp, W. S., Giedd, J. N., & Rapoport, J. L. (2007). Cerebellar development and clinical outcome in attention deficit hyperactivity disorder. *American Journal of Psychiatry, 164*, 647–655.

Mariani, M. A., & Barkley, R. A. (1997). Neuropsychological and academic functioning in preschool boys with attention deficit hyperactivity disorder. *Developmental Neuropsychology, 13*, 111–129.

Massetti, G. M., Lahey, B. B., Pelham, W. E., Loney, J., Ehrhardt, A., Lee, S. S.,...Kipp, H. (2007). Academic achievement over 8 years among children who met modified criteria for attention-deficit/hyperactivity disorder at 4-6 years of age. *Journal of Abnormal Child Psychology, 36*, 399–410.

McClure, F. D., & Gordon, M. (1984). Performance of disturbed hyperactive and nonhyperactive children on an objective measure of hyperactivity. *Journal of Abnormal Child Psychology, 12,* 561–571.

McGarney, S. B., & Arthaud, T. J. (2004). *Attention Deficit Disorders Evaluation Scale—Third Edition.* Columbia, MO: Hawthorne Educational Services, Inc.

McGoey, K. E., DuPaul, G. J., Haley, E., & Shleton, T. L. (2007). Parent and teacher ratings of attention deficit/hyperactivity disorder in preschool: The ADHD Rating Scale-IV Preschool Version. *Journal of Psychopathology Behavioral Assessment, 29,* 269–276.

McGrath, A. M., Handwerk, M. L., Armstrong, K. J., Lucas, C. P., & Friman, P. C. (2004). The validity of the ADHD section of the Diagnostic Interview for Children. *Behavioral Modification, 28,* 349–374.

Merrell, K. W. (1996). Social-emotional assessment in early childhood: The Preschool and Kindergarten Behavior Scales. *Journal of Early Intervention, 20,* 132–145.

Merrell, K. W. (2003). *Preschool and Kindergarten Behavior Scales—Second Edition.* Austin, TX: PRO-ED.

Muller, U., Kerns, K. A., & Konkin, K. (2012). Test-retest reliability and practice effects of executive function tasks in preschool children. *The Clinical Neuropsychologist, 26,* 271–287.

National Institutes of Health. (1998). *Diagnosis and treatment of attention deficit hyperactivity disorder: NIH Consensus Statement.* Washington, DC: NIH.

Nichols, P., & Chen, T. (1981). *Minimal brain dysfunction: a prospective study.* Hillside, NJ: Erlbaum Associates.

Nolan, E. E., Gadow, K. D., & Sprafkin, J. (2001). Teacher reports of DSM-IV ADHD, ODD, and CD symptoms in schoolchildren. *Journal of the American Academy of Child and Adolescent Psychiatry, 40,* 241–249.

Overgaard, K. R., Aase, H., Torgersen, S., & Zeiner, P. (2012). Co-Occurrence of ADHD and anxiety in preschool children. *Journal of Attention Disorders.* DOI: 10.1177/1087054712463063.

Palfrey, J. S., Levine, M. D., Walker, D. K., & Sullivan, M. (1985). The emergence of attention deficits in early childhood: a prospective study. *Journal of Developmental Behavioral Pediatrics, 6,* 339–348.

Pelham, W. E., Foster, E. M., & Robb, J. A. (2007). The economic impact of attention-deficit/hyperactivity disorder in children and adolescents. *Journal of Pediatric Psychology, 32,* 711–727.

Poblano, A., & Romero, E. (2006). ECI-4 Screening of attention deficit-hyperactivity disorder and co-morbidity in Mexican preschool children. *Arquivos de Neuro-Psiquiatria, 64,* 932–936.

Posner, K., Melvin, G. A., Murray, D. W., Gugga, S. S., Fisher, P., Skrobala, A., … Greenhill, L. L. (2007). Clinical presentation of attention-deficit/hyperactivity disorder in preschool children: The Preschoolers with Attention-Deficit/Hyperactivity Disorder Treatment Study (PATS). *Journal of Child and Adolescent Psychopharmacology, 17,* 547–562.

Rappley, M., Eneli, I., & Mullan, P. (2002). Patterns of psychotropic medication use in very young children with attention-deficit hyperactivity disorder. *Journal of Development and Behavioral Pediatrics, 23,* 23–30.

Rappley, M. D., Mullan, P. B., Alvarez, F. J., Eneli, I. U., Wang, J., & Gardiner, J. C. (1999). Diagnosis of attention-deficit/hyperactivity disorder and use of psychotropic medication in very young children. *Archives of Pediatrics and Adolescent Medicine, 153,* 1039–1045.

Reynolds, C., & Kamphaus, R. (2004). *Behavior assessment system for children-2.* Circle Pines, MN: American Guidance Systems, Inc.

Robb, J. A., Sibley, M. H., Pelham, W. E., Foster, E. M., Molina, B. S. G., Gnagy, E. M., … Kuriyan, A. B. (2011). The estimated annual cost of ADHD to the US education system. *School Mental Health, 3,* 169–177.

Shaffer, D., Fisher, P., Lucas, C. P., Dulcan, M. K., & Schwab-Stone, M. E. (2000). NIMH Diagnostic Interview Schedule for Children Version IV (NIMH DISC-IV): Description, differences from previous versions, and reliability of some common diagnoses. *Journal of the American Academy of Child and Adolescent Psychiatry, 39,* 28–38.

Shaw, P., Eckstrand, K., Sharp, W., Blumenthal, J., Lerch, J.P., Greenstein, D., Clasen, L., Evans, A., Giedd, J., & Rapoport, J.L. (2007) Attention-deficit/hyperactivity disorder is characterized by a delay in cortical maturation. *Proceedings of the National Academy of Sciences USA, 104,* 19649–19654.

Shaw, P., Malek, M., Watson, B., Sharp, W., Evans, A., & Greenstein, D. (2012). Development of cortical surface area and gyrification in attention-deficit/hyperactivity disorder. *Biological Psychiatry, 72,* 191–197.

Shelton, T., & Barkley, R. (1993). Assessment of attention deficit hyperactivity disorder in young children. In J. L. Culbertson & D. Willis (Eds.), *Testing young children* (pp. 290–318). Austin, TX: Pro-Ed.

Simon, H. A. (1975), The functional equivalence of problem solving skills. *Cognitive Psychology, 7,* 268–288

Sims, D. M., & Lonigan, C. J. (2012). Multi-method assessment of ADHD characteristics in pre-school children: relations between measures. *Early Childhood Research Quarterly, 27,* 329–337.

Smidts, D. P., Jacobs, R., & Anderson, V. (2004). The Object Classification Task for Children (OCTC): a measure of concept generation and mental flexibility in early childhood. *Developmental Neuropsychology, 26,* 385–401.

Snyder, J., Prichard, J., Schrepferman, L., Patrick, M. R., & Stoolmiller, M. (2004). Child impulsiveness-inattention, early peer experiences, and the development of early onset conduct problems. *Journal of Abnormal Child Psychology, 32,* 579–594.

Sonuga Barke, E. J. S., Koerting, J., Smith, E., McCann, D. C., & Thompson, M. (2011). Early detection and intervention for attention-deficit/hyperactivity disorder. *Expert Reviews Neurotherapeutics, 11,* 557–563.

Sonuga-Barke, E. J., Dalen, L., Daley, D., & Remington, B. (2002). Are planning, working memory, and inhibition associated with individual differences in preschool ADHD symptoms? *Developmental Neuropsychology, 21,* 255–272.

Sprafkin, J., & Gadow, K. D. (1996). *Early Childhood Symptom Inventories.* Stoney Brook, NY: Checkmate Plus.

Sprafkin, J., Volpe, R. J., Gadow, K. D., Nolan, E. E., & Kelly, K. (2002). A DSM-IV-Referenced screening instrument for preschool children: The early childhood inventory-4. *Journal of the American Academy of Child & Adolescent Psychiatry, 41,* 604–612.

Sterba, S., Egger, H. L., Angold, A. (2007). Diagnostic specificity and nonspecificity in the dimensions of preschool psychopathology. *Journal of Child Psychology and Psychiatry, 48,* 1005–1013.

Swanson, J., Greenhill, L., Wigal, T., Kollins, S., Stehli, A., Davies, M., ... Wigal, S. (2006). Stimulant-related reductions of growth rates in the PATS. *Journal of the American Academy of Child & Adolescent Psychiatry, 45,* 1304–1313.

Swanson, J. M. (1992). *School-based assessments and interventions for ADD students.* Irvine, CA: K.C. Publications

Tandon, M., Xuemei, S., & Luby, J. (2011). Preschool onset ADHD: Course and predictors of stability over 24m. *Journal of Child and Adolescent Psychopharmacology, 21,* 321–330.

Vitiello, B., Abikoff, H. B., Chuang, S. Z., Kollins, S. H., McCracken, J. T., Riddle, M. A., ... Greenhill, L. L. (2007). Effectiveness of methylphenidate in the 10-month continuation phase of the Preschoolers with Attention-Deficit/Hyperactivity Disorder Treatment Study (PATS). *Journal of Child & Adolescent Psychopharmacology, 17,* 593–604.

Von Stauffenberg, C., & Campbell, S. B. (2007). Predicting the early developmental course of symptoms of attention deficit hyperactivity disorder. *Journal of Applied Developmental Psychology, 28,* 536–552.

Wahlstedt, C., Thorell, L. B., & Bohlin, G. (2008). ADHD symptoms and executive function impairment: Early predictors of later behavior problems. *Developmental Psychology, 33,* 160–178.

Weiler, M. D., Bellinger, D., Marmor, J., Rancier, S., & Waber, D. (1999). Mother and teacher reports of ADHD symptoms: DSM-IV Questionnaire data. *Journal of the American Academy of Child and Adolescent Psychiatry, 38,* 1139–1147.

Weisen, S. (2008). Clinical use of the Differential Abilities Scales second edition (DAS-II) for children with attention deficit/hyperactivity disorder [Abstract]. *Section B: Sciences and Engineering, 69,* 3863.

Wilens, T. E., Biederman, J., Brown, S., Monuteaux, M., Prince, J., & Spencer, T. J. (2002a). Patterns of psychopathology and dysfunction in clinically referred preschoolers. *Journal of Developmental and Behavioral Pediatrics, 23*, S31–S36.

Wilens, T. E., Biederman, J., Brown, S., Tanguay, S., Monuteaux, M. C., Blake, C., et al. (2002b). Psychiatric comorbidity and functioning in clinically referred preschool children and school-age youths with ADHD. *Journal of the American Academy of Child and Adolescent Psychiatry, 41*, 262–268.

Yochman, A., Ornoy, A., & Parush, S. (2006). Co-occurrence of developmental delays among preschool children with attention-deficit-hyperactivity disorder. *Developmental Medicine and Child Neurology, 48*, 483–488.

Youngwirth, S. D., Harvey, E. A., Gates, E. C., Hashim, R. L., & Friedman-Weieneth, J. L. (2007). Neuropsychological abilities of preschool-aged children who display hyperactivity and/or oppositional defiant behavior problems. *Child Neuropsychology, 13*, 422–443.

4

Differential Diagnosis and Comorbidity

Primary Healthcare Provider Perspective

SYDNEY A. RICE AND

WILLIAM N. MARSHALL, JR.

Introduction

Primary healthcare providers encounter behavior problems and concerns in families with toddlers and preschool-aged children on a daily basis. Young active children can be both a great joy and a challenge to families; families often ask their primary healthcare provider for guidance for a varied combination of medical and behavioral concerns. Medical conditions can both mimic and exacerbate hyperactive and inattentive behaviors, and primary healthcare providers need to recognize when a medical condition is complicating behavioral patterns. Most primary healthcare clinicians are familiar with managing and giving direction regarding toddler and preschool behavioral issues and begin by establishing a relationship with the family, defining the behavioral concerns, and reviewing the parent's response to the undesired behaviors (Prugh, 1983).

Anticipatory guidance and problem-specific education will usually prevent escalation of the problem behaviors and lessen the stress of parenting. When the primary healthcare clinician has developed a relationship with the family, defined the behavioral concerns in the family context, and allowed adequate time for improvement through education and analysis of objective data, but no progress has taken place, further steps may be needed, including consultation and review of other diagnostic options.

The diagnosis of attention-deficit/hyperactivity disorder (ADHD) before school age and the use of medication to treat these young children is a relatively new practice for many pediatricians. The recent American Academy of Pediatrics (AAP) guideline has generated some controversy with its acknowledgment that these young children may indeed benefit from early diagnosis and treatment (AAP, 2011).

EARLIER DIAGNOSIS

Several factors may contribute to the current trend in earlier diagnosis and treatment. First, almost 60% of preschool children are cared for during the day in a childcare center

(U.S. Department of Education, 2012). Childcare workers have the opportunity to observe varied child behaviors and can alert parents and families to concerns that a child's behavior is out of the norm. Disruptive behaviors are usually less tolerated in group settings, and children often come to the attention of healthcare providers due to concerns for other children's safety.

Second, pediatricians are accustomed to the evaluation and treatment of school-aged children with ADHD. Guidelines and trainings through organizations such as the AAP have sensitized pediatricians to the diagnosis and treatment of school-aged children with ADHD. Since 1996, there has been a slow but steady increase in therapeutic stimulant use for ADHD, with the largest increase in adolescents.(Zuvekas & Vitiello, 2012). This increase in use of stimulant medication has not translated into the preschool population, but new guidelines from the AAP now include the use of stimulant medication for preschool-aged children (AAP, 2012).

Third, the use of diagnostic checklists and algorithms, the system of diagnostic coding, and the use of electronic medical record systems may tend to encourage categorization and certainty rather than postponing a definite diagnosis. The transition to the use of electronic health records has changed the interaction between clinician and patient from one of an evolving clinical narrative to a series of diagnostic observations. This may encourage movement toward diagnosis and intervention more quickly than in previous generations (Walsh, 2004).

The evaluation of ADHD symptoms includes observational assessments from both the home and the community settings and is more thoroughly described in Chapter 2. In preschoolers, there is more inconsistency in these observational assessments, with test–retest reliability coefficients showing more variability between observers than in school-age children (Thomas, Shapiro, DuPaul, Lutz, & Kern, 2011; Lakes, Swanson, & Riggs, 2011; Re & Cornoldi, 2009). This may be due to the wide variability in experiences among preschool children based on parental expectations and caregiving settings and situations (e.g., care by a parent at home with no other children, care by an elderly grandparent, care in a busy preschool setting or a family daycare). However, there are some DSM-based scales with validity and normative data in preschool children that can help with the diagnostic process in this population (McGoey, DuPaul, Haley, & Shelton, 2007).

CULTURAL AND SOCIETAL TRENDS SUPPORTING EARLY DIAGNOSIS

Cultural and societal trends influence parents, teachers, and clinicians. Publicity on television, Internet, or the print media about a certain diagnosis or medication may heighten parents' and professionals' concerns about children's behavior on one hand, but also deter seeking of treatment due to controversy and debate (e.g., use of psychostimulants for children).

Multiple factors have contributed to the increase in the rate of childhood diagnosis of ADHD over the past 20 years (Mayes, Bagwell, & Erkulwater, 2009, p. 2). Governmental recognition of ADHD as a disability has made financial payments and school accommodations available for children with ADHD. Professional trends such as the acceptance of the neurobiological basis of ADHD and the earlier diagnostic categorization of childhood behavior and mental health problems have accelerated the prevalence of ADHD diagnosis.

LABELING PRESCHOOL CHILDREN WITH PSYCHIATRIC DIAGNOSES

The anti-psychiatry movement and "labeling theory" of the 1970s set an initial tone of suspicion of psychiatry in general. The Scientology-funded groups in the 1990s garnered much media attention for the claim that normal children were being labeled and drugged because of intolerant schools, a powerful pharmaceutical industry, and compliant and/or incompetent doctors. Currently, social conservatives in political discussions and skeptical parents in school settings and social media on the Internet echo these concerns. Discovered links between pharmaceutical manufacturers and clinical researchers have compromised published research findings and created uncertainty for members of the medical profession. It is no wonder that some families are afraid of the ADHD diagnosis and its treatment (Mayes et al., 2009, pp. 139–173).

DIAGNOSTIC CHALLENGES

Many factors may cause parents and caregivers excessive worry about normal behaviors. New parents may have no frame of reference or may have unrealistic expectations about childhood behavior and development. Other stressors in their lives may make the child's developmentally normal behavior intolerable. Family situations may place the family at risk for inconsistent parenting; for example, parents may alternate work shifts to avoid the need for paid childcare. Each parent likely has a different parenting style and because they spend little time together as a family, they may not recognize the disparities in their parenting practices that may be exacerbating the typical preschool behavioral challenges. Parents' behavioral ratings and concerns about their child's behavior may be colored by their personal experiences, especially if the parents themselves or other family members have been diagnosed with ADHD or other psychiatric illness. The parents' personal experiences may result in behavior ratings that are more or less positive than those of an unbiased reporter. The fit between parent and child temperament also plays a role in the interaction between parent and child and a parent's ability to manage challenging, but typical, toddler and preschool behaviors. Changing family constellations, such as primary parenting by grandparents, can alter caregivers' behavioral expectations for young children. In addition, parents may receive criticism and mixed feedback from family members about their child's behavior and feel unprepared to process these comments and implement a consistent parenting practice.

Of concern to the clinician at the outset are these questions: Are the reported hyperactivity and inattentive behaviors simply normal for the child's age? Behaviors seen at age 4 years and above are more likely to persist than those in younger children. Is the child's behavior a reaction to family stress, or even abuse or neglect by the caretakers (Ouyang, Fang, Mercy, Perou, & Grosse, 2008)? Are the caretakers or reporting observers in the childcare setting or preschool reliable?

The difficulty of diagnosis in toddlers and preschool children is heightened by a number of factors, including limited expressive communication, limited behavioral repertoire, underconfident parents (especially first-time parents) with underdeveloped observational skills, fewer outside observers than in school-aged children, and less trained outside observers (many daycare workers). Information gathering is often done with one parent or caretaker, who may or may not spend the most time with the child, and who may not be able to provide an adequate family medical history, especially that of the other parent's (not present during the evaluation) family. The diagnostic problem is even more complex, or impossible, when foster children come to the clinic with a new foster parent and little information beyond the acute problems is available.

Reports from teachers or childcare center staff may also be biased. Inexperienced teachers in large preschool classrooms might feel overwhelmed by behaviors that a more experienced teacher might find manageable. On the other hand, some experienced teachers or staff may be overconfident that the child will respond to their discipline and be less likely to report problems. Often, personal and professional views of teachers and staff, molded by prior experiences, inform their observations of the child's behaviors. Parents may be blamed and social class differences in childrearing may go unrecognized.

The relative age effect (Morrow Garland, Wright, et al., 2012) makes ADHD diagnosis and treatment more likely in the younger children in any given classroom. A relatively immature child who has a birthdate immediately before the date cutoff for entering kindergarten will stand out behaviorally compared to a child almost a year older in the same classroom. In a study of British Columbia children ages 6 to 12 years (Morrow, Garland, Wright, et al., 2012), boys were 41% more likely and girls 77% more likely to be given a medication for ADHD if they were the youngest child in their grades; the effect could conceivably be even stronger in the preschool-age group. Due to concerns that their child's behavior will be compared to older (and hence more mature and less active) children in the classroom, some families chose to withhold their child from entering kindergarten, enrolling him or her in the following year.

Clinical Assessment

The primary healthcare provider is charged with investigating the underlying etiology of behavioral difficulties in children's presentations that may include ADHD in the differential diagnosis. It can be a challenging task to differentiate the medical and environmental factors from a behavioral situation in each child. After an initial assessment, the primary healthcare provider may then proceed with referral to a behavioral specialist or a child psychiatrist for further evaluation and recommendations.

The possibility of ADHD in a preschooler may be brought to the fore by the parents, other family members or friends, staff at a preschool or daycare center, another health professional, or a primary healthcare provider evaluating the child during a well-child visit or during an evaluation for behavioral problems. As always, a prior relationship with the child and family can be most helpful at the outset, putting the current concern in the context of known biopsychosocial factors affecting the child and the family. If the child and family are not well known to the clinician, then more extensive data gathering will be necessary. Reports from outside reporters are similarly evaluated, taking into account, if possible, the experience and understanding of the observer with regard to toddlers and preschoolers.

The first visit for a behavioral concern sets the stage for later success. If this is the family's first visit, a full history and physical examination should be performed at that visit or scheduled soon thereafter. If this is an established patient, a more focused review of basic history and physical elements is needed, including neurodevelopmental progress and growth. A history of the pregnancy should encompass prenatal care and events, including alcohol and drug use, infections, and fetal distress. Past medical history includes prior doctor visits for well-child care, illness, hospitalizations, surgeries, medications, and allergies. The well-child care history may reveal a pattern of concerns for tantrums, aggressive behavior, or parental over-concern; immunization history may find that the child has not received the proper vaccinations because of parental anxiety or parenting beliefs. For example, maternal depression is linked to lack of up-to-date immunization status in toddlers and preschool children, and parents who intentionally delay immunizations for their children are more likely to seek information on the Internet than from their physician (Minkovitz et al., 2005; Smith et al., 2010). History of illnesses in the child may be relevant in many ways, including conditions that predispose to ADHD or those leading to neurologic or developmental impairments. Medications—for example, antihistamines and barbiturates—may cause hyperactive behaviors.

SLEEP HISTORY

The daily routine and sleep pattern must be detailed—for example, parents may be asked to keep a detailed diary for the next visit. Sleep difficulties should be reviewed. Is there excessively loud or frequent snoring accompanied by respiratory pause or apnea? Does the child awaken during the night? Is the child refreshed and energetic in the morning or does he or she still require naps at age 3 or 4? The use of written questionnaires in the waiting room may be helpful. All of these data must be reviewed in the context of the family and sleep environment, since not all families follow a predicted sleep pattern. Working couples with different schedules may want to interact with their child at both late and early hours of the day, resulting in a "regularly irregular" schedule for the child. Some toddlers may be accustomed to staying awake with older siblings or parents; they may be sleepy if out-of-home childcare begins earlier in the day. If one or both caretakers do not sleep well, they may be more vigilant about their child's sleep pattern. Children who sleep in the same room or bed as their parents are more likely to be observed than those in another room.

FAMILY HISTORY

Family history must be reviewed in detail. If seeing the child for the first time, parents should be offered an opportunity to recall family medical history both at the initial visit, often by means of written forms, and during subsequent visits. Few patients and families are so well organized that all relevant details emerge at the outset. Psychiatric and behavioral histories are even more problematic. Do not expect "full disclosure" of embarrassing family history details like alcohol and drug abuse, incarcerations and criminal history, suicide attempts, marital failures, and domestic violence in families from parents who do not yet have a good relationship with the clinician.

PARENTS' EDUCATIONAL BACKGROUND

An understanding of the parents' educational background should be sought. Parental and second-degree relatives' educational accomplishments provide a window into the level of parental understanding and health literacy, the expectations of future educational success for the child, the specific concerns of the caretakers, and hereditary and environmental risks for the child. Because the approach to and understanding of educational problems continues to change, prior generations of children (parents and grandparents) may not have been given a firm reason for school or behavioral problems, and family understanding may attribute these difficulties to a spurious cause or a secondary cause such as substance abuse. Parents who graduated from high school may have been in special-education or resource-room programs, so their actual reading level, for example, should not be assumed.

PHYSICAL EXAMINATION

The physical examination of a new patient will assess general health and provide clues to underlying problems. Growth parameters may reveal evidence of abnormal head circumference leading to investigation of causes of microcephaly—for instance, congenital infections, intrauterine toxic exposures such as alcohol, genetic syndromes, or brain injury. The severely abused and malnourished infant will show evidence of growth delay; acquisition of old records is essential to adequately assess the growth pattern to account for abnormalities. Similarly, obesity, though rarely associated with genetic (Prader-Willi syndrome) or hormonal (hypothyroidism) conditions, can provide clues to family and community behavior, supervision, and standards regarding dietary patterns and habits.

The child's general appearance and demeanor are assessed throughout the examination. Pediatricians should not rely on an office-based assessment of behavior to establish a diagnosis of ADHD or other behavioral conditions; children, especially young children, exhibit a wide range of responses to the clinic or hospital environment that may be atypical of their usual actions. Some children may appear withdrawn and others may appear hyperactive in response to the stress of the examination room. Certainly the extremes must be investigated; the 4-year-old who hits the physician or parent or the 3-year-old who continuously screams in fright at the sight of the nurse or doctor is atypical. Similarly, a good understanding of developmental milestones will inform the overall assessment; a friendly office environment with toys and books will give the toddler and young child the chance to demonstrate their developmental progress. This is also the time to assess gait, gross and fine motor movements, and speech. The examiner should observe for abnormal or asymmetric movements, tremors, tics, and chorea.

Physical examination may uncover specific signs for underlying causes of behavioral conditions. Evidence of hearing impairment may be suggested by chronic otitis media with effusion; audiologic evaluation must follow. Central pallor may indicate iron deficiency. Evidence of abuse and neglect may be uncovered with the finding of bruising or old injury not accounted for or consistent with accidental injury, or the presence of severe dental caries and lack of basic hygiene. Thyromegaly or nodule must be evaluated with laboratory testing. On occasion, characteristic findings associated with known syndromes may have been unappreciated by previous examiners.

NEXT STEPS FOR A PRIMARY HEALTHCARE PROVIDER

Several other steps may be important here. Screening for hearing, vision, lead poisoning, and anemia should have been done in the recent past or be planned for the immediate future. The level of parental knowledge about the behavioral concerns should be assessed and information sources like books, websites, or office handouts given. Office contact information should be explicit, especially since frequent phone or email consultation may be useful. Finally, more global family issues must be recognized, since attention to and amelioration of household stressors like financial or marital problems may be the most important elements in treating the child. Primary healthcare providers who care for young children should be familiar with community resources to support children and their families and should be liberal in their use of community referrals. Pediatric clinic settings with onsite access to social workers or community lay workers offer early support that may avoid the need for more intensive family therapy interventions.

The first assessment visit is not the time for false reassurance ("This is normal behavior for some 3-year-olds") nor for immediate definitive diagnosis and treatment ("Your child has attention-deficit/hyperactivity disorder and needs psychostimulant treatment"). Rather, the visit may conclude with plans for further evaluation, including "homework" for the family, and discussion of future plans. Information from other caretakers or the preschool should be obtained. Basic pediatric advice should be offered, including suggestions for management of sleep problems, tantrums, and mealtime disruptions. If a crisis is present, such as a distraught parent or a child or parent who has been or seems likely to be abused, then immediate referral to an emergency center is, of course, warranted. A deliberative approach is all the more important for the younger child.

Several factors may influence how a primary healthcare provider proceeds with an evaluation for ADHD in preschoolers. A close relationship between the provider and the family may lead the provider to downplay symptoms and delay diagnosis due to concerns regarding labeling the child or to avoid worrying the parents. Often, children with ADHD may have distractible parents who may be inattentive during the visit, miss appointments, and be noncompliant with recommendations. Visits for behavioral concerns are less likely to end within the customary 20-minute appointments; providers may not feel a sense of accomplishment and often feel stressed with feelings of inadequacy for understanding of the behavioral problem and the knowledge that they are now behind schedule. The urge to "do something" is strong among providers, and parental frustration adds to the urgency; writing a prescription or making a referral, though premature in many cases, can satisfy this desire. Similarly, premature diagnosis can be made based on brief observations of the toddler or preschooler in the office setting, whereas the child may be distressed for other reasons, for example due to lack of a nap or needing a snack.

DISCUSSION OF TREATMENT OPTIONS

Once the clinician has made a diagnosis of ADHD in a preschool child, treatment options can be discussed with the family. Some pediatricians may wish to refer the family to a behavioral developmental pediatric subspecialist or a child psychiatrist at this point. Decisions about treatment may be deferred to these specialists. The decision to refer will vary based on the provider's experience with treatment of ADHD and the concern for comorbid developmental or psychiatric conditions. Several office sessions may be devoted to education and further exploration of family dynamics and can have an ameliorative effect. The new AAP guidelines (AAP, 2011) recommend parenting classes and support groups as primary therapy; families will vary as to their comfort with these and other options. Support groups specific to ADHD symptoms may be more acceptable to many families (e.g., Children and Adults with Attention Deficit/Hyperactivity Disorder [CHADD]). Social workers and other therapists may offer valuable help to the child and family; those of a support person therapist who visits the home and designs more effective parenting strategies to that of a support person who can assess the family's understanding and likelihood of adherence to the treatment plan. Whatever the treatment plan instituted, close follow-up is essential; if results are not positive, other options or referrals are indicated.

Alternatively, the pediatrician may decide to initiate medication, usually methylphenidate, though this is not the first option for treatment according to the new AAP guidelines (AAP, 2011). If ADHD medications are considered, a careful targeted cardiac history about any cardiovascular risks in the child should be obtained. Cardiac history should include previous history of cardiac problems, heart murmur, palpitations, increased heart rate, or extra or skipped heart beats, chest pain and/or shortness of breath with exercise, fainting or dizziness (particularly with exercise), syncope, unexplained and/or noticeable change in exercise tolerance, rheumatic fever, hypertension, diagnosis of hypertrophic cardiomyopathy (HCM), long-QT syndrome (LQTS), Wolff-Parkinson-White (WPW) syndrome or similar abnormal rhythm conditions, Marfan syndrome, and seizures. A detailed family cardiac history should also be obtained regarding any history of sudden death or heart attack, sudden death during exercise, cardiac arrhythmias, cardiomyopathy, LQTS, short-QT syndrome, or Brugada syndrome, WPW or similar abnormal rhythm conditions, and Marfan syndrome in children or young adults in the family (Ghuman & Ghuman, 2012; Perrin et al., 2008; Vetter et al., 2008).

CHALLENGES FOR THE PRIMARY HEALTHCARE PROVIDER IN PRESCHOOL POPULATIONS

Pediatricians are more comfortable with the management of ADHD than of other mental health problems (Garbutt, Leege, Sterkel, Gentry, & Strunk, 2012); this could shape diagnostic impressions, leading to overdiagnosis of ADHD. Many young families with young active children may be struggling with a combination of social and financial stresses (Brown, Ackerman,& Moore, 2013). Accurately identifying ADHD in preschoolers requires that environmental and family issues be recognized and addressed. This presents a significant challenge in a busy pediatric clinic setting, and assessment of many behavioral and psychosocial needs may be inadequate. Automated waiting room screening for ADHD, behavioral concerns, and family stress (Anand, Carroll, & Downs, 2012), may be an efficient way to enhance primary healthcare visits.

Parents or caretakers are the most important people in a child's life and usually the ultimate decision makers about seeking medical help and instituting treatment plans. It is vitally important, then, that the clinician be able to evaluate their personal and family history as it pertains to the care and support of the child. Parents who have already established a relationship with the clinician will tend to be more trusting and hence more able to give an accurate description of the child's behavior and their reactions to the child's behavior. The clinician, in turn, will have a better context and understanding of their story. Unfortunately, many encounters for behavioral concerns usually occur at the very first meeting when the child and the family are introduced to the clinician for the first time and trust and understanding have yet to be established.

Communication with the clinician may be hampered by many factors. Low print and oral literacy levels may compromise completion of behavior rating scales and the understanding of verbal and written materials about ADHD. Most individuals who struggle with reading literacy are unlikely to share information regarding their reading difficulty with healthcare providers. Even in individuals with adequate reading literacy, health literacy may be low and may be influenced by media, cultural tradition, and social structure (Heerman, Karpinos, & Rothman, 2012).

Evaluation of preschoolers with ADHD and other behavioral concerns is challenging in a busy primary healthcare setting. The child is often fearful of an examination and painful immunizations, making observation of the child's behavior less reliable. Parental concerns expressed about ADHD behaviors may lead the discussion rapidly toward a diagnosis of ADHD and may limit differential diagnosis. The primary healthcare provider may have little time to fully evaluate the child and feel pressured to treat with medications immediately, since counseling is time consuming and many pediatricians have not received adequate training in counseling and family therapy. In addition, other support services such as social work may be inadequate in many clinic and community settings.

Comorbidity and Differential Diagnosis

The differential diagnosis of the preschool child who presents for evaluation for possible ADHD includes most of the differential diagnoses considered for older children. A few of the diagnoses relevant for school-aged children, like dyslexia, are not yet recognizable; others, like conduct disorder, are by definition restricted to older children and adolescents, though antecedents may be supposed. Other problems, like tic disorders, are less common in this age group, presenting somewhat later.

MEDICAL COMORBIDITY AND DIFFERENTIAL DIAGNOSIS

Peri- and Prenatal Factors

The differential diagnosis is guided by results of the initial history and physical examination. Prenatal and birth history may reveal relevant toxic exposures like drugs and alcohol, although this information may not be forthcoming without a discussion of the importance of a full history. Gestational diabetes (Nomura et al., 2012) and low Apgar scores have also been correlated with ADHD, and this information is readily available in children's birth records (Li, Olsen, Vestergaard, & Obel, 2011). Universal hearing screening of newborns has helped with early identification of hearing loss at birth.

However, some forms of hearing loss are progressive and children may have a normal newborn hearing screening and then develop hearing impairment over the first several months to years of life. Formal audiologic or ophthalmologic examination should be performed with any suspicion of hearing or vision impairment; routine hearing and vision screenings are now recommended by the American Academy of Pediatrics for all preschool children (AAP, 2007). Parents should be asked about speech delay, a history of chronic otitis media, dysconjugate gaze, the need to view books or screens closely and about any concerns regarding vision or hearing.

Prematurity

Formerly extremely premature infants display inattention at school age characterized by attention lapses and decreased visuospatial working memory abilities (de Kieviet, van Elburg, Lafeber, & Oosterlaan, 2012). Preschool children who were born prematurely are frequently followed in neurodevelopmental clinics, as many have medical concerns for the first several years after birth. This close follow-up is very helpful in identifying symptoms of ADHD and guiding preschool interventions and therapies.

SENSORY IMPAIRMENT

Children who have hearing or vision impairment frequently present with severe inattention problems and hyperactivity. Children who have hearing impairment have associated receptive and expressive language delays that contribute to behavior issues. In addition, they may not hear behavioral prompts if they are unable to hear verbal redirection. Children who have vision impairment also miss visual behavioral cues, changes in caregiver's facial expressions, and modeling opportunities from family and typical peers. While children with sensory impairments may also have comorbid ADHD, it is important to include professionals who are experienced in evaluating children with sensory impairments.

FETAL ALCOHOL SPECTRUM DISORDERS

Fetal alcohol spectrum disorders (FASD) are the most common preventable developmental disorders in the United States, with a prevalence of 0.5 to 2.0 cases per 1,000 live births (NCBDDD, 2004). Children with FASD characteristically have abnormal facial characteristics (e.g., smooth philtrum and thin upper lip), lower-than-average height, weight, or both, and central nervous system problems (e.g., small head size, problems with attention and hyperactivity, poor coordination). Many children with FASD have ADHD as a characteristic of central nervous system dysfunctions (Fryer, McGee, Matt, Riley, & Mattson, 2007).

MEDICATIONS

It is important to take a complete medication history as part of a preschool evaluation for inattention, hyperactivity, and impulsivity. Several different medications for other conditions may make children inattentive and hyperactive. Behavioral side effects of oral steroid medications are well documented (e.g., restlessness, agitation, fussy, mood swings, hyperactivity, sleep problems) and easily recognized by pediatric practitioners. Behavioral side effects of some common asthma medications (e.g., albuterol) include restlessness, hyperactivity, and irritability. Allergy medications may cause sedation or hyperactivity. Medication reactions can be reliably differentiated from idiopathic ADHD based on resolution of symptoms when the medication is discontinued.

TOXINS

Environmental toxins have been associated with ADHD and recognition of these neurotoxins has changed commercial packaging and environmental surveillance practices for products used in the home. Identified neurotoxins predisposing young children to ADHD include lead, pesticides, and polychlorinated biphenyls (PCBs). Lead exposure in early childhood is associated with impaired executive functioning and inattention (Eubig, Aguiar, & Schantz, 2010; Nigg, 2008). Organophosphate pesticide exposure in utero and early childhood is associated with increased risk of ADHD (Eskanazi et al., 2007; Bouchard, Bellinger, Wright, et.al., 2010). Exposure to PCBs in infancy is associated with impaired working memory, response inhibition, and impaired cognitive flexibility (Eubig et al., 2010).

GENETIC SYNDROMES

Multiple genetic syndromes have been associated with an increased prevalence of ADHD, including neurofibromatosis type 1 (estimated prevalence 38%), 22q11 deletion syndromes, DiGeorge and velo-cardio-facial syndromes (estimated prevalence 40%), tuberous sclerosis (estimated prevalence 45%), Williams syndrome (estimated prevalence 65%), and sex chromosome syndromes, including fragile X (estimated prevalence 55%), XO (estimated prevalence 24%), and XXY (estimated prevalence 63%) (Lo-Castro, D'Agati, & Curatolo, 2011). The diagnosis of ADHD could be confused with cognitive impairment that is a part of some of these conditions; early recognition may be beneficial. Some of these syndromes (e.g., 22q11 deletion and Williams syndrome) are often recognized in infancy secondary to characteristic phenotypes including congenital cardiac disease; others may be recognized early because of family history (neurofibromatosis type 1) or prenatal findings (XO). However, sex chromosome disorders may not be recognized until puberty or later, so the clinician who finds ADHD in an otherwise normal preschooler may be in a position to make the diagnosis of the underlying syndrome using a variety of molecular genetic analysis tests.

Fragile X

Boys with fragile X frequently have behavior concerns consistent with autism, and many have behavioral characteristics of ADHD as well and have been shown to respond to stimulant medication for their ADHD symptoms (Roberts et al., 2011). In addition, premutation carriers of fragile X, with no significant difference in IQ from controls, have been shown to have an increased incidence of autism spectrum disorders (ASD) and ADHD (Farzin et al., 2006). Genetic analysis for fragile X is indicated when the phenotype is suspected on the basis of history (cognitive impairment, anxiety), examination (large ears, long face, soft skin, large testicles called "macroorchidism" in postpubertal males, ear infections, flat feet, high-arched palate, double-jointed fingers, and hyperflexible joints), and/or family history.

Klinefelter and XYY

Behavioral and cognitive profiles of Klinefelter syndrome (XXY) and XYY boys reveal an increased incidence of attentional problems and ADHD (Boada, Janusz, Hutaff-Lee, & Tartaglia, 2009; Ross et al., 2012). Most of these boys have IQs in the normal range, though the average is shifted toward the lower range, and autism may be more common as well, especially in the XYY population. Identification in the preschool child may be impossible without molecular genetic analysis since the phenotypic characteristics are not apparent until puberty, and may be missed even at puberty (Jones, 2006).

MUSCULAR DYSTROPHY

ADHD occurs commonly in boys who have Duchenne muscular dystrophy. Dystrophin mutations with isoforms that affect the brain are more likely to be associated with cognitive impairment and behavioral syndromes, including ADHD (Pane et al., 2012). The clinical diagnosis of Duchenne muscular dystrophy is confirmed with an elevated creatine kinase (CK) level found in presymptomatic and early symptomatic boys. Genetic studies for mutations of the dystrophin gene may be indicated.

SYDENHAM CHOREA, CANS, PANDAS

Sydenham chorea is a manifestation of rheumatic fever that may present weeks to months after streptococcal infection, and may present with behavioral manifestations including inattention and abnormal movements. It was the most common form of chorea at a referral center in Pittsburgh (Zomorrodi & Wald, 2006) and should be considered if the onset of difficulties appears abrupt.

Sydenham chorea may be the only major criterion of rheumatic fever in the child; evidence of streptococcal infection (antistreptococcal antibodies such as streptokinase and anti-DNAse B) must be sought. Because of the long interval between the infection and the onset of chorea, if other manifestations of rheumatic fever were not recognized by history, physical examination, or streptococcal testing, an echocardiogram should be obtained to look for carditis.

Singer, Gilbert, Wolf, Mink, and Kurlan (2012) propose the term "childhood acute neuropsychiatric symptoms" (CANS) to encompass both the pediatric autoimmune neuropsychiatric disorder associated with streptococcal infection (PANDAS) as well as other conditions such as Sydenham chorea, acute demyelinating encephalomyopathy (ADEM), the N-methyl-D-aspartate (NMDA) receptor antibody encephalitis, and Hashimoto's encephalitis. These conditions have an acute onset (which usually allows differentiation from Tourette syndrome) and early onset of obsessive compulsive disorder (OCD), and, in some cases, ADHD. In a study of 109 children (ages 4 to 17 years) with tics, OCD, or both (Murphy, Storch, Lewin, Edge, & Goodman, 2012), the average age of onset of disorder was 5.7 ± 2.5 years; the incidence of ADHD was not statistically significant between those with PANDAS and those without PANDAS (61% vs. 46%). Specific antibody studies may be done to confirm NMDA or Hashimoto's encephalitis.

THYROID DYSFUNCTION

Hyperthyroidism and hypothyroidism in preschool children may present with behavioral changes only, but more commonly the broader clinical picture includes both behavioral and developmental manifestations. In most developed countries, thyroid screening is done in neonates, so most cases of congenital hypothyroidism are detected and treated early. Preschoolers who are hypothyroid have poor growth and development as the primary signs; other physical signs and behavioral concerns include constipation, fatigue, and decreased activity. The hyperthyroid child may show a decreased attention span, emotional lability, and signs of nervousness and restlessness (which may be confused with being fidgety as in ADHD). Screening for thyroid-stimulating hormone (TSH) and T4 is indicated when these behavioral indicators occur in the setting of goiter, tachycardia, a familial pattern of inheritance of thyroid dysfunction (thyroid hormone resistance often includes ADHD symptoms), or other markers of possible hyperthyroidism. Even though routine thyroid testing is not recommended in ADHD, it should be obtained if thyroid dysfunction is suspected.

ADRENOLEUKODYSTROPHY

Concern for a neurodegenerative condition is heightened when there is a decline in function in a previously healthy child. X-linked adrenoleukodystrophy (X-ALD) is characterized by progressive cerebral white matter demyelination and affects boys. However, female carriers of the condition may have symptoms in adulthood. The childhood cerebral form is the most severe, with onset between ages 4 and 10. Boys with X-ALD may present with behavioral changes such as abnormal withdrawal or aggression, poor memory, poor school performance, and learning disabilities and are frequently diagnosed with ADHD. They have a progressive course with increasing inattention and behavior concerns as well as an abnormal neurologic examination that may include hearing impairment, vision impairment, hypertonia, ataxia, and seizures. It is important that the clinician be alert for changes in behavior, complete a thorough neurologic examination, and refer the child to a neurologist for definitive testing (Prasun & Misra, 2012).

SEIZURES

Absence seizures are brief staring episodes lasting usually a few seconds accompanied by behavioral arrest and may be commonly confused with inattentive symptoms and misdiagnosed as ADHD. The spells are often accompanied by eye blinking but are usually without other motor manifestations. An EEG should be done if history and/or observation reveals such episodes, and the tracing is usually diagnostic. Video EEG may be indicated if the described events are atypical or infrequent.

Children with seizures are at a higher risk for mental health and behavioral comorbidities, including ADHD (Davis, Katusic, Barbaresi, et.al., 2010; Dunn & Kronenberger, 2006). Children with epilepsy and intellectual disability are more likely to meet the diagnostic criteria for ADHD (Emerson & Hatton, 2007; Hastings et al., 2005).

CONGENITAL HEART DISEASE

Congenital heart disease is a risk factor for neurocognitive impairment due to the risk for hypoxic brain injury from a multitude of reasons, including the need for hospitalization and surgical intervention (Allen & Milstein, 2012). Often children with congenital heart disease have altered cerebral oxygen delivery in utero and after birth, experience hypoxic brain injury at a very sensitive period in their development, and are at a higher risk for poor neurodevelopmental outcome. Children with hypoplastic left heart syndrome, transposition of the great arteries, and tetralogy of Fallot are at the highest risk for cognitive impairment, including ADHD. In addition, cardiac bypass or deep hypothermic circulatory arrest used to support vital organs during surgery in children may cause cerebral emboli or a period of global cerebral hypoxic ischemia (Marino et al., 2012). Such serious congenital cardiac disorders will likely have already been recognized and treated surgically.

PSYCHIATRIC COMORBIDITY AND DIFFERENTIAL DIAGNOSIS

Comorbid psychiatric disorders are very common in preschool children with ADHD. In the Preschool ADHD Treatment Study sample, 72% of the preschoolers with ADHD had one or more comorbid disorders, approximately two fifths had one comorbid disorder, one fifth had two comorbid disorders, and one tenth had three or more comorbid disorders. The most common comorbid disorder, oppositional defiant disorder (ODD), was present in 54.5% of the participants, 20% had communication disorders, 17% had anxiety disorders, 8% had elimination disorders, and 4% had developmental coordination disorder (DCD; Ghuman et al., 2007). Preschoolers with ADHD and comorbid psychiatric disorders have a poorer long-term prognosis compared to ADHD preschoolers without psychiatric comorbidity.

At the initial evaluation for ADHD, it is important to determine not only if the preschooler has a comorbid psychiatric disorder in addition to ADHD, but also whether symptoms from the comorbid disorder might be the underlying cause of the preschooler's "seeming hyperactivity and inattentive" symptoms. For example, restlessness in an anxious child may be confused with hyperactivity. A preschooler with learning difficulties may appear inattentive. For a comorbid disorder to be diagnosed, the preschooler needs to meet the full DSM criteria for both ADHD and the comorbid disorder.

Oppositional Defiant Disorder
ADHD and ODD are frequently comorbid conditions, with symptoms of both disorders frequently seen early in childhood. Both conditions may present with increased physical activity levels, risk-taking, and inattention to caregiver directions. Preschoolers with ODD present with frequent defiant behaviors that can be mistaken as inattention. These children have frequent temper tantrums and are argumentative, angry, and resentful. They blame others for their mistakes. They annoy others, get easily annoyed themselves, and can appear impulsive. Children may meet the criteria for both diagnoses, and interventions should be designed for each condition.

Anxiety Disorders

School-aged children who have ADHD are at a much higher risk of having anxiety disorders (Jarrett et al., 2012). Separation anxiety disorder is the most common anxiety disorder in preschoolers. Preschoolers with separation anxiety disorder are clingy, shadowing the parents, and have excessive anxiety regarding separation from attachment figures, with unrealistic and persistent worries, somatic complaints, difficulty sleeping alone, and nightmares with themes of separation. Anxious children may appear restless and inattentive, but their anxiety is usually more pervasive. Evidence suggests that preschool psychiatric disorders, such as anxiety, are stable as children move into the school-age population, and therefore both conditions will need to be addressed when they are identified in the preschool child (Bufferd, Dougherty, Carlson, & Rose, 2012). Managing a comorbid diagnosis of anxiety with ADHD can be challenging for both the family and the medical care provider as they try to discern which of the diagnoses is affecting the child's behavior more at a certain time.

Mood Disorders

Children who have mood disorders can present with symptoms that overlap with the symptoms of ADHD—for example, problems with attention and concentration. Angry and agitated behavior in children with mood disorders can be misinterpreted as hyperactivity due to ADHD. Additionally, preschoolers with mood disorders present with sad and irritable mood, low self-esteem, and sleep and appetite disturbances. Preschool children may meet the diagnostic criteria for both conditions. Familiarity with the criteria for mood disorders will help the primary care provider recognize these symptoms and help with the transition to appropriate psychiatric care (Arnold, 2011; Chilakamarri, Fiilkowski, & Ghaemi, 2011).

Communication Disorders

Communication disorders are very common in preschool children with ADHD. Preschoolers with communication disorders are easily frustrated and have tantrums frequently because they are unable to express themselves. Preschoolers with receptive language deficits may appear inattentive as they may not understand verbal instructions or verbal interchanges. Often improvement in a child's speech and communicative abilities with appropriate intervention results in a dramatic improvement in the child's behavior.

Specific Learning Disability

Children will be inattentive if they do not understand the task instructions presented. For example, children who will later be diagnosed with reading learning disability may be easily distracted from learning to identify sight words and/or learning the alphabet because it is difficult for them. They may act out in classroom-like settings since they may not engage in the activity because they do not understand it. On the other hand, children with learning disabilities may also have comorbid ADHD with inattention, impulsivity, and hyperactivity noted consistently in varied settings, not only in specific situations that require them to use skills that are impaired because of their learning disability.

Developmental Coordination Disorder

Approximately one third of children with ADHD also have DCD; the motor impairment can exacerbate symptoms of ADHD, especially in the classroom, where writing and sitting up are required at the same time as attention to discussion (Fliers et al., 2008). Children with DCD have motor incoordination and mild hypotonia that affects their daily functioning but otherwise have a normal physical examination and neuroimaging studies. Children with DCD have poor execution of motor tasks and difficulty with proprioception, sensory integration, and visual processing. The motor delays are usually recognized early and parents complain about their child's clumsiness and motor delays compared to their peers.

Intellectual Disability

Children who have intellectual disability frequently have associated behavior issues. One of the challenges in caring for children with intellectual disability is that behavioral expectations in some settings are consistent with a child's chronological age rather than the child's cognitive skills. However, some children who have intellectual disability have symptoms consistent with ADHD in addition to their cognitive disability, and management of their ADHD symptoms improves their functional and academic outcomes (Bigam, Hastings, Beck, Daley, & Hill, 2013). Children and toddlers who have cognitive impairment are generally diagnosed with developmental delay rather than a specific cognitive disability. Since cognitive testing results are also less reliable and stable in this age group, children may be diagnosed with ADHD instead of a cognitive disability, making it important that these diagnoses be reevaluated throughout the preschool years (Simonoff et al., 2007).

Autism Spectrum Disorders

Children with ASD have overlapping signs and symptoms with ADHD and may be initially diagnosed as having ADHD rather than an ASD. Children with both ASD and ADHD exhibit attention deficit, overactivity, behavior problems, and social skills impairment. Children with ASD show impaired reciprocal social interaction, deviant communication, repetitive behaviors, and restricted interests. If a child is suspected to have ASD, expert evaluation using a thorough history, physical examination, play-interactive observation (such as through Autism Diagnostic Observation Schedule administration), observations from teachers and caretakers, and a variety of standardized rating scales should be obtained.

Tourette Syndrome

ADHD is a frequent comorbid condition with Tourette syndrome. Tourette syndrome is a tic disorder in which tics occur many times a day nearly every day or intermittently over a period of more than 1 year and with a tic-free period of no more than 3 consecutive months during that time. Both multiple motor tics and one or more vocal tics must have been present at some time over the course of the illness but do not necessarily occur concurrently. The disorder onset is younger than 18 years, and it must not be directly caused by a medical condition or the effect of a medication (American Psychiatric Association, 2000). Tics usually develop between age 5 and 7 years but have been identified in preschool children.

Adjustment Disorders

Stressful life situations and sudden changes in life circumstances can result in transient ADHD-like symptoms (Anthony, 1998) but can be distinguished by the onset of ADHD symptoms after the stressful situation.

Sleep Disorders
Sleep disorders may mimic or exacerbate symptoms of ADHD. See Chapter 9 for more information.

Treatment Implications

Diagnosis and treatment of ADHD at earlier ages can result in positive behavioral changes, increased capacity for learning and a subsequent better start to school, and improved family dynamics. Maladaptive parental reactions to the hyperactive preschooler can be remediated or avoided with early initiation of treatment.

The initial approach to treatment must be guided by a shared understanding of diagnosis and goals so that parents, other caretakers, and the professional team are knowledgeable participants in efforts to help the child. Knowledge and trust may be attained through interviews and visits with the family and might be aided through use of a standardized instrument for parental preference and goals for ADHD treatment (Fiks et al., 2011). A behavioral and parent training approach is an effective first-line therapy in preschool ADHD (Davis & Williams, 2011). A home-based program may include games that include the need for inhibitory control (e.g., "Simon Says"), working memory (e.g., remembering a list), motor control (e.g., jumping rope), and visuospatial skills (e.g., puzzles) (Halperin et al., 2012).

Preschool children with ADHD may receive a variety of services in treatment (physical therapy, speech and language therapy, occupational therapy) at a substantial cost (Marks et al., 2009). For example, preschool children with ADHD may require increased staffing in the classroom to maintain their safety and the safety of their peers. Preschool therapy services to improve focus while sitting, such as use of a therapy (stability) ball (Fedewa & Erwin, 2011), requires the intervention of an occupational therapist in the school setting. Children with ADHD and comorbid DCD may receive physical therapy to remediate their motor delays. Speech and language therapy may need to focus on pragmatic language skills that are frequently difficult for the very active and inattentive child.

If the preschooler still has impairing ADHD symptoms despite behavior therapy and other therapy and remedial services, pharmacologic treatment may be considered (as described in detail in Chapters 7 and 8). When pharmacologic success occurs, the results can be dramatic in transforming the life of the family and child; if little or no positive change occurs, a number of possibilities must be considered. One, the medication may not have been given; some caretakers are reluctant to challenge a doctor's prescription but do not feel that medication is the answer. In this case, a calm, nonjudgmental approach will often uncover the parental fears and lead to reformulation of the plan, sometimes including medication. The possibility that the child is not swallowing the medication must also be explored. Incorrect time of administration (i.e., at bedtime) may be another problem that a treatment plan review will uncover, resulting in appropriate recommendations and education. Refer to Chapters 7 and 8 for further details regarding pharmacologic intervention practice.

Two, the diagnosis may be wrong and more history and a repeat examination for further diagnostic clarification must be done. A young child's stress in the setting of domestic violence or alcoholism, for example, may lead to consideration of attentional problems.

Methylphenidate may have an initial placebo effect, but improvement will be limited. Unfortunately, many caretakers may still hesitate to reveal these family stressors and many visits may be required to obtain the trust necessary for the disclosure. Other times the history and behavioral reporting forms are colored by the assumption that the child has ADHD. Families with a number of children being treated for ADHD may indeed be examples of a hereditary effect, but some may instead be fitting the child into a diagnosis that is desired by the caretaker. Foster families with multiple biologically unrelated children being treated for ADHD may attribute the preschooler's initial disruptive behavior (when the preschooler is first placed in the foster home) to ADHD. Hence, each child's psychosocial stresses and changes in living situation must be judiciously and carefully evaluated.

Three, comorbid conditions may be obscuring the success of the psychostimulant medication in improving attention and controlling hyperactivity. Here again, a careful review of the child's behavior pattern with family and caretakers and reevaluation of the treatment plan to include treatment of comorbid disorders is essential.

Four, the diagnosis may be correct but the psychostimulant dose isn't effective. A change in psychostimulant dosage or a change in medication, first to another psychostimulant prior to switching to a non-stimulant medication, is indicated.

Appreciation of the benefits of earlier diagnosis and treatment of ADHD must be balanced with recognition of the risks involved. The risks of medication side effects are probably similar to those seen in older children, but extensive experience is lacking. Because treatment of preschoolers with psychostimulants does not have a long history, long-term benefits, if any, are not known. The developing brain is a moving target and untoward effects on development are possible (Davis & Williams, 2011). The MTA study of 7- to 10-year-old children with ADHD who received medication, behavior therapy, combination therapy, or community care during the 14-month study period has been reviewed for longer-term outcomes (Molina et al., 2009). Molina and colleagues found that, 6 to 8 years later, only 32.5% of the subjects had received medication treatment for 50% or more days during the past year. Long-term outcomes were predicted by early symptom trajectory and did not differ by treatment group.

Although changes in parent–child interactions would seem to be positive if medication is successful, these changes, especially if pretreatment family dynamics were relatively benign, have not been assessed for long-term implications. Earlier diagnosis also categorizes the child during what may be a transient developmental interval; once the diagnosis is made, parents, clinicians, and school personnel will tend to continue the diagnosis even if it is no longer warranted. Diagnostic precision and routine reevaluation can lessen these potential risks.

Some parents and families elect an integrative approach that includes dietary changes, herbal remedies, and other alternative modalities. These interventions are discussed in more depth in recent reviews (Chan, 2008; Newmark, 2010; Weber et al., 2008) and in Chapter 9.

Summary

Earlier recognition of children with ADHD allows early intervention to prevent the consequences of educational failure and development of an untoward behavioral repertoire and family dysfunction. Preschool children are challenging to diagnose, however, and a broad differential diagnosis is essential. Since precise diagnosis is not yet possible and long-term outcomes of therapy are not certain, caution is indicated. A systematic, comprehensive, and unhurried approach will best clarify the nature of the preschooler's difficulties.

In the future, research can further clarify the genetic and environmental antecedents of ADHD; development of clinically useful structured interviews, computer-based screening questionnaires, and advanced biometric techniques may add to our diagnostic capabilities. Advances in cognitive-behavioral therapies and pharmacologic interventions will continue, ideally with greatly enhanced long-term outcome studies to guide clinical judgment.

Disclosures

Sydney A. Rice, M.D., has no conflicts to disclose and is funded by CDC (1U01DD000691-01) and HRSA (T73MC20662-03-00).

William N. Marshall, Jr., M.D., has no conflicts to disclose.

References

Allen, H. D., & Milstein, J. A. (2012). IQ may be normal, but are there future neurocognitive implications for infants with d-TGA? *Journal of Pediatrics, 161*(1), 7–9.

American Academy of Pediatrics Committee on Practice and Ambulatory Medicine and Bright Futures Steering Committee. (2007). Recommendations for preventive pediatric health care. *Pediatrics, 120*, 1376.

American Academy of Pediatrics Committee on Quality Improvement and the Subcommittee on Attention-Deficit/Hyperactivity Disorder, & Steering Committee on Quality Improvement and Management. (2011). ADHD: Clinical practice guideline for the diagnosis, evaluation, and treatment of attention-deficit/hyperactivity disorder in children and adolescents. *Pediatrics, 128*, 1007–1022.

American Psychiatric Association. (2000). *Diagnostic and statistical manual of mental disorders* (4th ed., text rev.). Washington, DC: Author.

Anand, V., Carroll, A. E., & Downs, S. M. (2012). Automated primary care screening in pediatric waiting rooms. *Pediatrics, 129*(5), e1275–e1281. Advance online publication April 16, 2012. doi:10.1542/peds.2011-2875.

Anthony, B. J. (1998). Attention deficit/hyperactivity disorder. In H. S. Ghuman & R. M. Sarles (Eds.), *Handbook of child and adolescent outpatient, day treatment and community psychiatry* (pp. 159–174). Philadelphia, PA: Brunner/Mazel

Arnold, L. E. (2011). Pediatric bipolar spectrum disorder and ADHD: comparison and comorbidity in the LAMS clinical sample. *Bipolar Disorders, 13*(5–6), 509–521.

Bigam, K., Daley, D. M., Hastings, R. P., & Jones, R. S. P. (2013). Association between parent reports of attention deficit hyperactivity disorder behaviours and child impulsivity in children with severe intellectual disability. *Journal of Intellectual Disability Research, 57*(2), 191–197.

Boada, R., Janusz, J., Hutaff-Lee, C., & Tartaglia, N. (2009). The cognitive phenotype in Klinefelter syndrome: A review of the literature including genetic and hormonal factors. *Developmental Disabilities Research Review, 15*(4), 284–294.

Bouchard, M. F., Bellinger, D. C., Wright, R. O., & Weisskopf, M. G. (2010). Attention-deficit/hyperactivity disorder and urinary metabolites of organophosphate pesticides. *Pediatrics, 125*(6), e1270–e1277.

Brown, E. D., Ackerman, B. P., & Moore, C. A. (2012). Family adversity and inhibitory control for economically disadvantaged children: Preschool relations and associations with school readiness. *Journal of Family Psychology, 27*(3), 443–452.

Bufferd, S. J., Dougherty, L. R., Carlson, G. A., & Rose, S. (2012). Psychiatric disorders in preschoolers: continuity from ages 3 to 6. *American Journal of Psychiatry, 169*(11), 1157–1164.

Chan, E. (2008). St. John's wort does not show benefit for ADHD in short trial. *Journal of Pediatrics, 153*(5), 724. doi:10.1016/j.jpeds.2008.09.002.

Chilakamarri, J. K., Fiilkowski, M., & Ghaemi, S.N. (2011). Misdiagnosis of bipolar disorder in children and adolescents: A comparison with ADHD and major depressive disorder. *Annals of Clinical Psychiatry, 23*(1), 25–29.

Davis, S. M., Katusic, S. K., Barbaresi, W. J., Killian, J., Weaver, A. L., Ottman, R., Wirrel, E. C. (2010). Epilepsy in children with attention deficit hyperactivity disorder. Pediatr Neurol, 42, 325-330.

Davis, D. W., & Williams, P. G. (2011). Attention deficit/hyperactivity disorder in preschool-age children: Issues and concerns. *Clinical Pediatrics, 50*, 144–152.

de Kieviet, J. F., van Elburg, R. M., Lafeber, H. N., & Oosterlaan, J. (2012). Attention problems of very preterm children compared with age-matched term controls at school-age. *Journal of Pediatrics*, Advance online publication June 14, 2012. doi:10.1016/j.jpeds.2012.05.010.

Dunn, D. W. & Kronenberger, W. G. (2006). Childhood epilepsy, attention problems, and ADHD: Review and practical considerations. *Seminars in Pediatric Neurology, 12*, 222–228.

Eskenazi, B., Marks, A. R., Bradman, A., Harley, K., Barr, D. B., Johnson, C., Morga, N., Jewll, N. P. (2007). Organophosphate Pesticide Exposure and Neurodevelopment in Young Mexican-American Children. *Environ Health Perspect* 115(5), 792–798. doi:10.1289/ehp.9828

Eubig, P. A., Aguiar, A., Schantz, S. L. (2010). Lead and PCBs as risk factors for attention deficit/ hyperactivity disorder. *Environ Health Perspect, 118*, 1654–1667.

Farzin, F., Perry, H., Hessl, D., Loesch, D., Cohen, J., Bacalman, S., . . . Hagerman, R. (2006). Autism spectrum disorders and attention-deficit/hyperactivity disorder in boys with the fragile X premutation. *Developmental Behavioral Pediatrics* (2 Suppl), S137–S144.

Fedewa, A. L., & Erwin, H. E. (2011). Stability balls and students with attention and hyperactivity concerns: implications for on-task and in-seat behavior. *American Journal of Occupational Therapy, 65*(4), 393–399.

Fiks, A. G., Hughes, C. C., Gafen, A., Guevara, J. P., & Barg, F. K. (2011). Contrasting parents' and pediatricians' perspectives on shared decision-making in ADHD. *Pediatrics, 127*, e188–e196.

Fliers, E., Rommelse, N., Vermeulen, S. H., et al. (2008). Motor coordination problems in children and adolescents with ADHD rated by parents and teachers: effects of age and gender. *Journal of Neural Transmission, 115*, 211.

Fryer, S. L., McGee, C. L., Matt, G. E., Riley, E. P., & Mattson, S. N. (2007). Evaluation of psychopathological conditions in children with heavy prenatal alcohol exposure. *Pediatrics, 119*, e733–734.

Garbutt, J. M., Leege, E., Sterkel, R., Gentry, S., & Strunk, R. C. (2012). Providing depression care in the medical home: what can we learn from attention-deficit/ hyperactivity disorder? *Archives Pediatrics Adolescent Med, 166*(7), 672–673.

Ghuman, J. K., & Ghuman, H. S. (2012). Pharmacologic intervention for attention-deficit hyperactivity disorder in preschoolers: is it justified? *Paediatric Drugs, 15*(1), 1–8.

Ghuman, J. K., Riddle, M. A., Vitiello, B., Greenhill, L. L., Chuang, S. Z., Wigal, S. B., . . . Skrobala, A. M. (2007). Comorbidity moderates response to methylphenidate in the Preschoolers with Attention Deficit/Hyperactivity Disorder Treatment Study (PATS). *Journal of Child and Adolescent Psychopharmacology, 17*, 563–580.

Halperin, J. M., Marks, D. J., Bedard, A-C. V., Chacko, A., Curchack, J. T., Yoon C. A., & Healey, D. M. (2012). Training executive, attention, and motor skills: A proof-of-concept study in preschool children with ADHD. *Journal of Attention Disorders*.doi:10.1177/1087054711435681.

Heerman, W. J., Karpinos, A. R., & Rothman, R. L. (2012). Mastering the language: Communicating with parents who have low health literacy. *Contemporary Pediatrics*, April, 32–37.

Jarrett, M. A., Wolff, J. C., Davis, T. E., Cowart, M. J., & Ollendick, T. H. (2012), Characteristics of children with ADHD and comorbid anxiety. *Journal of Attention Disorders, 20*(10), 1–9.

Jones, K. L. (2006). *Recognizable patterns of human malformation* (6th ed.). Philadelphia, PA: Elsevier.

Lakes, K. D., Swanson, J. M., & Riggs, M. (2011). The reliability and validity of the English and Spanish strengths and weaknesses of ADHD and normal behavior rating scales in a preschool sample: Continuum measures of hyperactivity and inattention. *Journal of Attention Disorders.* doi:10.1177/1087054711413550.

Li, J., Olsen, J., Vestergaard, M., & Obel, C. (2011). Low Apgar scores and risk of childhood attention deficit hyperactivity disorder. *Journal of Pediatrics, 158*(5), 775–779. doi:10.1016/j.jpeds.2010.10.041.

Lo-Castro, A., D'Agati, E., & Curatolo, P. (2011). ADHD and genetic syndromes. *Brain Development, 33*(6), 456–461.

Marino, B. S., Lipkin, P. H. Newburger, J. W., Peacokc, G., Gerdes, Gaynor, J. W.,…Mahle, W. T. (2012). Neurodevelopmental outcomes in children with congenital heart disease: Evaluation and management. A Scientific Statement from the American Heart Association. *Circulation.* Advance online publication July 30, 2012. doi: 10.1161/CIR.0b013e318265ee8a. Retrieved from http://circ.ahajournals.org/content/early/2012/07/30/CIR.0b013e318265ee8a.full.pdf+html

Marks, D. J., Mlodnicka, A., Bernstein, M, Chacko, A., Rose, S., & Halperin, J. M. (2009). Profiles of service utilization and the resultant economic impact in preschoolers with attention deficit/hyperactivity disorder. *Journal of Pediatric Psychology, 34,* 681–689.

Mayes, R., Bagwell, C., & Erkulwater, J. (2009). In *Medicating children: ADHD and pediatric mental health.* Cambridge, MA: Harvard University Press.

McGoey, K., DuPaul, G., Haley, E., & Shelton, T. (2007). Parent and teacher ratings of attention-deficit/hyperactivity disorder in preschool: The ADHD Rating Scale-IV Preschool Version. *Journal of Psychopathology and Behavioral Assessment, 29*(4), 269–276. doi:10.1007/s10862-007-9048-y.

Minkovitz, C. S., Strobino, D., Scharfstein, D., Hou, W., Miller, T., & Mistry, K. B. (2005). Maternal depressive symptoms and children's receipt of health care in the first 3 years of life. *Pediatrics, 115,* 306–314.

Molina, B. S. G, Hinshaw, S. F., Swanson, J. M., Arnold, I. E., Vitiello, B., Jensen, P. S.,…Houck, P. R. & the MTA Cooperative Group (2009). The MTA at 8 years: Prospective follow-up of children treated for combined–type ADHD in a multisite study. *Journal of the American Academy of Child & Adolescent Psychiatry, 48,* 484–500.

Morrow, R. M., Garland, J., Wright, J. M., Maclure, M. Taylor, S, & Dormuth, C. R. (2012). Influence of relative age on diagnosis and treatment of attention-deficit/hyperactivity disorder in children. *Canadian Medical Association Journal.* doi:10.1503/cmaj.111619.

Murphy, T. A., Storch, E. A., Lewin, A. B., Edge, P. J., & Goodman, W. K. (2012). Clinical factors associated with pediatric autoimmune neuropsychiatric disorders associated with streptococcal infections. *Journal of Pediatrics, 160*(2), 314–319. doi:10.1016/j.jpeds.2011.07.012.

National Center on Birth Defects and Developmental Disabilities, Centers for Disease Control and Prevention, Department of Health and Human Services. (2004). *Fetal alcohol syndrome: guidelines for referral and diagnosis.* www.cdc.gov/ncbddd/fasd/documents/fas_guidelines_accessible.pdf

Newmark, S. C. (2010). *ADHD without drugs: a guide to the natural care of children with ADHD.* Tucson, AZ: Nurtured Heart Publications.

Nigg, J. T., Knottnerus, G. M., Martel, M. M., Nikolas, M., Cavanagh, K., Karmaus, W., Rappley, M. D. (2008). Low blood levels associated with clinically diagnosed attention deficit /hyperactivity disorder and mediated by weak cognitive control. *Biol Psychiatry 63,* 325–331.

Nomura, Y., Marks, D. J., Grossman, B., Yoon, M., Loudon, H., Stone, J., & Halperin, J. M. (2012). Exposure to gestational diabetes mellitus and low socioeconomic status: Effects on neurocognitive development and risk of attention-deficit/hyperactivity disorder in offspring. *Archives of Pediatric Adolescent Medicine, 166*(4), 337–343.

Ouyang, L., Fang, X., Mercy, J., Perou, R., & Grosse S. D. (2008). Attention-deficit/hyperactivity disorder symptoms and child maltreatment: A population-based study. *Journal of Pediatrics, 153*(6), 851–856.

Pane, M., Lombardo, M. E., Alfieri, P., D'Amico, A., Bianco, F., Vasco, G.,...Mercuri, E. (2012). Attention deficit hyperactivity disorder and cognitive function in Duchenne muscular dystrophy: Phenotype-genotype correlation. *Journal of Pediatrics, 161*(4), 705–709e1. Advance online publication October 2012.

Perrin, J. M., Friedman, R. A., & Knilans, T. K. (2008). Cardiovascular monitoring and stimulant drugs for attention-deficit/hyperactivity disorder. *Pediatrics, 122*(2), 451–453.

Prasun, P., & Misra, V. K. (2012). Declining school performance as a harbinger of a treatable neurodegenerative condition. *Journal of Pediatrics, 160*(6), 1062–1062. e1. doi:10.1016/j.jpeds.2011.12.040.

Prugh D. (1983). *The psychosocial aspects of pediatrics.* Philadelphia, PA: Lea and Febiger.

Re, A. M., & Cornoldi, C. (2009). Two new rating scales for assessment of ADHD symptoms in Italian preschool children: A comparison between parent and teacher ratings. *Journal of Attention Disorders, 12*, 532–539.

Roberts, J. E., Miranda, M., Boccia, M., Janes, H., Tonnsen, B. L., & Hatton, D. D. (2011). Treatment effects of stimulant medication in young boys with fragile X syndrome, *Journal of Neurodevelopmental Disorders, 3*(3), 175–184.

Ross, J. L., Roeltgen, D. P., Kushner, H., Zinn, A. R., Zegar Bardsley, M., McCauley, E., & Tartaglia, N. (2012). Behavioral and social phenotypes in boys with 47,XYY syndrome or 47,XXY Klinefelter syndrome. *Pediatrics, 129*(4), 769–778.

Simonoff, E., Pickles, A., Wood, N., Gringras, P., & Chadwick, O. (2007). ADHD symptoms in children with mild intellectual disability. *Journal of the American Academy of Child and Adolescent Psychiatry, 48*(5), 591–600.

Smith, P. J., Humiston, S. G., Parnell, T., Vannice, K. S., & Salmon, D. (2010). The association between intentional delay ov vaccine administration and timely childhood vaccination coverage. *Public Health Reports, 125*(4), 534–541.

Stein, D. S., Blum, N. J., & Barbaresi, W. J. (2011). Developmental and behavioral disorders through the life span. *Pediatrics, 128*(2), 364–373.

Thomas, L. B., Shapiro, E. S., DuPaul, G. J., Lutz, J. G., & Kern, L. (2011). Predictors of social skills for preschool children at risk for ADHD: The relationship between direct and indirect measurements. *Journal of Psychoeducational Assessment, 29*, 114–124.

U.S. Department of Education, National Center for Education Statistics. (2012). *Digest of Education Statistics, 2011* (NCES 2012-001), Chapter 2.

Vetter, V., Elia, J., Erickson, C., Berger, S., Blum, N., Uzark, K., et al. (2008). Cardiovascular monitoring of children and adolescents with heart disease receiving medications for attention deficit/hyperactivity disorder [corrected]: a scientific statement from the American Heart Association Council on Cardiovascular Disease in the Young Congenital Cardiac Defects Committee and the Council on Cardiovascular Nursing. *Circulation, 117*(8), 2407–2423.

Walsh, S. T. (2004). The clinician's perspective on electronic health records and how they can affect patient care. *British Medical Journal, 328*(7449), 1184–1187. Doi:10.1136/bmj.328.7449.1184.

Weber, W., Vander Stoep, A., McCarty, R. L., Weiss, N. S., Biederman, J., & McClellan J. (2008). *Hypericum perforatum* (St. John's Wort) for attention-deficit/hyperactivity disorder in children and adolescents: A randomized controlled trial. *Journal of the American Medical Association, 299*(22), 2633–2641. doi:10.1001/jama.299.22.2633

Zomorrodi, A., & Wald, E. R. (2006). Sydenham chorea in Western Pennsylvania. *Pediatrics, 117*(4), e675–e679.

Zuvekas, S. H., & Vitiello, B. (2012). Stimulant medication use in children: a 12-year perspective. *American Journal of Psychiatry, 169*(2), 160–166.

Section 2

TREATMENT INTERVENTIONS

5

Psychosocial and Behavioral Interventions with a Focus on Parent–Child Interaction Therapy

Theory and Clinical Practice

REGINA BUSSING AND DESIREE W. MURRAY

Overview of Psychosocial and Behavioral Interventions

This chapter provides an overview of psychosocial and behavioral interventions for preschoolers with attention-deficit/hyperactivity disorder (ADHD) based upon recent evidence reviews (Charach et al., 2011; Eyberg, Nelson, & Boggs, 2008; Pearl, 2009), emphasizing information that will be most useful for practitioners. We include non-ADHD-specific interventions addressing disruptive behavior in young children in order to provide a broad yet relevant perspective. We also briefly address combination treatments of parent and classroom interventions and behavioral interventions directly targeting young children with disruptive behaviors. As most treatment research in this area has focused on parent management training (PMT), we review the background, theory, and common elements of parent training approaches and then briefly describe several specific PMT programs. Detailed information will be provided for the two empirically supported parenting programs most accessible to U.S. clinicians, namely Parent–Child Interaction Therapy (PCIT) and the Incredible Years (IY) program (covered in the next chapter).

BACKGROUND AND RATIONALE FOR PSYCHOSOCIAL AND BEHAVIORAL INTERVENTIONS

Parent training and other behavioral therapies are endorsed as the first-line intervention for preschoolers with ADHD by several independent entities. The American Academy of Child and Adolescent Psychiatry (AACAP) Preschool Psychopharmacology

Working Group (Gleason et al., 2007) and the American Academy of Pediatrics (AAP, 2011) recommend parent training with the highest level of evidence based upon algorithms that considered the quality of research and balance of benefit versus harm. The Agency for Healthcare Research and Quality (AHRQ) reached similar conclusions based on a comprehensive comparative effectiveness review (Charach et al., 2011), as did the National Institute for Health and Clinical Excellence in the United Kingdom (Kendall, Taylor, Perez, & Taylor, 2009) based on a review process that also emphasized expert consensus.

There is clear clinical consensus that psychosocial interventions should be initiated before considering ADHD medications in younger children, because although medications can be effective (see Chapter 7), the evidence base is smaller than for behavioral interventions and the current strength of evidence for medication is considered low (Charach et al., 2011). In addition, the side-effect profile of medication treatment is more adverse than for behavioral interventions and the long-term neurodevelopmental effects are largely unknown (AAP, 2011; Gleason et al., 2007). Moreover, it is unlikely that medication alone can address the multiple and pervasive impairments of ADHD in preschoolers. However, some clinicians may consider medication as an adjunctive treatment when behavioral interventions alone are not adequate or where evidence-based psychosocial treatments are not available (AAP, 2011).

There are several reasons to think that the preschool years are an optimal time to initiate psychosocial interventions for ADHD. Although preschoolers with ADHD symptoms demonstrate delays in response inhibition and delay aversion that can interfere with emotion regulation and impulse control (Pauli-Pott & Becker, 2011), they also experience rapid brain growth, suggesting a neurodevelopmental elasticity and potential receptivity to intervention (Shonkoff & Phillips, 2000). Theoretically, interventions may also be more effective when implemented before negative behavior patterns become ingrained in parent–child interactions and before children have repeated experiences of school failure and peer conflict. Such early intervention may interrupt the negative developmental trajectory seen in youngsters with ADHD, including the development of comorbid difficulties and impairments in additional domains (Connor et al., 2003; Lahey et al., 2004).

The rationale for parenting interventions is derived from research demonstrating that parents of preschoolers with ADHD exhibit ineffective parenting strategies such as inconsistent and controlling management strategies, poor maternal coping, and decreased encouragement (Cunningham & Boyle, 2002; Keown & Woodward, 2002). These findings are generally consistent with patterns of parenting and parent–child interactions for young children with disruptive behavior (Campbell, Shaw, & Gilliom, 2000; DuPaul et al., 2001) and may not be unique to ADHD. However, these findings suggest that a coercive interaction pattern (Patterson, 1982) begins at an early age in this population and that specific parenting interventions are indicated.

THEORETICAL GROUNDING OF PMT

PMT is well grounded theoretically and empirically in literature that links positive child outcomes to firm discipline in the context of a secure relationship. The theoretical model underlying PMT draws from social learning, social interaction, and behavioral perspectives and has been referred to as social interaction learning (Patterson, Forgatch, & DeGarmo, 2010). Most PMT programs seek to teach "authoritative parenting," characterized by a combination of nurturance, good communication, and firm control, in accordance with Baumrind's developmental theory of parenting (Baumrind, 1968, 1991). Baumrind's research has demonstrated that parents who provide both nurturance and limit-setting are more likely to raise healthy adolescents (Baumrind, Larzelere, & Owens, 2010). Most PMT programs are also informed by attachment theory and social learning theory as well as Patterson's coercion hypothesis. Attachment theory purports that parental warmth and responsiveness to the emotional needs of young children contribute to the development of a secure parent–child relationship, which in turn leads to greater emotional regulation and enhances the child's desire to please and willingness to comply (Bowlby, 1979). Social learning theory (Bandura, 1977) posits that people learn in a social context through observation and modeling, which are important teaching strategies seen in many PMT programs. Finally, PMT is informed by Patterson's (1982) coercion hypothesis in which maladaptive parent–child interactions are believed to shape and maintain child noncompliance and aggression (Dishion, Patterson, & Kavanagh, 1992). PMT seeks to interrupt the coercive cycle by helping parents incorporate clear limit-setting in the context of a nurturing relationship (Patterson, 1982). Successful PMT interventions produce significant reductions in coercive parenting and significant increases in positive parenting, with emerging evidence that these improvements not only persist but can increase in magnitude over time amidst a "cascade" of collateral other changes that were not necessarily targeted as initial outcomes, such as effects on maternal and sibling mental health (Patterson, Forgatch, & DeGarmo, 2010).

COMMON ELEMENTS OF PMT

Although originally developed in the 1960s for children with oppositional behavior, since the early 1980s PMT has been recommended for children with ADHD since they also have difficulty following directions and rules (Barkley, 1981). Many PMT programs have roots in Constance Hanf's two-stage model of parent training (Hanf, 1969; Reitman & McMahon, 2012), in which parents first learn to give positive attention to desirable behaviors ("Child's Game") through "attending" (i.e., targeted positive attention) and praise, and then to decrease inappropriate behaviors ("Mother's Game") using strategies such as planned ignoring, providing clear instructions, and time-out from positive reinforcement. A recent meta-analysis of PMT components validated the effectiveness of several specific strategies consistent with the Hanf model, including positive parent–child interactions, responding sensitively to the child's emotional needs, responding consistently to child behavior, and time-out (Kaminski, Valle, Filene, & Boyle, 2008).

Although PMT content is similar across many programs (which achieve comparable results), there is considerable variability in their format, delivery, and teaching methods. Programs may be delivered individually by a therapist or using self-directed materials, they may be delivered in groups, or variations in or combinations of these formats may be used for different levels of intervention. Additional program variations include the extent to which instruction is provided in a didactic versus a more collaborative manner, the location of the training (e.g., community, clinic, or home), and the level of intervention (universal, targeted or preventive, and indicated or treatment). To date, there is little evidence of differential efficacy of these different formats. Specific methods that are associated with statistically better outcomes are modeling through live or video-recorded demonstrations of parenting behaviors and practicing with the child in session (Kaminski et al., 2008).

EFFICACY OF PMT

For preschoolers with ADHD symptoms or disruptive behavior (considered to be at risk for ADHD), a recent systematic literature review shows 28 high-quality randomized controlled trials (RCTs) of behavioral parent training with positive effects in reducing the number and intensity of problem behaviors (Charach et al., 2011). Several studies identified improvement in ADHD symptoms, with five of six studies specifically targeting ADHD symptoms finding significant effects. Overall, the average effect size for intervention completers was .68 (considered moderate to large), with a high degree of consistency across studies with varying intervention and outcome measures. Although methodologically rigorous follow-up studies are limited, particularly by lack of a control group, some evidence supports maintenance of effects up to 6 years (Drugli, Larsson, Fossom, & Morch, 2009; Hood & Eyberg, 2003). Importantly, parent training appears to be equally efficacious for young children with conduct problems both with and without attention difficulties (Hartman, Stage, & Webster-Stratton, 2003).

Despite the benefits of PMT, there are some limitations to its effectiveness, including lower attendance rates and decreased efficacy for higher-risk families (i.e., those with socioeconomic disadvantage, single-parent family status, younger maternal age, and higher parental stress; Werba, Eyberg, Boggs, & Algina, 2006). Parental ADHD may also have a negative impact on parent training outcomes (Sonuga-Barke, Daley, & Thompson, 2002). Some programs seek to increase access to and engagement in PMT by providing treatment in community settings (Cunningham, Bremner, & Boyle, 1995) and use of more collaborative intervention approaches (Webster-Stratton, 2005). Others have developed more intensive adjunctive interventions (Sanders, Bor, & Morawska, 2007). Recent work has also explored treating ADHD in parents with stimulants prior to parent training, although additional supports or modification of parent-training protocols may also be needed (Chronis-Tuscano & Stein, 2012).

COMBINATION TREATMENTS AND OTHER BEHAVIORAL INTERVENTIONS

Seven studies meeting AHRQ review criteria have evaluated the combination of PMT or parent education with classroom interventions (primarily teacher training or consultation) for preschoolers with significant ADHD symptoms and disruptive behavior (Charach et al., 2011). Most show some evidence of improvement in children's disruptive behavior at school as well as in teachers' classroom management skills. However, the maintenance of these effects past one school year is unclear. In addition, poor parent attendance at school-based PMT was a concern in more than one study (perhaps because not all children were formally diagnosed or referred for services), which appeared to have a negative impact on outcomes. Most importantly, it remains unclear whether combination treatments improve outcomes above and beyond parent training: some studies report additional benefits (Webster-Stratton, Reid, & Hammond, 2004), while others don't (e.g., Kern et al., 2007). With regard to specific school intervention programs showing promise, three well-conducted studies (Webster-Stratton et al., 2004, 2011; Williford & Shelton, 2008) have used the IY Teacher Classroom Management program or the IY child-directed intervention (aka "Dinosaur School"), described further in the next chapter.

There is limited support for behavioral interventions directly targeting young children with disruptive behavior without concurrent parent training (Eyberg, Nelson, & Boggs, 2008). However, a few case studies of preschoolers with ADHD symptoms suggest that specific behavior management techniques implemented by teachers may be effective (McCain & Kelly, 1993; McGoey et al., 2000). Strategies showing promise include use of daily report cards, token reinforcement, and response cost procedures (e.g., awarding and removing buttons that could be exchanged for prizes and privileges). The unique effects of a kindergarten classroom intervention including direct child instruction in self-control and anger management and behavior management procedures were evaluated by Barkley and colleagues (2000), who found some benefits at the end of the school year, although these were not maintained (Shelton et al., 2000).

One well-conducted combination treatment study found some benefit for a social-emotional child training program when implemented as a single intervention for 4- to 8-year-olds with ODD (Webster-Stratton et al., 2004). This program was also included in a combination study of PMT and child training showing positive effects for 4- to 6-year-olds with ADHD (Webster-Stratton et al., 2011). Given the age span in these studies, the specific impact for preschoolers cannot be evaluated, nor have long-term outcomes been evaluated for the child intervention alone. Thus at this time, additional research is needed to support either teacher training alone or child skills training as a single intervention for preschoolers with ADHD.

Description of and Empirical Evidence for Specific PMT Interventions

WELL-ESTABLISHED PMT PROGRAMS

There are three well-established PMT programs recognized as effective with preschoolers with disruptive behavior difficulties (including ADHD): PCIT, IY, and Positive Parenting of Preschoolers (Triple P). Specific research studies supporting their efficacy have been reviewed extensively elsewhere (Charach et al., 2011; Eyberg et al., 2008; Pearl, 2009); therefore, our focus is on summarizing the level of evidence and ADHD-specific data. Other PMT programs such as the Oregon model may also be considered evidence-based but have not been evaluated specifically for preschoolers and are therefore not included here. An overview of programs with the greatest evidence is provided in Table 5.1.

Table 5.1 **Overview of PMT Programs with Greatest Evidence of Support for Preschoolers**

	PCIT	IY- Parent	Triple P	NFPP
Level of Evidence	Well established	Well established	Well established	Promising
Defining Feature	Assessment- driven direct coaching of parent–child interactions	Video-modeling with collaborative discussion	Multilevel system for population-based intervention	Parents taught to be child's "self-regulation trainer"
Unique Characteristic	Criterion-based parent skill performance	Multicomponent program series (parent, teacher, child)	Flexible delivery modalities tailored to meet family need	Developed specifically for preschoolers with ADHD
Focus of curriculum	Parent–child relationship Behavior management	Parent–child relationship Behavior management Home–school collaboration Social-emotional competence	Parent–child relationship Behavior management	Parent–child relationship Behavior management Attention training
Theoretical Orientation	Behavioral and social-learning	Relational and social-learning	Social-learning Public health	Social-learning Cognitive- developmental
Method	1:1 in clinic (group option, primary care version and anticipatory guidance version available)	Clinic or community groups (self-directed option available)	Ranges from psychoeducation to group to 1:1 (self-directed option available)	In-home
Length (for ADHD)	12–16 weeks	20–24 weeks	10 (standard)–15 (enhanced)	8 weeks
Level of Intervention	Indicated (clinical)	Targeted (at-risk) Indicated (clinical)	Universal (prevention) Targeted (at-risk) Indicated (clinical)	Indicated (clinical)

PCIT, Parent–Child Interaction Therapy; IY, Incredible Years; Triple P, Positive Parenting Program; NFPP, New Forest Parenting Program.

PCIT was developed by Sheila Eyberg in the 1970s for children aged 2 to 7 years with disruptive behavior (Eyberg & Bussing, 2011). PCIT has demonstrated efficacy in eight studies meeting rigorous review criteria by the AHRQ (Charach et al., 2011), with maintenance effects (without a control group) documented up to 6 years (Hood & Eyberg, 2003). Children with ADHD symptoms or comorbid diagnoses have been included in research at high rates, and there is evidence of reduction in ADHD symptoms with treatment in several studies (Wagner & McNeil, 2008). A large-scale NIMH-funded RCT targeting an ADHD-specific population and comparing a group versus individual treatment approach in 4- to 6-year-old children with ADHD, with and without ODD, is ongoing (Eyberg, 2008). Furthermore, promising findings were reported for two abbreviated versions of PCIT for primary care, a group preventive intervention called Primary Care PCIT (PC-PCIT) and a self-directed program called PCIT Anticipatory Guidance (PCIT-AG; Berkovits et al. 2010). To date, standard PCIT is being used for preschoolers with ADHD without particular modifications; however, examples of tailoring PCIT for ADHD may be found in the PCIT treatment manual, accessible at www.pcit.org. More specific details of PCIT's core features and implementation are provided later in this chapter.

IY is a comprehensive series of programs for parents, teachers, and children developed by Carolyn Webster-Stratton (2005) for children ages 3 to 8 years at risk for social-emotional difficulties or exhibiting conduct problem behavior (with recent extension down to babies and up to age 12). Like PCIT, it is based on the Hanf model and is well grounded in relationship and social learning theory, as well as social-cognitive learning models. IY is video-mediated with over 200 vignettes for the parent program that demonstrate effective and ineffective ways of interacting with young children and handling different behavior concerns. It is a collaborative model in which the group leader "facilitates" rather than teaches parents using a set of core principles. Additional details on IY are provided in the next chapter.

The IY Parent program has since been extensively researched, with five IY Parent studies meeting AHRQ review criteria supporting its efficacy in reducing children's behavior problems and improving parenting skills (Charach et al., 2011), with maintenance of benefits (without comparison to a control group) documented for up to 6 years (Drugli et al., 2009). In addition to including high rates of children with ADHD in IY research, studies of IY Parent have demonstrated a reduction in ADHD symptoms (Jones, Daley, Hutchings, Bywater, & Eames, 2007) and a greater decrease in disruptive behavior in boys with significant ADHD symptoms compared to those without (Hartman, Stage, & Webster-Stratton, 2003). More importantly, a recently published RCT of the combination of IY Parent and Child Training for 4- to 6-year-olds diagnosed with ADHD (half of whom also met criteria for oppositional defiant disorder) found significant improvements in child behavior and social-emotional skills as well as in parenting skills for mothers (Webster-Stratton et al., 2011).

Triple P is a multileveled treatment system with five levels to match the intensity of child behavior problems and parent need. Development of the program began in Australia in the late 1970s by Sanders and colleagues. Level 1 is a universal media-based psychoeducational strategy appropriate for all parents; Level 2 provides specific advice and parenting tips through a few brief consultations; Level 3 provides brief consultation in four 20-minute sessions that teach parents how to handle mild to moderate behavior difficulties, typically in a primary care setting; Level 4 (referred to as Standard Triple P) is an intensive program for children with more severe difficulties (such as ADHD) delivered in a combination of 10 individual and group sessions; Level 5 (known as Enhanced Triple P) is a behavioral family intervention provided through three to five individual sessions focused on partner support and coping skills for families experiencing distress. Standard Triple P teaches 17 child management strategies and conducts planned activities training through a variety of methods, including didactic presentation, modeling, role-plays, feedback, problem solving exercises, recommended readings, and use of a workbook. Three in-home sessions are provided where parent skill implementation is supported directly with the child, and parents are encouraged to bring their child to other sessions to facilitate skill practice.

Across different program versions for young children with disruptive behavior, seven Triple P studies meeting AHRQ review criteria support its efficacy, and there are uncontrolled data suggesting maintenance of effects up to 3 years (Sanders, Bor, & Morawska, 2007). One study demonstrated improvements in ADHD symptoms as well as oppositional behavior in a sample of preschoolers with clinically significant difficulties using the Standard Triple P program, with no additional gains observed from the Enhanced program (Bor, Sanders, & Markie-Dadds, 2002). Compared to PCIT and IY, fewer studies have been conducted on Triple P by independent investigative teams. The unique systemic design of Triple P (and its extension to the age of 16 and use with a variety of target populations) has supported its large-scale adoption internationally (see triplep-america.com).

OTHER PMT PROGRAMS WITH EVIDENCE OF BENEFIT

Although the evidence base is not as extensive, several other PMT programs have shown benefit for preschoolers with ADHD and/or disruptive behavior. including the Community Parent Education Program (COPE), Helping the Noncompliant Child (HNC), and the New Forest Parenting Program (NFPP), each of which will be reviewed briefly. Barkley's Defiant Children program (Barkley, 1997) has had elements included in other parent training studies with young children (Pisterman et al., 1989; van den Hoofdakker et al. 2007) and was evaluated in one large RCT. However, it did not demonstrate efficacy with preschoolers with disruptive behavior in that study (Barkley et al., 2000), likely due to poor attendance in a school-based setting.

COPE is a large-group–based preventive program developed by Cunningham (Cunningham, Bremner, & Secord, 1998) using a Coping Modeling Problem Solving approach in which parents formulate solutions to videotapes depicting exaggerated parenting errors and role-play alternative strategies. Parents work in small groups with larger group discussions that allow significantly more parents to participate (i.e., 20 to 25) than typical group-based PMT programs. The content of the program is based on the Hanf model, although it also includes social-cognitive strategies and group problem solving to enhance attitude change and commitment. There is a child activity group curriculum supporting social skill development in children whose parents attend the groups. The program is implemented in 10 to 16 weekly sessions, each lasting 2 hours, and is intended to be provided in community settings.

COPE has demonstrated positive effects on parent report of problem behaviors in one RCT with preschoolers with disruptive behavior (Cunningham et al., 1995).

A large program evaluation also suggested that it may be beneficial for Hispanic families with preschoolers at risk for ADHD (Tamm et al., 2005). Although it was provided to all parents participating in the multisite NIMH-funded Preschool ADHD Treatment Study (Kollins et al., 2006), parent training outcomes were not evaluated.

HNC, which was developed by Forehand and McMahon (1981) for children aged 3 to 8 years with noncompliant behavior, is based on the Hanf model with an explicit focus on modifying coercive parent–child interactions. Individual treatment occurs in 8 to 10 clinic-based sessions of 60 to 90 minutes during which parents are taught positive interaction and management skills through demonstration, role-plays, and in vivo practice with their child. Similar to PCIT, therapists provide immediate and direct feedback to parents during the sessions and skill progression is paced according to parents' behavioral performance (McMahon & Forehand, 2003). HNC has demonstrated benefits for preschoolers with oppositional behavior in at least one well-conducted study (Wells & Egan, 1988), and components of it were included in an early RCT of behavioral parent training for preschoolers with ADHD (Pisterman et al., 1989). A comparative efficacy trial with HNC and the New Forest Parenting Program is being conducted in preschoolers with ADHD (Abikoff, 2008).

Unlike the previous programs described, **NFPP** was designed specifically for preschoolers with ADHD. It was developed in the 1990s by Thompson and colleagues in England and has since been formally revised. It is based on a novel therapeutic model that intervenes directly in parent–child processes thought to underlie the development of attention and self-regulation by having parents become their child's self-regulation trainer. In addition to taking a social-cognitive developmental approach, it also has roots in social-learning and relationship theory. Revised NFPP teaches "constructive parenting" to directly address core ADHD symptoms. More specifically, parents use therapeutic games to help scaffold children's abilities to attend, take turns, wait, enhance working memory, and self-regulate. Oppositional behavior is also targeted through behavior management strategies. Key methods include psychoeducation and skills practice using a naturalistic behavioral teaching approach that can address individual family needs, including parental ADHD.

Results of two relatively small but well-conducted RCTs indicate substantial reductions in ADHD symptoms, with less-marked improvement in oppositional behavior (Sonuga-Barke, Daley, Thompson, Laver-Bradbury, & Weeks, 2001; Thompson et al., 2009). One study where the original NFPP was administered by non-specialist nurses was found not to be effective (Sonuga-Barke et al., 2004). As noted, a larger NIMH-funded RCT of this program as compared to HNC is ongoing.

PCIT for Preschool Children with ADHD

As noted, PCIT is an empirically supported treatment originally developed for preschool children with disruptive behavior disorders. PCIT seeks to improve the quality of the parent–child relationship and to achieve lasting behavior change in both parent and child. In PCIT, parents are taught specific skills to establish a nurturing and secure relationship with their child while increasing their child's pro-social behavior and decreasing negative behavior. PCIT focuses on two basic interactions. Child Directed

Interaction (CDI) is similar to play therapy in that parents engage their child in a play situation with the goal of strengthening the parent–child relationship and shaping child behavior through differential social attention. Parent Directed Interaction (PDI) resembles clinical behavior therapy in that parents learn to use specific behavior management techniques as they play with their child and to establish consistent contingencies for child behavior. PCIT aims to bring children's behavior within the normal range through use of the core features and treatment structure outlined below, which contains several components identified as effective in a recent meta-analysis of PMTs (Kaminski et al., 2008).

CORE FEATURES AND TREATMENT STRUCTURE

Assessment driven. PCIT relies on multiple informants (parent, therapist, and teacher, if applicable) and multiple assessment methods (parent and teacher questionnaires, direct observation) to define treatment needs, guide the course of therapy, assess progress through treatment, and evaluate outcomes. During the pretreatment assessment, and weekly throughout treatment, parents complete the 36-item Eyberg Child Behavior Inventory (ECBI) Intensity Scale to quantify the frequency of the child's behavior problems (Eyberg & Pincus, 1999). If the child also exhibits problems in the school setting, the child's teacher is asked to complete the Sutter-Eyberg Student Behavior Inventory-Revised (SESBI-R), which is similar in format to the ECBI and assesses disruptive behavior at school (Eyberg & Pincus, 1999). Both measures can be obtained from Psychological Assessment Resources (PARinc.com). Furthermore, direct observations of parent–child interactions are conducted at baseline and the beginning of most therapy sessions in the clinic using the Dyadic Parent–Child Interaction Coding System-III (DPICS-III), which permits coding of important parental antecedents (e.g., direct or indirect commands) and consequences (e.g., praise, criticism) of child behavior (Eyberg, Nelson, Duke, & Boggs, 2009). For clinical purposes, an abridged version of the DPICS is used that contains fewer coding categories than the full version (which is mostly employed for intervention research); during the PCIT training process, therapists learn to code parent–child interactions to a performance standard of at least 80% interrater agreement with their trainer.

Parent and child together. Except during two didactic sessions, parent and child are seen together in PCIT play sessions. This approach allows direct observation with immediate feedback, which facilitates parental behavior change and interrupts the coercive cycling. Joint sessions also have other desirable effects: children do not resist therapy sessions because they look forward to their parents' positive playtime attention, and parents feel validated when therapists witness difficult child behavior and praise parents for applying their new skills.

Coding. PCIT sessions usually start out with 5-minute segments of direct observation using the abridged DPICS. Therapists specifically code desirable parenting skills (e.g., number of labeled praises, reflections, and behavioral descriptions during CDI coding, or number of correctly provided commands and follow-through in case of child noncompliance during PDI coding) and of undesirable parenting habits (e.g., questions, commands, and criticism during CDI coding, or incorrectly provided commands or follow-through during PDI coding). The coding results are communicated to parents via the bug-in-the-ear device and serve to set coaching goals for the subsequent therapy session. Through this feedback process parents learn to actively monitor their own progress toward mastery criteria. Coding results are also graphed visually and shared at appropriate points in therapy to review progress.

Coaching. PCIT sessions represent an active skills training intervention, with therapists coaching the parents in their play with the child. Coaching consists of frequent, brief statements that give parents immediate feedback on their CDI or PDI skills (e.g., "Nice labeled praise," "Good direct command"), their manner (e.g., "Good job staying calm"), or their effect (e.g., "He stays on task longer when you describe what he is doing"). The therapist also offers suggestions (e.g., "Give her as many praises as you can when she's playing so quietly and gently with the toys"). This coaching ideally occurs through a one-way mirror system and a bug-in-the-ear device but can also be successfully implemented through in-room coaching.

CDI. The primary goal for parents during CDI is to follow their child's lead; during CDI parents also learn to shape child behavior through differential social attention. Parents learn five important skills—labeled praises (P), reflections (R), behavioral imitation (I) and descriptions (D) delivered with expressed enjoyment (E)—to give positive attention to their child's desired behaviors as they play together. These parental "do skills" are referred by their acronyms as "PRIDE" skills. Parents also learn not to use commands, questions, or criticisms during child-led play because they take away the child's lead; these parent behaviors are referred to as "don't skills." Parents learn to ignore mild negative child behaviors. By giving attention only to positive child behaviors, parents learn to use the technique of *differential social attention* to shape their child's behavior in this phase of treatment. During a CDI teaching session parents are instructed on the "do" and "don't skills," then are given a chance to observe and participate in role-modeled skill play. Therapists provide parents with a skill summary handout along with a homework recording sheet and ask parents to practice for 5 minutes ("Special Time") each day. Just as the parent learns to follow the child in CDI, the therapist "follows" the parent and shapes parental skill building through differential social attention. In the first CDI coaching session, therapists provide only positive reinforcement by focusing exclusively on parents' use of any CDI skill and ignore parental "don't skills." In subsequent sessions, therapists may also give suggestions or directions as the parents become more comfortable and trusting of their therapist. For example, a therapist might focus on increasing labeled praise, and whenever the parent gives an unlabeled praise (e.g., "Good job"), the therapist might cue the parent to label it by saying "Good job of what?" or just "Of what?" The therapist would also reinforce the parent for each use of labeled praise (e.g., "Great labeling that praise!").

If the child becomes disruptive during a CDI session, parents are coached to ignore the child by looking away and not talking or gesturing to the child. Parents are advised that the ignored behavior is likely to get worse before it gets better and that they must follow through with ignoring until the child's behavior improves. Parents are then coached to return to the positive CDI skills when their child is again behaving appropriately. Parents are also taught to stop the interaction for negative behaviors that cannot be ignored, such as aggressive or destructive behaviors like hitting, biting, or breaking toys. Therapists coach the parent to state that Special Time is over because of the destructive or aggressive behavior, and parents are encouraged to reengage in the

CDI after the child has calmed down. Therapists continue to coach parents in using the CDI skills until parents meet the criteria for mastery during the 5-minute observation: (a) 10 behavioral descriptions; (b) 10 reflective statements; (c) 10 labeled praises; and (d) no more than 3 total questions, commands, and criticisms. Once parents have met these criteria, they move into the second phase of treatment, the PDI. Because the CDI skills form an important foundation for establishing and maintaining effective discipline, however, the therapist continues to code 5 minutes of CDI at the beginning of subsequent therapy sessions. If a parent falls below criterion on any of the CDI skills, the therapist will coach these skills before beginning the PDI. The 5-minute CDI home practice sessions also continue.

PDI. Primary goals of PDI include decreasing noncompliance and other negative behaviors that are not extinguished by active ignoring. Parents continue to give positive attention to appropriate behaviors, but rather than exclusively following the child's lead, parents learn to give effective directions and follow through consistently with calm, predictable responses to their child's behavior. In between practicing commands the parent and child return to CDI sequences and have fun together.

In the PDI teaching session parents learn to give clear, positively stated, direct commands rather than criticisms (e.g., "Walk by my side" rather than "Stop running") or indirect commands that suggest optional compliance (e.g., "Please give me the car" rather than "Will you give me the car?"). Parents also learn about the timing of giving reasons to children; they are taught to explain before giving commands ("It is time for us to go. It is cold and rainy outside. Please put your shoes on.") or after the child has obeyed ("Good job of putting on your shoes! Your feet will stay warm and dry even though it is cold outside.") but not in between those times, to avoid arguments and reinforcement of delay tactics.

Next, parents are taught consistent steps to follow once a command has been given. If the child obeys, the parent praises the child for compliance (e.g., "Thank you for listening!"). If the child disobeys, the parent initiates the time-out sequence. Parents learn to follow through on all commands, because noncompliant behavior is reinforced if children are permitted to disobey. The time-out procedure provides concrete steps to follow after disobedience, with three levels: warning, chair, and room. At each level, the child may choose to obey the parent and end the time-out. Children are not allowed to use time-out as a way to evade compliance, and the procedure does not end until the child obeys the original command. Because children receive their own developmentally appropriate explanation of time-out procedures, both parents and children know what consequences will occur, which reduces parental anxiety and helps parents to feel more in control of their child's behavior.

The Warning. The warning is given after the child first disobeys a direct command. The warning repeats the original command: "If you don't [original command], then you have to go to the time-out chair." If the child complies after receiving a warning, the parent praises him or her for listening and the play continues.

The Chair. If the child has not started to obey the warning within 5 seconds, the parent calmly and quickly takes the child to the time-out chair while saying, "You didn't do what I told you to do, so you have to sit on the time-out chair." This statement reminds the child of the reason for the time-out and reiterates the connection between noncompliance to a direct command and a negative consequence. After placing the child on the chair, the parent says only, "Stay here until I say you can get off." Therapists teach parents to ignore all negative behavior as long as the child stays on the chair. The child must stay on the chair for 3 minutes, plus 5 seconds of quiet at the end of 3 minutes. These 5 seconds of quiet ensure that the child does not leave the chair with the impression that whatever he or she said or did on the chair immediately before the end of time-out caused the parent to end time-out. As long as the child continues to whine or argue, the 5-second count of quiet can't start and the time-out will last longer.

Once the child's time on the chair is up, the parent is instructed to walk over to the child and say, "You are sitting quietly on the chair. Are you ready to [original command]? If the child says "No," begins to argue, or ignores the parent, the parent says, "Then stay on the chair until I say you can get off." The parent then walks away and begins the 3-minute-plus-5-seconds-of-quiet time period again. If the child indicates that he or she is ready, either by saying, "Yes" or by getting off of the chair in a compliant manner, the parent walks the child back to the task. The parent then indicates that the child should obey the original command (e.g., pointing to the block that the child was originally instructed to hand to the parent). A child rarely refuses to obey at this point, but if the child did disobey, the parent would say again, "You didn't do what I told you to do, so you have to sit on the chair," and then follow through as before.

When the child does obey the original command, the parent gives only a brief acknowledgement, such as "Fine." The parent does not give the child extensive labeled praise at this point because the child did not comply until he or she was sent to time-out. Instead the parent immediately gives the child another similar but very simple command. The child will very likely obey this command, and at this point the parent gives the child highly enthusiastic labeled praise for minding and returns to some CDI play before practicing the next command. This way, the child begins to distinguish between the positive responses that follow immediate compliance and the less-reinforcing responses that follow compliance that required time-out.

The Room. When time-out is necessary, the time-out chair alone may not be sufficient in the beginning of treatment if the child gets off the chair without permission. For this reason, parents are taught to use a time-out room as a backup to teach their child to stay on the chair. Parents rarely need to use the time-out room after the first 2 or 3 weeks of PDI because children learn quickly to stay seated once they realize they will have to go to the time-out room if they get off of the chair without permission.

Parents practice their first command sequence in the therapy session, not at home. Therefore, the time-out room procedure is usually accompanied by coaching. The first time a child gets off the time-out chair without permission, the parent gives a time-out room warning, places the child back on the chair, and starts the 3-minute timing again. After one warning, whenever a child gets off the time-out chair without permission, the parent leads or carries the child to the time-out room while saying, "You got off the chair before I said you could, so you have to go to the time-out room." Once the child is in the time-out room, the parent stays just outside the door and keeps track of the time. The child stays in the room for 1 minute plus 5 seconds of quiet. The parent then leads the child back to the time-out chair and says, "Stay on the chair until I say you can get off." The child's 3-minute time-out on the chair then starts over. This process may need to be repeated several times during the first time-out, so it is essential that parents and therapists allow adequate time in the initial PDI coaching sessions to follow through until the child learns to stay on the chair.

Whereas therapists "follow" parents in CDI with gradual introduction of directive coaching, in PDI therapists "lead" parents concisely in the initial sessions, giving direct instructions and praising follow-through, gradual lessening their directiveness as parents gain mastery. Through active coaching during the initial PDI sessions therapists support parents in the difficult process of learning consistency, and they use the time-out periods to teach parents about their own and their child's behavior. Therapists can convey accurate attributions about the reasons for the child's behavior (e.g., "He doesn't like not getting his way") and can provide behavioral interpretations of the change as it is occurring (e.g., "He can tell a direct command means business"). They can coach parents in relaxation or anger-control techniques in vivo, if indicated. If the child makes many journeys between the time-out chair and time-out room, they can assure parents that their child does understand the process, is choosing time-out over obeying, but will complete the procedure and obey the original command within the session.

As PDI progresses, generalization of PDI skills from practice sessions to real life is emphasized. Parents learn to use commands for behaviors that are incompatible with problem behaviors (called "positive opposites"), such as, "Use your indoor voice" and "Pet the cat gently." Parents are coached to use direct commands with correct follow-through at the clinic at all times, including in the waiting room and during the parent–therapist wrap-up at the conclusion of sessions if indicated by child disruptive behavior. After children learn to respond to the running commands of PDI, parents may be taught to develop "House Rules" to address aggressive or destructive behaviors that have not responded to praise for positive opposite behavior. Before setting up a house rule (e.g., no jumping on furniture), parents will spend a day or two labeling the specific undesirable behavior explicitly for the child when it occurs, to avoid any confusion and reduce debating once the rule is in place. The parent then explains to the child that he or she will be taken to the time-out chair immediately any time the rule is broken.

In the latter treatment sessions, parents learn and practice other variations of PCIT as needed to achieve treatment completion criteria, such as managing their child's behavior in public situations or with siblings. For example, therapists may coach during an in vivo session in a public area, such as a hospital gift shop, in preparation for parents' practice of PDI in community settings. If sibling conflict remains a problem after the parents and child have mastered the PDI procedure, the therapist would schedule a sibling-attended session and coach the parents in how to alternate their CDI skills between children, with emphasis on their positive interactions with one another, and how to insert targeted commands to each child for specific cooperative behaviors, particularly those that resolve a conflict, followed by targeted labeled praises.

Throughout PDI, therapists teach and coach parents toward mastery level for PDI skills, defined as (a) making at least 75% of their commands "effective" during the DPICS-III observation of PDI at the beginning of the session (i.e., direct, positively stated, single commands that provide opportunity for compliance); (b) at least 75% correct follow-through (labeled praise after obey; warning after disobey); and (c) if the child requires a time-out during the PDI coding, successful follow-through, so that the interaction ends with a labeled praise for compliance to the original command. Some parents achieve mastery of PDI skills within four PDI sessions; however, for children with significant disruptive symptoms, parents usually require the detailed teaching and coaching offered in PDI sessions to achieve a normalization of child behavior.

Performance based. PCIT completion is not time-limited but based on the families' progress in three ways. First, the observation and DPICS-III coding of parent–child interactions at the start of each session determine whether parents have reached mastery criteria for CDI and PDI. Secondly, the therapist graphs the parents' weekly ratings of child behavior via the ECBI intensity score toward the treatment completion goal of scores within one half of a standard deviation of the normal mean (ECBI intensity score of 114 or lower). Thirdly, parents determine whether they feel ready to handle the child's behavioral issues by themselves in the future.

TAILORING CDI SKILLS TO ADHD BEHAVIORS

During CDI parents learn to use *differential social attention* to shape their child's behavior. To tailor treatment to preschoolers with ADHD, therapists can teach parents to identify incompatible positive opposite behaviors for unwanted ADHD behaviors. Because common ADHD behaviors occur so frequently, CDI sessions are well suited to coach parents in ignoring these behaviors (e.g., grabbing toys from parents, playing roughly with toys, or running around the room during playtime), catching the child performing the positive opposite behavior (e.g., asking nicely for a toy, playing gently, or sitting calmly at the table), and then providing enthusiastic labeled praises for these behaviors. Parents' generalization skills can be further enhanced through a supplemental parent handout on managing ADHD behaviors with CDI skills. Differential parental social attention and parental modeling of desired play behavior during PCIT appear to contribute to the reduction of core symptoms of ADHD, including inattention, hyperactivity, and impulsivity (Matos, Bauermeister & Bernal, 2009; Wagner & McNeil, 2008).

PCIT Case Illustration

Amy was a 5-year-old kindergarten student whose pediatrician referred her for PCIT with concerns about ADHD, combined type, with significant behavior problems at home and in school. Amy lived with her biological parents and 3-year-old brother Andrew. Amy was "always on the go" and routinely butted into conversations and was oppositional with her mom and jealous of Andrew, refusing to share and hitting when he took her things. She minded her dad better than her mom, who complained that Amy seemed angry and did not care for mom's affection. Both parents worked full time and felt strained by their differences in parenting style, with mom being strict and dad more permissive. Dad viewed mom's insistence on professional help for Amy as unwarranted because he "had similar problems as a child, never received any intervention, yet turned out okay." Even though Amy appeared bright, learned quickly, and already read fluently, she had significant behavioral problems in school. She frequently interrupted the teacher, bossed around and hit other children, and constantly got out of her seat, resulting in repeated referrals to the office at school and social isolation.

Mom came without dad for the initial PCIT orientation session; her ECBI ratings showed Amy's behaviors to be clinically elevated in intensity (T-score 76) and problem count (T-score 71). Mom was informed that PCIT could be successful whether one or both parents were participating, but that brief daily homework practice ("Special Time") would be essential. The parents decided that joint participation would foster more unified parenting and arranged babysitting for Andrew. During the CDI teaching session, mom voiced concerns that Amy would be too uninterested in mom's positive attention for CDI to work; however, she was willing to try, especially because discipline strategies would be addressed in therapy as well. The parents planned how to fit homework practice into their busy evening routine and opted to conduct Special Time with Andrew as well. They were instructed that it was important to give each child his or her own separate Special Time with a parent, because it is too difficult to begin practicing the parenting skills with two children at once. They were told that toward the end of therapy there would be opportunities to practice Special Time with both children together, assisted by the coach. For now, they were told to split up with one child per parent in Special Time, and switch after 5 minutes.

Despite high motivation, the parents returned for the first coaching session reporting problems with their 5-minute homework plan. They had practiced only twice because they "were too busy" getting the children ready for bed. The therapist helped to process solutions; best results were achieved with moving homework practice to the morning. Having homework "playtime" set a positive mood and actually helped getting everyone ready to leave the house. In CDI coaching sessions Amy initially insisted on playing only with dad and acted sullen during mom's playtime. Mom was coached to ignore these behaviors; instead she enthusiastically imitated Amy's creative pursuits, delivered labeled praises for pro-social play, and expressed enjoyment over their joint activities. The parents observed each other's coaching efforts and quickly adopted the therapist's style of positive feedback to each other. Mom reached CDI mastery criteria after five sessions. She learned to "catch Amy being good" and enthusiastically praised positive opposites of impulsive grabbing ("I love it when you ask so politely"), running around ("you are doing a great job walking by my side"), or not finishing an activity ("great job sticking with something that is hard to do; I am proud of you").

Dad's progress was slowed because he immersed in his own play rather than following Amy's lead. He recognized that his skill building progress was slowed because he talked too much and had difficulties staying focused on the PRIDE skills. This insight prompted him to obtain his own ADHD assessment, during which he was diagnosed with adult ADHD, inattentive subtype, and started stimulant medication. Treatment of dad's ADHD symptoms appeared to facilitate his PCIT progress. By the time he reached CDI mastery (CDI coaching session 7), Amy's ECBI score had already dropped to 131 (T-score 60), with remaining concerns about ADHD symptoms, defiance, and hitting her brother.

The parents had become supportive of each other's parenting efforts and completed the PDI teaching session without voicing any concerns. They jointly identified best solutions for placement of the time-out chair (hallway) and time-out room (guest bathroom, emptied of toiletries for the period of habituation to chair). The first PDI coaching session required three time-out chair/time-out room sequences until Amy complied with mom's command to hand her a specific toy; however, for the remainder of mom's coaching instructions were followed immediately or after the warning.

Parents expressed the desire to extend the PDI practice to Andrew, who had received CDI homework along with Amy. This was deemed a workable plan; the parents had moved PDI practice time to the evening so that they could follow through on a command sequence even if repeated time-out sequences were needed. Both children quickly learned to mind parental commands during the initial weeks of play-based PDI homework; subsequently commands were generalized throughout the day as needed. After a time-limited extinction burst in response to starting PDI, Amy's ECBI scores continued to drop into the normative range by PDI session 4. Both parents quickly reached PDI competencies and also maintained their CDI skills; the only remaining concern was handling sibling rivalry. The therapist initiated teaching of house rules (no hitting) along with increased labeled praises of positive opposites (sharing, using nice words), and within 2 weeks, daily episodes decreased from four to zero.

To further enhance the parents' ability to foster pro-social sibling behavior, the therapist offered a sibling session with both Amy and Andrew present for play time to practice CDI and PDI with two children at once. In this session parents were coached to alternate their attention between children, focusing on the children's positive behaviors while ignoring minor misbehaviors or addressing them with competing commands (positive opposites). Through coaching support the parents consolidated their sense of mastery of using differential social attention to support their children's pro-social behavior and provide them with needed structure, including time-out sequences if indicated. The parents felt confident that they would be able to handle future concerns without further assistance. Thus, after seven CDI and six PDI coaching sessions termination criteria were reached (normalized ECBI intensity score, parenting competencies in CDI and PDI skills, parental readiness). At the exit assessment Amy no longer met DSM-IV criteria for ADHD or ODD; however, she still displayed occasional hyperactivity in classroom settings. The parents were encouraged to continue their daily Special Time practice and their generalized use of CDI and PDI skills. The therapist cautioned that Amy remained at risk for ADHD recurrence and advised episodic follow-up assessments.

Amy's case illustrates the use of PCIT to improve the parent–child relationship, convey practical skills in reducing core ADHD symptoms through differential social attention, reduce oppositional defiant child behavior (which confers increased risk for poor outcomes in children with ADHD), and model positive problem solving approaches.

Suggestions and Guidelines for Everyday Practice

As with most childhood mental health interventions, treatment for ADHD in preschoolers should be tailored to the individual child and family's specific needs and should consider supports and adaptations necessary to address children's comorbid difficulties as well as psychosocial adversity and parental ADHD. Strength of evidence is high for PMT, and therefore PMT should be the first-line intervention in this age group. For practitioners who seek to implement evidence-based PMT programs, several options have been shown to be effective. Selection may therefore depend on local program availability as well as particular characteristics of each program that might represent a good fit for a particular family. Cost-effectiveness may be enhanced by large-group–based approaches (e.g., IY, COPE), although some parents with significant needs may warrant a more intensive one-on-one intervention with in vivo coaching (e.g., PCIT). Options are also available for abbreviated, preventive interventions of some evidence-based programs (e.g., PCIT Anticipatory Guidance/Primary Care or Triple P Levels 2 or 3) as valuable adjunctive services in primary care settings for families whose youngsters may be demonstrating some disruptive behavior or ADHD symptoms but have not yet been formally diagnosed.

Consideration of program differences in educational, training, and certification requirements for treatment providers may also be relevant. For example, PCIT training requires a minimum of a master's degree in a mental health field, while IY and Triple P only specify having a professional background in relevant areas such as child development and behavior management. Therefore, complicated cases may benefit from referral to interventions delivered by skilled clinicians with relevant expertise. Training in all three of these programs begins with 3- to 5-day workshops, offered at various sites by certified trainers. As noted previously, IY and PCIT appear to have more U.S.-based training sites than Triple P. All three programs outline a competency-based certification process for treatment providers, and both PCIT and IY require a minimum number of cases/groups to qualify for certification. PCIT uses a specific supervision and consultation structure as therapists learn to implement the therapy with integrity, and IY employs a mentoring process as well as peer coaching to support implementation fidelity locally.

Summary

Given that ADHD is the most commonly diagnosed condition among young children referred for mental health services (Wilens et al., 2002), effective interventions are greatly needed. Substantial progress has been made in the last decade in evaluating PMT programs for this population in rigorous studies using experimental designs, with several interventions showing strong evidence of efficacy for preschoolers with disruptive behavior, including ADHD. This has resulted in the identification of PMT as a first-line treatment for preschoolers with ADHD by several major professional organizations and in well-conducted research reviews. The majority of manualized PMT programs available utilize approaches based in social interaction learning and relationship theories, although more direct skills-development approaches for children are also being studied (i.e., NFPP). Among the remaining significant challenges of PMT are low participation and decreased efficacy rates for those families most in need, warranting further investigation and development of specific accommodations or supplemental interventions. In addition, further development and testing of classroom-based and multimodal ADHD interventions for preschoolers appear indicated. A final challenge is increasing the availability of evidence-based PMT delivered with high fidelity, so that the impressive effectiveness of PMT generalizes as broadly as possible. For now, practitioners should familiarize themselves with their local and regional referral options for evidence-based PMT and develop collaborative professional relationships. Practitioners can then advise families of preschoolers with ADHD of the indication for PMT, provide psychoeducation regarding the developmentally appropriate sequencing of interventions (i.e., PMT and not medications as a first-line approach), and make effective referrals.

Disclosures

Regina Bussing, M.D., receives grant support from NIMH and AHQR. She has received study drug for an NIMH-funded study from Pfizer, and research support from Otsuka. She has received honoraria as a consultant for Shire.

Desiree Murray, Ph.D., receives research support from the Institute of Educational Sciences (IES) and National Institute of Drug Abuse Prevention (NIDA). She has also received compensation from Incredible Years, Inc. for providing teacher training.

References

Abikoff, H. (2008). *Home-based parent training in ADHD preschoolers* (5R01MH074556-02). Retrieved from http://crisp.cit.nih.gov/crisp/CRISP_LIB.

American Academy of Pediatrics. (2011) ADHD: Clinical practice guideline for the diagnosis, evaluation, and treatment of Attention-Deficit/Hyperactivity Disorder in children and adolescents. *Pediatrics*; originally published online October 16, 2011; DOI: 10.1542/peds.2011-2654

Bandura, A. (1977). *Social learning theory*. New York: General Learning Press.

Barkley, R. A (1981). *Hyperactive children: A handbook for diagnosis and treatment*. New York: Guilford Press.

Barkley, R. A. (1997). *Defiant children: A clinician's manual for parent training* (2nd ed.) New York: Guilford Press.

Barkley, R. A., Shelton, T. L., Crosswait, C., Moorehouse, M., Fletcher, K., Barrett, S., et al. (2000). Multi-method psycho-educational intervention for preschool children with disruptive behavior: preliminary results at post-treatment. *Journal of Child Psychology and Psychiatry, 41*, 319–332.

Baumrind, D. (1968). Authoritarian vs. authoritative parental control. *Adolescence, 3*(11), 255–272.

Baumrind, D. (1991). The influence of parenting style on adolescent competence and substance use. *Journal of Early Adolescence, 11*, 56–96.

Baumrind, D., Larzelere, R. E., & Owens, E. B. (2010). Effects of preschool parents' power assertive patterns and practices on adolescent development. *Parenting-Science and Practice, 10*(3), 157–201. doi: 10.1080/15295190903290790

Berkovits, M.D., O'Brien, K.A., Carter, C.G., & Eyberg, S.M. (2010). Early identification and intervention for behavior problems in primary care: A comparison of two abbreviated versions of parent-child interaction therapy. *Behavior Therapy, 41*, 375–387. doi: 10.1016/j.beth.2009.11.002

Bor, W., Sanders, M.R., & Markie-Dadds, C. (2002). The effects of the Triple P-Positive Parenting Program on preschool children with co-occurring disruptive behavior and attentional/hyperactive difficulties. *Journal of Abnormal Child Psychology, 30*(6):571–587.

Bowlby, J. (1979). The Bowlby-Ainsworth attachment theory. *Behavioral and Brain Sciences, 2*(4), 637–638.

Campbell, S. B., Shaw, D. S., & Gilliom, M. (2000). Externalizing behavior problems: Toddlers and preschoolers at risk for later maladjustment. *Development and Psychopathology, 12*, 467–488.

Charach, A., Dashti, B., Carson, P., Booker, L., Lim, C.G., Lillie, E., ... Schachar, R. (2011). *Attention deficit hyperactivity disorder: Effectiveness of treatment in at-risk preschoolers; long-term effectiveness in all ages; and variability in prevalence, diagnosis, and treatment*. Comparative Effectiveness Review No. 44. AHRQ Publication No. 12-EHC003-EF. Rockville, MD: Agency for Healthcare Research and Quality. Retrieved from www.effectivehealthcare.ahrq.gov/reports/final.cfm.

Chronis-Tuscano, A. & Stein, M. A. (2012). Pharmacotherapy for parents with attention-deficit hyperactivity disorder (ADHD): impact on maternal ADHD and parenting. *CNS Drugs,26*(9). 725–732. DOI: 10.2165/11633910-000000000-00000.

Connor, D. F., Edwards, G., Fletcher K. E., Baird, J., Barkley, R. A., & Steingard, R. J. (2003). Correlates of comorbid psychopathology in children with ADHD. *Journal of the American Academy of Child and Adolescent Psychiatry, 42,* 193–200.

Cunningham, C. E., & Boyle, M. H. (2002). Preschoolers at risk for attention-deficit hyperactivity disorder and oppositional defiant disorder: family, parenting, and behavioral correlates. *Journal of Abnormal Child Psychology, 30,* 555–569.

Cunningham, C. E., Bremner, R., & Boyle, M. (1995). Large group community-based parenting programs for families of preschoolers at risk for disruptive behavior disorders: utilization, cost effectiveness, and outcome. *Journal of Child Psychology and Psychiatry, 36*(7), 1141–1159.

Cunningham, C. E., Bremner, R., & Secord, M. (1998). *COPE, the Community Parent Education Program: a school-based family systems oriented workshop for parents of children with disruptive behavior disorders.* Hamilton, ON: COPE Works.

Dishion, T. J., Patterson, G. R., & Kavanagh, K. A. (1992). An experimental test of the coercion model: Linking theory, measurement, and intervention. In J. M. R. E. Tremblay (Ed.), *Preventing antisocial behavior: Interventions from birth through adolescence* (pp. 253–282). New York: Guilford Press.

Drugli, M. B., Larsson, S., Fossom, B., & Morch, W. (2009). Characteristics of young children with persistent conduct problems 1 year after treatment with the Incredible Years Program. *European Child Adolescent Psychiatry.* Doi:10.1007/s00787-009-0083.

DuPaul, G. J., McGoey, K., Eckert, T. L., & Vanbrakle, J. (2001). Preschool children with attention-deficit/hyperactivity disorder: Impairments in behavioral, social, and school functioning. *Journal of the American Academy of Child and Adolescent Psychiatry, 40,* 508–515.

Eyberg, S. (2008). *Group versus individual PCIT for preschoolers with ADHD* (5R01MH072780-02). Retrieved from http://crisp.cit.nih.gov/crisp/CRISP_LIB

Eyberg, S. M., & Bussing, R. (2011): Parent child interaction therapy for preschool children with conduct problems. In R. C. Murrihy, A. D. Kidman, & T. H. Ollendick (Eds.), *A clinician's handbook for the assessment and treatment of conduct problems in youth* (pp. 139–162). Springer Press.

Eyberg, S. M., Nelson, M. M., & Boggs, S.R. (2008). Evidence-based treatments for child and adolescent disruptive behavior disorders. *Journal of Clinical Child and Adolescent Psychology, 37,* 213–235.

Eyberg, S. M., Nelson, M. M., Duke, M., & Boggs, S. R. (2009). *Manual for the Dyadic Parent-Child Interaction Coding System* (3rd ed.). Retrieved from http://pcit.phhp.ufl.edu/measures/dpics%20(3rd%20edition)%20manual%20version%203.07.pdf

Eyberg, S. M., & Pincus, D. (1999). *Eyberg Child Behavior Inventory and Sutter–Eyberg Behavior Inventory–revised: Professional Manual.* Odessa, FL: Psychological Assessment Resources.

Forehand, R. & McMahon, R.J. (1981). *Helping the noncompliant child: A clinician's guide to parent training.* New York: Guilford.

Gleason, M. M., Egger, H. L., Emslie, G. J., Greenhill, L., Kowatch, R. A., Lieberman, A.F.,… Zeanah, C. H. (2007). Psychopharmacological treatment for very young children: Contexts and guidelines. *Journal of the American Academy of Child and Adolescent Psychiatry, 46*(12), 1532–1572. Retrieved from http://resources.childhealthcare.org/resources/

Hanf, C. (1969, April). *A two-stage program for modifying maternal controlling during mother-child interaction.* Paper presented at the meeting of the Western Psychological Association, Vancouver, British Columbia.

Hartman, R. R., Stage, S., & Webster-Stratton, C. (2003). A growth curve analysis of parent training outcomes: Examining the influence of child factors (inattention. impulsivity, and hyperactivity problems), parental and family risk factors. *Child Psychology and Psychiatry, 44*(3), 388–398.

Hood, K. K., & Eyberg, S. M. (2003). Outcomes of parent-child interaction therapy: mothers' reports of maintenance three to six years after treatment. *Journal of Clinical Child and Adolescent Psychology, 32*(3), 419–429.

Jones, K., Daley, D., Hutchings, J., Bywater, T. & Eames, C. (2007). Efficacy of the Incredible Years Basic Parent Training Programme as an early intervention for children with conduct problems and ADHD. *Child Care Health and Development, 33*(6), 749–756. DOI:10.1111/j.1365-2214.2007.00747.x

Kaminski, J. W., Valle, L. A., Filene, J. H., & Boyle, C. L. (2008). A meta-analytic review of components associated with parent training effectiveness. *Journal of Abnormal Child Psychology,* 36(4), 567–589.

Kendall, T., Taylor, E., Perez, A. & Taylor, C. (2009). Diagnosis and management of attention-deficit/ hyperactivity disorder in children, young people, and adults: Summary of NICE Guidance. *British Medical Journal,* 337(7672), 751–753.

Keown, L. J., & Wooward, L. J. (2002). Early parent-child relations and family functioning of preschool boys with pervasive hyperactivity. *Journal of Abnormal Child Psychology, 30,* 541–553.

Kern, L., DuPaul, G. J., Volpe, R. J., Sokol, N. G., Lutz, G., Arbolino, L. A.,... VanBrakle, J.D. (2007). Multi-setting assessment-based intervention for young children at risk for attention deficit hyperactivity disorder: Initial effects on academic and behavioral functioning. *School Psychology Review, 36*(2), 237–255.

Kollins, S. K., Greenhill, L., Swanson, J., et al. (2006). Rationale, design, and methods of the Preschool ADHD Treatment Study (PATS). *Journal of the American Academy of Child and Adolescent Psychiatry, 45,* 1275–1283.

Lahey, B. B., Pelham, W. P., Loney, J., et al. (2004). Three-year predictive validity of DSM-IV attention deficit hyperactivity disorder in children diagnosed at 4–6 years of age. *American Journal of Psychiatry, 161,* 2014–2020. 10.1176/appi.ajp.161.11.2014

Matos, M., Bauermeister, J. J., & Bernal, G. (2009). Parent-child interaction therapy for Puerto Rican preschool children with ADHD and behavior problems: a pilot efficacy study. *Family Process, 48,* 232–252.

McCain, A. P., & Kelley, M. L. (1993). Managing the classroom behavior of an ADHD preschooler: The efficacy of a school-home note intervention. *Child and Family Behavior Therapy, 15,* 33– 44.

McGoey, K. E., & DuPaul, G. J. (2000). Token reinforcement and response cost procedures: Reducing the disruptive behavior of preschool children with ADHD. *School Psychology Quarterly, 15,* 330–343.

McMahon, R. J., & Forehand, R. (2003). *Helping the noncompliant child: Family-based treatment for oppositional behavior* (2nd ed.). New York: Guilford.

Patterson, G. R. (1982). *A social learning approach to family intervention. III. Coercive Family Process.* Eugene, OR: Castalia.

Patterson, G. R., Forgatch, M. S., & DeGarmo, D. S. (2010). Cascading effects following intervention. *Development and Psychopathology, 22*(4), 949–970. doi: 10.1017/s0954579410000568

Pauli-Pott, U., & Becker, K. (2011). Neuropsychological basic deficits in preschoolers at risk for ADHD: A meta-analysis. *Clinical Psychology Review, 31*(4), 626–637.

Pearl, E. S. (2009). Parent management training for reducing oppositional and aggressive behavior in preschoolers. *Aggression and Violent Behavior, 14,* 295–305.

Pisterman, S., McGrath, P., Firestone, J. T., et al. (1989). Outcome of parent-mediated treatment of preschoolers with attention deficit disorder with hyperactivity. *Journal of Consulting and Clinical Psychology, 57,* 628–635.

Reitman, D., & McMahon, R. J. (2012). Constance "Connie" Hanf (1917–2002): The mentor and the model. *Cognitive and Behavioral Practice.* doi: 10.1016/j.cbpra.2012.02.005

Sanders, M. R., Bor, W., & Morawska, A. (2007). Maintenance of treatment gains: a comparison of enhanced, standard, and self-directed Triple P-Positive Parenting Program. *Journal of Abnormal Child Psychology, 35*(6), 983–998.

Shelton, T. L., Barkley, R. A., Crosswait, C., et al. (2000). Multimethod psychoeducational intervention for preschool children with disruptive behavior: Two year post-treatment follow-up. *Journal of Abnormal Child Psychology,28,* 253–266.

Shonkoff, J., & Phillips, D. A. (Eds.) (2000). *From Neurons to Neighborhoods.* Washington, DC: National Academy of Sciences.

Sonuga-Barke, E. J. S., Daley, D., & Thompson, M. (2002). Does maternal ADHD reduce the effectiveness of parent training for preschool children's ADHD? *Journal of the American Academy of Child and Adolescent Psychiatry, 41,* 696–702.

Sonuga-Barke, E. J. S., Daley, D., Thompson, M., Laver-Bradbury, C., & Weeks, A. (2001). Parent-based therapies for preschool attention-deficit/hyperactivity disorder: A randomized, controlled trial with a community sample. *Journal of the American Academy of Child and Adolescent Psychiatry,40,* 402–408.

Sonuga-Barke, E. J. S., Thompson, M., Daley, D., et al. (2004). Parent training for attention-deficit/hyperactivity disorder. Is it as effective when delivered as routine rather than as specialist care? *British Journal of Clinical Psychology, 43,* 449–457.

Tamm, L., Swanson, J., Lerner, M., Childress, C., Patterson, B., Lakes, K., ... Cunningham, C. (2005). Intervention for preschoolers at risk for Attention-Deficit/Hyperactivity Disorder (ADHD): Service before diagnosis. *Clinical Neuroscience Research, 5,* 247–253.

Thompson, M. J., Laver-Bradbury, C., Ayres, M., et al. (2009). A small-scale randomized controlled trial of the revised New Forest Parenting Programme for preschoolers with attention deficit hyperactivity disorder. *European Child and Adolescent Psychiatry, 18*(10). 605–616.

van den Hoofdakker, B. J., van der Veen-Mulders, L., Sytema, S., Emmelkamp, P. M., et al. (2007). Effectiveness of behavioral parent training for children with ADHD in routine clinical practice: a randomized controlled study. *Journal of the American Academy of Child and Adolescent Psychiatry, 46*(10). 1263–1271.

Wagner, S., & McNeil, C. B. (2008). Parent-Child Interaction Therapy for ADHD: A conceptual overview and critical literature review. *Child and Family Behavior Therapy,30,* 231–256.

Webster-Stratton, C. (2005). The Incredible Years parents, teacher, and child training series: Early intervention and prevention programs for young children. In P. S. Jensen & E. D. Hibbs (Eds.), *Psychosocial treatments for child and adolescent disorders: Empirically based approaches.* Washington, DC: American Psychological Association.

Webster-Stratton, C., Reid, M. J., & Beauchaine, T. (2011) Combining parent and child training for young children with ADHD. *Journal of Clinical and Adolescent Psychology, 40*(2), 1–13.

Webster-Stratton, C., Reid, M., & Hammond, M. (2004). Treating children with early-onset conduct problems: Intervention outcomes for parent, child, and teacher training. *Journal of Clinical Child and Adolescent Psychology, 33,* 105–124.

Wells, K. C., & Egan, J. (1988). Social learning and systems family therapy for childhood oppositional disorder: Comparative treatment outcome. *Comprehensive Psychiatry, 29,* 138–146.

Werba, B., Eyberg, S. M., Boggs, S. R., & Algina, J. (2006). Predicting outcome in parent-child interaction therapy: Success and attrition. *Behavior Modification, 30,* 618–646.

Wilens, T. E., Biederman, J., Brown, S., Monuteaux, M., Prince, J., & Spencer, T. J. (2002). Patterns of psychopathology and dysfunction in clinically referred preschoolers. *Journal of Developmental and Behavioral Pediatrics, 23,* S31–S37.

Williford, A. P., & Shelton, T. L. (2008). Using mental health consultation to decrease disruptive behaviors in preschoolers: Adapting an empirically-supported intervention. *Journal of Child Psychology and Psychiatry, 49*(2), 191–200.

6

Tailoring the Incredible Years™

Parent, Teacher, and Child Interventions

for Young Children with ADHD

CAROLYN WEBSTER-STRATTON

AND JAMILA REID

Attention-deficit/hyperactivity disorder (ADHD) in young children marks a significant risk for later development of oppositional defiant disorder (ODD), conduct disorder (CD), and more serious antisocial behavior in adolescence (Beauchaine, Hinshaw, & Pang, 2010; Campbell, Shaw, & Gilliom, 2000). Children with ADHD are impulsive, inattentive, distractible, and hyperactive. They have difficulty attending to, hearing, or remembering parental or teacher requests and anticipating consequences and therefore don't seem to be cooperative or to learn from negative consequences. Because of their distractibility, they have difficulty completing tasks such as schoolwork, homework, chores, or other activities that require sustained concentration. Many children with ADHD have difficulties with peers (Coie, 1990; Coie, Dodge, & Kupersmidt, 1990; Coie & Koepple, 1990; Menting, Van Lier, & Koot, 2011). Because of their impulsivity, it is hard for them to wait for a turn when playing, use their words to ask for what they want, or concentrate long enough to complete a game or make a better decision. They are more likely to grab things away from other children or disrupt an ongoing activity because of their impulsivity and lack of patience. In fact, research has shown these children are delayed in their play and social skills (Barkley, 1996; Webster-Stratton & Lindsay, 1999). For example, a 5-year-old with ADHD plays more like a 3-year-old and will have difficulty with sharing, waiting, taking turns, and focusing on a play activity for more than a few minutes and is more likely to be engaged in solitary play. Because these children are annoying to play with, they have few same-age friends, and other children frequently reject them. They are usually the children who are not invited to birthday parties or play dates, a problem that compounds their social difficulties by reducing their social learning opportunities and lowering their self-esteem.

Between 20% and 60% of children with ADHD have a comorbid diagnosis such as ODD, language delays, or learning disabilities (Beauchaine, et al., 2010; Beauchaine & Waters, in press; Ghuman, Arnold, & Anthony, 2008; Ghuman, et al., 2007). ADHD symptoms, externalizing behaviors, and academic and developmental problems are intertwined with social and emotional problems. For example, impulsive and/or oppositional behaviors make it difficult for children to function in a school setting with peers and teachers. Poor attention, hyperactivity, and language or reading difficulties limit children's ability to engage in academic learning and also result in less encouragement and instruction from teachers as well as parents. Thus children with ADHD are likely receiving negative feedback from their peers, parents, and teachers, creating a cycle whereby one problem exacerbates the other (Barkley, 1996; Dishion & Piehler, 2007).

Behavioral Interventions for Young Children with ADHD

Behavioral treatment research for preschoolers (ages 4 to 6 years) with ADHD is not extensive; however, parent training for young children diagnosed with ADHD has shown some preliminary promising outcomes. For example, Pisterman and colleagues (Pisterman, McGrath, Firestone, & Goodman, 1989) reported improvements in mother–child interaction quality and rates of child compliance among preschoolers with ADHD following parent training. Effects were maintained 3 months post-treatment and were replicated in a subsequent study (Pisterman et al., 1992). Sonuga-Barke and colleagues (Sonuga-Barke, Daley, Thompson, Laver-Bradbury, & Weeks, 2001) reported similar findings, which extended to ADHD behaviors and were maintained at the 6-month follow-up. In a notable exception to this prevailing pattern, Barkley and colleagues (Barkley et al., 2000) recruited 158 kindergarteners who exhibited high levels of ADHD, ODD, and CD behaviors and assigned them to parent training only, classroom day treatment only, a combined condition, or a control group. In general, treatment response was poor, and effects did not persist at a 2-year follow-up (Shelton et al., 2000) and did not generalize beyond the classroom. The parent training intervention produced no added effects. Null effects for the parent intervention are probably attributable to lack of parental attendance and low program dosage, as only 25% of the sample attended more than 4 of 14 sessions. Further research is needed with a more comprehensive and higher-dosage parent intervention.

Research on the Incredible Years™ Interventions

The Incredible Years™ (IY) parent, teacher, and child interventions have proven efficacious in reducing conduct problems in multiple randomized control studies for young children with the primary diagnosis of ODD or CD (Menting, Orobio de Castro, & Matthys, 2013; Webster-Stratton & Hammond, 1997; Webster-Stratton, Reid, & Hammond, 2004). Studies have shown that adding the child and/or teacher program to the parent treatment program has resulted in greater improvement in children's conduct problems in the classroom setting and more sustained results at follow-up assessments (Webster-Stratton & Reid, 2007; Webster-Stratton, Reid, & Hammond, 2001a; Webster-Stratton et al., 2004; Webster-Stratton, Reid, & Stoolmiller, 2008). In these studies, approximately one third of children also had high levels of inattentive and hyperactive symptoms (Hartman, Stage, & Webster-Stratton, 2003; Webster-Stratton & Reid, 2010). Analyses of predictors of treatment outcomes, including child attention problems, indicated that both the IY parent and child programs were equally as effective for children with ODD with and without comorbid hyperactivity-impulsive-attention problems (Hartman et al., 2003; Webster-Stratton, Reid, & Hammond, 2001b). Moreover, a subsequent analysis indicated that including the IY teacher classroom management (TCM) program in the treatment plan enhanced treatment efficacy for boys with hyperactive and attention symptoms (Beauchaine, Webster-Stratton, & Reid, 2005). However, until recently, the efficacy of the IY programs had not been evaluated among children whose primary diagnosis was ADHD (Webster-Stratton, Reid, & Beauchaine, 2011). This randomized control trial found positive post-treatment effects for a 20-week IY parent and child intervention condition compared to a waitlist control condition for 4- to 6-year-old children diagnosed with ADHD. Results showed intervention effects for (1) mother and father reports of child problem behavior, ADHD symptoms, and social competence; (2) mother reports of positive parenting and discipline strategies; (3) teacher reports of externalizing behavior; (4) independent observations of mother's parenting and coaching, children's behavior problems with mothers, and social contact at school; and (5) children's feelings vocabulary and problem-solving skills. At 1-year follow-up, most of these results were sustained in the intervention group with no significant deterioration in parent or child behaviors from post-treatment to 1-year follow-up. Families in the waitlist control group had received intervention by the 1-year follow-up, so there was no longer an untreated control group for comparison (Webster-Stratton, Reid, & Beauchaine, 2013).

IY Interventions for an ADHD Population

When working with preschool children with ADHD, it is recommended that parents be offered the treatment version of the IY parenting program. This program is 20 to 24 weeks and combines the BASIC 16-week parent program with a minimum of four additional sessions taken from the ADVANCE IY parent program. It is also recommended that children receive the Children's Small Group Training Series: Dina Dinosaur's Social Skills, Emotion and Problem Solving Small Group Therapy Curriculum. The Dinosaur School curriculum results in generalization of behavior changes to the school setting and sustained improvement at follow-up (Webster-Stratton & Hammond, 1997; Webster-Stratton et al., 2004) and is effective with children with an ADHD diagnosis (Webster-Stratton et al., 2011). These parent and child programs are offered concurrently and weekly for 20 to 24 weeks in 2-hour sessions. Parents meet with therapists in a parent group at the same time that children meet in groups of six children with two or three child therapists.

For therapists to begin tailoring the program for children with ADHD diagnoses, it is extremely important to understand the core content of the IY treatment programs and the methods and therapeutic process of program delivery. The parent and child programs are described in great detail in each program leader's manuals and in summary chapters (Webster-Stratton & Reid, 2005, 2008, 2009). Although some modifications are made in each program when treating children with ADHD, the core content, methods, and process are relevant and crucial to implementation of the programs with fidelity. Therapists with a thorough training and understanding of the program quickly see that it is designed to allow for tailoring the teaching and learning process, as well as the emotional and behavioral goals for the individual parents and developmental stage of children. Below, we will provide a brief outline of the program objectives for the IY parent and child programs along with additional areas of focus or program tailoring for children with ADHD.

Tailoring the Core IY Parent Treatment Program for the Child with ADHD

Table 6.1 shows the content and objectives of the core IY parenting treatment program.

One of the core methods for the IY parent program is that therapists work collabora-tively with parents to develop individual goals for each parent and child. IY therapists collaborate with parents to tailor the program content to each parent and child's particu-lar situation. For parents of children with ADHD, this tailoring process often involves helping parents understand ADHD and how it affects children's social, emotional, and academic development, setting developmentally appropriate goals around increasing children's attention and focus and reducing misbehavior, strengthening children's emo-tion regulation skills, and also changing the environment to support children's need for movement, structure, predictable routines, scaffolding, and immediate feedback. Below are outlined some of the ways that therapists work with parents in each major area of the program to address the special needs of families who have children with ADHD.

Parents Learning How to Coach Their Children's Friendship Skills and Help Sustain Their Attention on Play Activities. It is critical that parents of children with ADHD become highly skilled as academic, persistence, social, and emotional coaches. The academic and persistence coaching during child-directed parent play interactions helps the par-ents scaffold their children's play so that the children can sustain their play activities for longer periods of time. During *persistence coaching,* the parent is commenting on the child's attention and focus regarding the task. For example, a parent might say to his child who is working with blocks, *"You are really concentrating on building that tower; you are staying patient; you are trying again and really focusing on getting it as high as you can; you are staying so calm; you are focused; there, you did it all by yourself."* With this persis-tence coaching the child begins to be aware of the internal state that is associated with being calm, focused, and patient and persisting with an activity even when it is frustrat-ing. Next the parents learn how to do *emotion and social coaching* during child-directed play. During social coaching, the parents describe the child's behavior when he takes turns, waits, shares, makes a suggestion, follows another's ideas, or gives a compliment. During emotion coaching, parents describe children's feelings, giving more attention to positive emotions than negative emotions. When they do label uncomfortable feel-ings, they combine this with persistence coaching to help them stay calm. For example, a parent might say to a child who is trying to do a puzzle and getting frustrated, *"That is frustrating and hard work to get the right puzzle piece, but you keep trying and staying patient. I think you are going to find the right one."* Parents begin practicing this coaching

Table 6.1 **Core Content and Objectives of IY Parenting Treatment Program (BASIC plus ADVANCE)**

Objectives	
Strengthen Parent-Child Relationships and Bonding (BASIC Program)	• Increase parents' understanding, empathy, and acceptance of their child's temperament and developmental stage. • Increase parents' positive and decrease negative attributions about their child and promote realistic expectations for his development. • Teach parents how to use persistence, social, emotion, and academic coaching methods during child-directed play interactions. • Encourage parents to give more effective praise and encouragement for targeted prosocial behaviors and for their children's efforts to self-regulate and stay calm. • Strengthen positive parent–child relationships and attachment.
Promote Effective Limit Setting, Nonpunitive Discipline, and Systematic Behavior Plans (BASIC Program)	• Help parents develop salient rewards for targeted prosocial behaviors. • Help parents set up predictable and safe household routines and schedules and clear rules for their children. • Help parents use nonpunitive and proactive discipline approaches for misbehavior. • Teach parents anger-management skills so they can stay calm and controlled when disciplining their children. • Teach parents how to do compliance training with their children. • Teach parents how to help their children emotionally self-regulate, manage their anger, and problem solve. • Help parents learn how to provide children with joyful and happy experiences and memories and reduce exposure to violent TV, computer games, and a diet of fear or depression.
Strengthen Parents' Interpersonal Skills and Supportive Networks (ADVANCE Program)	• Teach parents coping skills, such as depression, stress and anger management, effective communication skills, and problem solving strategies. • Teach parents ways to work with teachers to develop home–school behavior plans focused on social, emotional, and academic outcomes. • Teach parents how to give and get support in order to enhance peer supportive networks.

during dyadic play with their children; they model appropriate social skills and feelings language and prompt their children's use of appropriate social skills. Later, they are encouraged to arrange scaffolded play dates with other children and to provide peer coaching during these visits to further their children's social and emotional learning experiences. Parents in the group discuss the unique developmental, temperament, and biological differences in their children, such as variation in distractibility, impulsiveness, and hyperactivity. Through role-play practices in the group and weekly home practice assignments with their children, they learn to provide the extra scaffolding and support to their children so they can be successful during these peer play interactions.

Parents Learn to Increase the Saliency of Their Praise and Tangible Rewards. Children with ADHD get less praise and encouragement from adults than children without the diagnosis. When children with ADHD do get praise, they are less likely to notice or even comprehend that they were praised. In fact, frequently parents of these children remark that their children are unresponsive to their praise and encouragement. Because of their inattentiveness, distractibility, and failure to read nonverbal facial cues, children with ADHD need praise that is highly pronounced, salient, and combined with visual and tactile cues. For example, before giving praise to a distractible child, the parent needs to move close and establish eye contact and a physical connection in order to capture his attention. Next, the parent must give the praise with a genuine smile, lots of emotional enthusiasm, and a pat on the back or hug. Finally, the parent clearly describes the social behavior that is being encouraged. For these children, behaviors targeted for praise may include concentrating hard on an activity, waiting a turn, problem solving, asking for something (rather than grabbing), staying calm, and politely asking to be part of a game. Because it is not normal to praise in such an exaggerated way, parents of these children need extra training in these coaching skills and language as well as extra encouragement to keep praising even when their children don't seem to be responsive to or notice their praise.

Parents of children with ADHD often need to break down tasks into smaller parts and praise each part of the process rather than waiting for the completion of a particular activity. For instance, a kindergartner without ADHD may be organized enough to quickly learn a routine for coming home from school: take off shoes at the door and hang up coat and backpack. For this child, it may be reasonable for the parents to praise compliance after all three tasks are completed, and the tasks may quickly become a habit that will no longer need to be elaborately praised each day. For a child with ADHD, however, even this seemingly simple set of behaviors may be too hard to remember. Parents are taught to initially coach and describe each small step with a labeled praise that describes exactly what the child did: *"Thank you so much for taking off your shoes right when you came in the door." "You hung up your coat on the hook! That is so helpful." "I appreciate that you put your backpack away. Now you will be all ready for tomorrow. I am so proud of you for remembering everything."* Initially parents may be reluctant to describe and praise behaviors that are seemingly so simple and are expected. Through the process of the group, parents are helped to understand that for many children with ADHD, this detailed praise and coaching helps them to organize their behavior and helps keep them focused on completing a complex task without distractions.

Many parents of children with ADHD complain that their children do not seem to have the intrinsic motivation to complete tasks such as chores or homework. Parents would like their children to complete these tasks out of an internal sense of pride in their accomplishments or an understanding that these tasks are important to contribute to the family functioning or to learn at school. The parent group discusses normal developmental progression of intrinsic motivation and the fact that intrinsic motivation develops over time, often after behaviors have been extrinsically motivated. Moreover, children with ADHD are usually on a slower developmental schedule and it is extremely difficult for them to stay focused on homework or chores and not be distracted by many other things that may be going on in the family. They will take much longer than typical children to develop intrinsic motivation because this requires the ability to take the time to reflect on one's behavior and its consequences. Self-reflection is difficult for any preschooler, but for these children it is even more difficult because of their inability to focus and think ahead to future consequences or back to prior successes or failures. Developmentally they are more like toddlers, still in the stage of individual exploration and discovery. Sticker charts and behavior plans with clearly established behavioral goals and incentives can help children remember the behaviors they are working on and also serve as concrete markers depicting their success. Incentive systems provide salient and immediate rewards as well as a visual reminder to the children of their accomplishments and a continual reminder of the positive consequences of working toward their goal. Behavior charts and incentive programs are covered in detail when working with parents of children with ADHD and refined over time so that parents are able to continually motivate and challenge their children in novel ways. Charts also offer a kind of structure and positive scaffolding that provides a sense of safety and security for distractible and inattentive children.

Parents Learn About Clear Limit Setting and Predictable Schedules. Just as children with ADHD frequently fail to hear vague praise statements, they also fail to focus upon or remember parental instructions. They may not comprehend the parental request if it is unclear, negatively stated, or embedded in a great deal of distracting verbal content and negative emotion or if too many commands are strung together. Therefore, parents of such children need to learn how to make a positive request that is clear, calm, and specific. As when giving praise, parents must get their child's attention before making the request. Moreover, because children with ADHD live in the present moment and have difficulty thinking ahead to future consequences (positive or negative), they are not motivated by delayed consequences. Therefore they need consequences that are immediate and as closely related to the misbehavior as possible. This means that child compliance to a parental request requires immediate praise, and noncompliance needs immediate follow-through.

Because these children are frequently disruptive and don't seem to respond to commands, adults are more likely to speak loudly, yell, and repeat a great many commands. Parents need help reducing their commands to those that are the most important, giving them in a positive, clear, and respectful manner, and then being prepared to follow through if the command is not obeyed. When this is achieved, children will learn that when their parents make a request they are expected to and helped to comply.

Another way to help children follow the rules and to limit the number of commands given is to have clearly articulated schedules for the children. For example, therapists help parents set up a predictable afterschool routine such as hanging up their coat, having a snack, reading together, having a play activity, and eating dinner, and predictable morning and bedtime routines such as getting dressed (or putting on pajamas), eating, brushing teeth, and washing face and hands. Group leaders work these schedules out with parents and then help them use picture cues for each activity on laminated boards (or magnets for the refrigerator) so children can move each activity to the "done" side of the board. These visual cues and schedules help children know what is required of them during these difficult transition times. The difficulty for young children with ADHD is they forget what they are to do next and get distracted easily. These schedule boards with pictures describing each step, which can be moved or checked by the child himself, help them to remember what to do, thereby increasing their independence and reducing parents' need to remind them. Parents can also add chores to these picture boards, contributing to their children's sense of responsibility in the family.

Parents Learn About Immediacy of Consequences. Children with ADHD need immediate consequences for their misbehavior. However, it is important that parents have developmentally appropriate expectations for their children's behavior. Since children with ADHD are about one-third delayed in their social and emotional development (Barkley et al., 2000), the 5-year-old with ADHD cannot be expected to wait easily for a turn, sit still at a table for any extended period of time, or concentrate on a complex puzzle or Lego set. Parents will need to plan for activities that are developmentally appropriate for their child's abilities and learn to ignore distractible, hyperactive, fidgety, and noisy behaviors as long as they are not hurtful to others. Parents also learn the value of redirecting distractible children to another task in order to keep them from losing their interest or from disrupting others. However, aggressive and oppositional behavior requires time-out so that the behavior is not reinforced. Parents learn the entire compliance training regimen to help their children be more cooperative. However, before doing this training, several sessions will be spent on setting up predictable schedules and reducing commands to those that are most important. Other discipline strategies that work well for children with ADHD are consequences that are immediately tied to the misbehavior. For example, scissors are removed for a brief period if children are using them inappropriately, or children must clean up the floor because they made a mess with the paint.

Problem Solving with Children. In addition to focusing on helping parents understand developmentally appropriate discipline strategies such as reminders, ignoring and redirecting, using brief logical and natural consequences, and giving time-out to calm down for aggression, parents also learn how to teach their children beginning problem solving strategies and to practice more appropriate solutions. Parents help their children learn and practice a variety of prosocial and self-regulating solutions (e.g., trade, ask first, wait patiently, get parent, take a deep breath, share, help another, apologize, use words, tell yourself to calm down, ignore, use positive imagery) using *Wally's Detective Books for Solving Problems at School and at Home* (Webster-Stratton, 1998). These books present children with hypothetical problem situations such as wanting for a turn on the computer, being excluded from play, or being teased for children to solve. Parents and children talk about solutions and act them out with puppets. The advantage of using hypothetical problem situations is that children can practice appropriate solutions when they are calm before trying to use these solutions during real conflict. Then when problems really do occur with siblings or friends, parents help scaffold their interactions and problem solving through the use of social and emotional coaching.

Promoting Positive Adult Communication Between Parents and Teachers. Families of children with ADHD and conduct problems often experience parental depression, marital conflict, high levels of stress, anger-management problems, and a sense of isolation or stigma because of their children's behavior problems and a lack of family, school, or community support (Webster-Stratton, 2012a). Elements of the ADVANCE program focus on helping the parents learn effective communication skills with partners and with teachers, ways to cope with discouraging and depressive thoughts, anger-management strategies, ways to give and get support from family members and other parents, and effective problem solving strategies.

As part of this unit, parents are helped to work together with their child's teachers to develop a behavior plan that supports specific positive goals for the child in the classroom. In the parent group, parents discuss the most effective ways to communicate with teachers, practice how to bring up concerns in a positive, proactive way, and learn how to encourage and support teachers. While the parents are in their parent group, the children are in the small group dinosaur therapy program. The child group therapists for these groups work with parents to develop a behavior plan based on goals that are set by the child group therapists, parents, and teachers. Parents are encouraged to take the lead on working on these plans with the teachers. Parents also problem solve ways to support their child and their child's teachers during the yearly transition from one grade to another.

Tailoring the Core Child Program for Children with ADHD

Table 6.2 includes the core content and objectives for the Children's Small Group Treatment Series: Dina Dinosaur's Social Skills, Emotion and Problem Solving Small Group Therapy Curriculum.

Child Small Group Methods. The core methods of group teaching and therapy are similar regardless of the makeup of the child group. All groups use music, DVD vignettes specific to each content area, role-play practices, child-size puppets, hands-on practice activities, coached play interactions, homework assignments, session summary letters, and phone calls to parents and teachers. Within these methods, the therapists make adjustments according to the unique needs of the children in their groups. For example, the puppets frequently bring in problem scenarios and ask the children to help them problem solve. These problems are formulated to directly reflect the reality of children's issues in the group. For example, Wally (one of the puppets) could be unhappy because his mother yells at him each morning because he starts to play in his room when he is supposed to get dressed (inattention/distractibility), frustrated because circle time at school is long and his body wants to wiggle (impulsivity), angry because a boy took his ball and he got mad and hit him (emotion regulation problems), or sad because his parents are divorcing.

Child Small Group Process. Each treatment group is set up with clear and contingent behavioral expectations that are necessary to manage and teach children with oppositional and aggressive conduct problems. During the first group sessions, rules and expectations are reviewed and role played. Children participate actively in this process

Table 6.2. **Content and Objectives of Dina Dinosaur Social Skills, Emotion and Problem Solving Program**

	Objectives
Making Friends and Learning School Rules	• Understanding the importance of rules • Participating in the process of rule making • Understanding consequences if rules are broken • Learning how to earn rewards for good behavior • Learning to build friendships
Dina Teaches How to Do Your Best in School	• Learning to listen, wait, avoid interruptions, and put up a quiet hand to ask questions in class • Learning to handle other children who tease or interfere with the child's ability to work at school • Learning to stop, think, and check work • Learning the importance of cooperation with the teacher and other children • Practicing concentrating and good classroom skills
Wally Teaches About Understanding and Detecting Feelings	• Learning words for different feelings • Learning how to tell how someone is feeling from verbal and nonverbal expressions • Increasing awareness of nonverbal facial communication used to portray feelings • Learning different ways to relax such as using the calm down thermometer, deep breathing, and positive imagery. • Understanding feelings from different perspectives • Practicing talking about feelings
Detective Wally Teaches Problem Solving Steps	• Learning to identify a problem • Thinking of solutions to hypothetical problems • Learning verbal assertive skills • Learning to inhibit impulsive reactions • Understanding what apology means • Thinking of alternative solutions to problem situations such as being teased and hit or rejected • Learning to understand that solutions have consequences • Learning to critically evaluate solutions
Tiny Turtle Teaches Anger Management	• Recognizing that anger can interfere with good problem solving • Using the Turtle Technique to manage anger • Understanding when apologies are helpful • Recognizing anger in oneself and others • Understanding that feeling anger is okay but acting on it by hitting or hurting someone else is not • Learning to control anger reactions • Practicing alternative responses to being teased, bullied, or yelled at by an angry adult or peer • Learning skills to cope with another person's anger

(continued)

Table 6.2 (**Continued**)

	Objectives
Molly Manners Teaches How to be Friendly	• Learning what friendship means and how to be friendly • Understanding ways to help others • Learning the concepts of sharing and helping • Learning what teamwork means • Understanding the benefits of sharing, helping, and teamwork • Practicing friendship skills
Molly Explains How to Talk with Friends	• Learning to ask questions and tell something to a friend • Learning to listen carefully to what a friend is saying • Learning to speak up about something that is bothering you • Understanding how to give an apology or compliment • Learning to enter into a group of children who are already playing • Learning to make a suggestion rather than give a command

and help to establish the classroom rules. A token system is used whereby children earn tokens ("dinosaur chips") for appropriate behavior. These chips are exchanged for stickers and small prizes at the end of the group. Children receive very high levels of praise and the chip reinforcement. As little attention as possible is given to negative behaviors. Much off-task behavior is ignored, and children are redirected or prompted with nonverbal cues. When necessary, children are given warnings of a consequence (loss of privilege) for disruptive behavior, and leaders follow through with the consequence if the misbehavior continues. Aggressive behavior receives an automatic brief time-out for children to calm down.

Methods and Process for Working with Children with ADHD. The structure of the group is modified for children with ADHD because of their more limited capacity for sustained attention during circle time and their need for more movement than other children. Therapists introduce more songs, more role-play practices and physical activities, and more coaching experiences and hands-on group activities to keep the attention of the children. If the entire group comprises children diagnosed with ADHD the 2-hour format is revised to include three shorter circle-time lessons lasting 10 to 15 minutes instead of two 20- to 30-minute circle-time lessons. In addition, three small group activities are planned instead of the standard two activities, and sessions begin and end with some coached play times to facilitate appropriate peer play.

Once therapists have tailored the schedule to meet the developmental needs, attention span, and activity level of the group, it is important to help children understand and follow the schedule. Therapists use a pocket chart with pictures paired with words showing each segment of the group (play time, circle time, small group time, snack time, etc.). Children take turns using a moveable arrow to show what activity is happening next. A predictable and routine schedule helps these children feel safe in this environment and know what is expected of them. The visual reminder helps to keep them focused if they are unable to think ahead to what is coming next. Even within each segment (e.g., circle time) it is helpful to have a predictable routine. For example, every circle-time lesson is started with some familiar songs and the puppets make a predictable entrance and greet each student. Video vignettes are always introduced with the "ready, set, action" statement to ensure children are focused.

Therapists will have somewhat different behavioral expectations for each child in the group and therefore will set different limits accordingly. Children with ADHD may be given slightly more physical space than other children, with visible boundaries used to delineate the space. For example, a masking-tape "box" might be placed around the child's chair, and as long as the child is within the tape boundaries he would not be required to be seated with both feet on the floor at all times. It may also be helpful to give the child a sanctioned "wiggle space" to use if it becomes too difficult to stay in the group. This is not a punishment, but rather a self-regulation space so that the child has a place to go to re-regulate and then come back to the group. This space should also have the physical boundary marked out with tape and might have nearby a picture of the puppet Wally relaxing or taking deep breaths as signal to remind children of the calm-down steps. Another approach is to ask the child with ADHD who is becoming very distracted to go over to an area of the room where there is a "Show Me Five" hand posted on the wall and to briefly put his hand on the poster to help him regain focus. This "Show Me Five" hand cue is a signal with a picture for each finger that indicates the following: eyes on the teacher, ears open, mouth closed, hands to self, and body quiet.

The token system is also manipulated to meet the individual needs of the children in the group. For instance, not all children are earning chips for the same behaviors. For a very young child who has ADHD, chips may be given every 30 seconds if she is sitting with her bottom on the chair, or every time she remembers to raise a quiet hand. For another child who has difficulties with peer relationships, leaders will focus on giving praise and tokens for prosocial interactions (helping, sharing, giving a suggestion, listening, problem solving with a friend, complimenting). Leaders look for ways to make sure that children who are working hard at their individual goals are earning chips at relatively equal rates. In this way, each child in the group is working on target goals within a system that is clear and developmentally appropriate, has been negotiated ahead of time, and feels fair to all children.

Therapists are coaching, praising, labeling, and reinforcing (with dinosaur chips) targeted child behaviors such as waiting, managing impulsivity (e.g., remembering to raise a quiet hand rather than blurting out), staying calm, staying in seat, concentrating, following directions, appropriately using wiggle space, and respecting physical boundaries. At first, therapists notice even very short periods of attention, waiting, and calm behavior, and a child might receive a tangible reward such as a token along with praise for sitting in his chair for as short a period of time as 30 seconds. One goal for these children, however, is to help them learn to sustain this kind of attention for longer and longer periods of time. Gradually over the course of treatment, therapists will tailor their rewards, rate of praise, and expectations to extend the children's ability to focus, wait, concentrate, and attend. Very young or extremely impulsive children may have difficulty connecting the tokens with a reward given at the end of the 2-hour session. For these children there may need to be even more frequent opportunities to earn more immediate rewards such as stickers or hand stamps.

Content Focus for Children with ADHD. For children with ADHD, there is a special focus on the content topics of Doing Your Best in School, Emotion Regulation, and

Friendship Skills. These three areas address the key skills deficits experienced by most children with ADHD. In the school unit, for preschool children there is a focus on listening, following directions, and persisting with a difficult play activity. Therapists use "persistence coaching" to coach them to stay focused and to keep trying when something is difficult. In the Feelings and Anger Management units, the focus for these children is on emotion regulation. They learn to relax, recognize signs of dysregulation, and learn to calm down by taking deep breaths, thinking of their happy place, and using positive self-talk. In the Friendship units, these children are taught specific social sequences for situations such as how to enter a group of children who are already playing, waiting for a turn, playing cooperatively with a peer, negotiating the decision-making process with other children, and practicing friendly communication skills.

Doing Your Best in School: School Readiness. Approximately 30% of children with ADHD and ODD also have academic problems such as language or reading delays or learning disabilities (Bennett, Brown, Boyle, Racine, & Offord, 2003; Sturge, 1982). For children with ADHD, the link between written and oral language should be emphasized throughout the curriculum. Each visual cue card that presents a new social, emotional, or problem solving concept has both a picture and a word that describes the concept. Having the children practice "reading" the word on the picture by repeating it aloud, pointing to the word as it is said, and acting out the word at the same time that it is spoken will help children with language delays to associate printed words with spoken words. Small group activities can also be chosen that will reinforce particular academic goals. There are many activities that involve reading and writing that can be adjusted for children's developmental level. These therapist-coached activities provide a low-pressure time for children to experience success with academic tasks that may be difficult for them at school.

Therapists focus special effort on coaching, praising, and encouraging academic behaviors and persistent efforts for children with learning problems. Raising a quiet hand, concentrating on work, checking something again, correcting a mistake, trying again, and persisting on a hard task are all examples of behaviors to reinforce. Cognitive processes are also recognized by therapists. Examples of this are, "*I can see you are really thinking hard about your answer.*" "*You are thinking about the sound that letter makes!*" "*It's great that you stayed calm and asked for help on that project. Did you tell yourself, I can stay calm when someone grabs the ball?*"

Therapists also use an interactive or dialogic reading approach. This reading style encourages exploration of a book without the sole focus on reading the words accurately. Therapists discuss the pictures with the child by taking turns labeling objects, feelings, or other aspects of the picture, follow the child's lead and interest in the story, and help the child make up alternate endings to the stories, or even act out parts of the story with hand puppets. As children become familiar with particular stories, they may become the storyteller and will read or recite the story back to the therapist. Research has shown that when preschool teachers and parents read dialogically with their children, the children's vocabulary increases significantly (Whitehurst et al., 1999) as well as their word recognition and motivation to read.

Teaching Self-Regulation. It is important to begin to teach children with ADHD to self-regulate and use cognitive strategies and positive self-talk. Initially, adult prompting and visual cues are used to achieve this. Picture cue cards are used as a signal to use a self-regulation strategy (relaxation or calm down thermometer, stop sign). Children practice simple external self-talk (*"I can do it. I can calm down."*). All children in the group rehearse using these words out loud and are praised for their efforts. They practice using these words in hypothetical situations (pretend that you are feeling mad), and teachers also prompt the self-talk at times when children are beginning to dysregulate.

Part of teaching children self-regulation is also teaching them how to manage their anger when conflict occurs. In the problem-solving and anger unit, the precise steps for how to identify a problem and generate possible solutions are taught, modeled, and rehearsed. For example, specific behaviors that children learn to manage anger are taking three deep breaths, counting to 10, and practicing making their bodies tense and relaxed. Cognitive strategies they learn range from simple statements such as *"I can do it, I can calm down"* to more complex cognitions such as *"I'm feeling mad because my sister took my truck, but I'm going to be strong and use my ignore muscles. Then I won't get in trouble and I will feel better."* Cognitive strategies involve thinking of happy thoughts or places, positive imagery, giving a compliment to yourself, or telling yourself that feelings can change and even though you're mad now, you will feel better later.

Friendship Unit. In the friendship unit, the precise steps for learning how to play with another child are taught, modeled, prompted, and practiced extensively. First, children watch the DVD vignettes of children playing with a variety of toys (blocks, make-believe, puzzles, art projects, etc.) and in a variety of settings (playground, classroom). While viewing these vignettes the children are prompted by the therapists to notice how the children on the video vignettes wait, take turns, and share. One or two of these friendship skills are modeled by the puppet in interaction with the therapist or children. Then each child practices one or two friendship skills with one of the puppets and is reinforced for using these behaviors. Next, each child is paired up with another child (the "buddy") to play with, and the therapist prompts, coaches, and reinforces them for using these friendly play behaviors. Sometimes it is helpful to break up the group by taking pairs of children out of the large group to practice their play skills without the distractions of other children in their peer group. After these dyadic practice sessions, the children return to the group for a circle-time lesson focused on learning and practicing a particular social skill. Children with significant play delays may need to practice the social skills one on one with the puppet before doing this with a peer.

Collaborating with Teachers. Therapists communicating with the child's classroom teacher is particularly important for children with ADHD because attention and behavioral problems interfere with their academic learning. Therapists begin developing their relationships with teachers by asking them to complete standard behavior inventories regarding the child during the initial assessment phase. They also ask teachers to share their concerns regarding the child in the classroom and obtain their input regarding the specific behaviors they think the child needs help with and their priorities for goals. Once dinosaur group therapy sessions begin, therapists provide teachers with summaries regarding the goals for every topic being covered in the program. They call teachers every 2 or 3 weeks to share strategies that are working for them and refine goals. About halfway through the program, child and parent therapists begin to develop behavior plans for children and outline the strategies they believe are helpful. Parents and teachers meet with the child or parent therapists (usually at the school) to discuss these behavior plans, to collaborate on goals for the child, and to share strategies that they have found particularly helpful. For example, therapists share with teachers how to use Tiny's calm down thermometer, or Wally's solution kit, or some of Dina's reward charts in the classroom. This coordinated team approach to the child's behavior plan builds a support network between all those working with the child and helps promote consistency of approaches and language used across settings.

Moreover, involving teachers in IY TCM training or providing them with training in aspects of the Dinosaur School curriculum enhances what children are learning in the small group dinosaur treatment program. Research suggests this coordinated approach will improve outcomes even more (Webster-Stratton & Reid, 2007; Webster-Stratton et al., 2001a, 2004, 2008). More information regarding the IY TCM program can be found elsewhere (Webster-Stratton, 1999, 2012b).

Clinical Recommendations

- Parents, teachers, and therapists should use social, emotional, academic, and persistence coaching methods when interacting with children.
- Parent IY group interventions should be dovetailed with IY child social, emotional, and problem solving programs.
- Teacher and parent collaboration should be encouraged regarding goals and methods used to manage children's behavior.
- Intervention requires teamwork between therapists, parents, and teachers who are involved in training, consultations, and behavior plans.
- Parents, therapists, and teachers should offer salient and immediate praise and rewards for children's prosocial behaviors.
- Parents, therapists, and teachers should use clear and predictable schedules and positive, specific limit-setting methods.
- Consequences for misbehavior should be immediate and provide new learning experiences.

Summary

In this chapter, we have shown how the IY parent and child programs have been used effectively for children with ADHD. The basic IY parent and child program methods, content, and process are relevant for this population and need only minor tailoring to be effective for children with ADHD. Therapists must understand the rationale for presenting each content component as well as the cognitive, emotional, and behavioral principles and methods that are important for working therapeutically with parents and children (e.g., frequent positive attention for behaviors they would like to see increase and minimal attention for behaviors they would like to see decrease). With this in mind, the parent and child therapists, in collaboration with the parents and classroom teachers, can set individual parent goals and develop a specific behavior plan for each child in the group. Central to this treatment model is the idea that while a specific set of skills are taught in a specific order, the way the skills are taught, the level of sophistication with which they are presented, and the amount of time spent on each content area must depend on each family's situation, knowledge level, and culture as well as the child's behavioral and emotional needs and developmental level. In this way, the programs can be individualized while at the same time providing parents and children with a support group.

In addition to the parent and child programs, which are described in detail above, it is recommended that teachers of children with ADHD receive the IY TCM program. This program provides teachers with proactive strategies for supporting children's learning and classroom behavior, tailoring their approach to specific developmental needs of all children, including those with ADHD, using positive classroom management strategies, developing individual behavior plans that address children's specific social-emotional goals and partnering with parents to promote strong school and home connections. This program has been shown to be effective for teachers of preschool and school-aged children, improving both teaching practices (Webster-Stratton et al., 2001a) and children's school readiness behaviors and social skills (Webster-Stratton et al., 2008) and strengthening the impact of the IY parent and child programs in reducing externalizing problems at school as well as at home (Webster-Stratton, et al., 2004).

In conclusion, research on the importance of effective parenting on mediating longer-term outcomes for these children provides the hope that consistent, positive, and contingent parenting may help prevent children with ADHD from going on to develop more serious conduct problems. In addition, improvements in children's social and problem solving skills and ability to regulate their emotions provide a protective factor for their success in school and peer relationships.

It is important to note, however, that while the IY parent and child treatment programs have been shown to be effective in helping parents to manage challenging behaviors of children with ADHD and in helping children to use strategies to improve self-regulation and friendship skills, treatment does not change the core developmental deficits that these children experience. These children and their families are likely to need ongoing support in managing the impulsive, inattentive, and hyperactive behaviors over time, particularly during transition times such as moving from one grade to another or from one school to another. As children grow older and develop more self-awareness, they will need and will be able to take advantage of more sophisticated self-management strategies to help them compensate for their lack of natural internal self-control. Thus, treatment beginning in preschool is an important start to supporting these families and children with ADHD but will need to be supported over time.

Disclosures

Carolyn Webster-Stratton, Ph.D., has disclosed a potential financial conflict of interest because she disseminates these treatments and stands to gain from favorable reports. Because of this, she has voluntarily agreed to distance herself from certain critical research activities, including recruitment, consenting, primary data handling, and data analysis. The University of Washington has approved these arrangements.

The US research was supported by grant # MH067192 from the National Institute of Mental Health (ADHD).

M. Jamila Reid, Ph.D., is hired by the Incredible Years to train other practitioners in the programs.

References

Barkley, R. A. (1996). Attention deficit/hyperactivity disorder. In E. J. Mash & R. A. Barkley (Eds.), *Child psychopathology* (pp. 63–112). New York: Guilford Press.

Barkley, R. A., Shelton, T. L., Crosswait, C., Moorehouse, M., Fletcher, K., Barrett, S., et al. (2000). Multi-method psycho-educational intervention for preschool children with disruptive behavior. *Journal of Child Psychology and Psychiatry, 41*, 319–332.

Beauchaine, T. P., Hinshaw, S. P., & Pang, K. L. (2010). Comorbidity of attention-deficit/hyperactivity disorder and early-onset conduct disorder: Biological, environmental, and developmental mechanisms. *Clinical Psychology: Science and Practice, 17*, 327–336.

Beauchaine, T. P., & Waters, E. (2003). Pseudotaxonicity in MAMBAC and MAXCOV analyses of rating scale data: Turning continua into classes by manipulating observers' expectations. *Psychological Methods, 8*(1), 3–15.

Beauchaine, T. P., Webster-Stratton, C., & Reid, M. J. (2005). Mediators, moderators, and predictors of one-year outcomes among children treated for early-onset conduct problems: A latent growth curve analysis. *Journal of Consulting and Clinical Psychology, 73*(3), 371–388.

Bennett, K. J., Brown, K. S., Boyle, M., Racine, Y., & Offord, D. (2003). Does low reading achievement at school entry cause conduct problems? *Social Science and Medicine, 56*(2443–2448).

Campbell, S. B., Shaw, D. S., & Gilliom, M. (2000). Early externalizing behavior problems: Toddlers and preschoolers at risk for later maladjustment. *Development and Psychopathology, 12*, 467–488.

Coie, J. D. (1990). Toward a theory of peer rejection. In S. R. Asher & J. D. Coie (Eds.), *Peer rejection in childhood* (pp. 365–398). Cambridge: Cambridge University Press.

Coie, J. D., & Koepple, G. K. (1990). Adapting intervention to the problems of addressive and disruptive rejected children. In S. R. Asher & J. D. Coie (Eds.), *Peer rejection in childhood* (Vol. xii, 417, pp. 309–337). New York: Cambridge University Press.

Coie, J. D., Dodge, K. A., & Kupersmidt, J. B. (1990). Peer group behavior and social status. In S. R. Asher & J. D. Coie (Eds.), *Peer rejection in childhood* (pp. 17–59). New York: Cambridge University Press.

Dishion, T. J., & Piehler, T. F. (2007). Peer dynamics in the development and change of child and adolescent problem behavior. In A. S. Masten (Ed.), *Multilevel dynamics in development psychopathology: Pathways to the future* (pp. 151–180). Mahwah, NJ: Erlbaum

Ghuman, J. K., Arnold, E., & Anthony, B. J. (2008). Psychopharmacological and other treatments in preschool children with Attention-Deficit/Hyperactivity Disorder: Current evidence and practice. *Journal of Child and Adolescent Psychopharmacology, 18*(5), 413–447.

Ghuman, J. K., Riddle, M. A., Vitiello, B., Greenhill, L. L., Chuang, S. Z., & Wigal, S. B. (2007). Comorbidity moderates response to methylphenidate in the preschoolers with Attention-Deficit/Hyperactivity Disorder Treatment Study (PATS). *Journal of Child and Adolescent Psychopharmacology, 17*(5).

Hartman, R. R., Stage, S., & Webster-Stratton, C. (2003). A growth curve analysis of parent training outcomes: Examining the influence of child factors (inattention, impulsivity, and hyperactivity problems), parental and family risk factors. *The Child Psychology and Psychiatry Journal, 44*(3), 388–398.

Menting, A. T. A., Orobio de Castro, B., & Matthys, W. (2013). Effectiveness of the Incredible Years Parent Training to Modify Disruptive and Prosocial Child Behavior: A Meta-Analytic Review. *Clinical Psychology Review, 33*, 901–913.

Menting, B., Van Lier, P. A. C., & Koot, H. M. (2011). Language skills, peer rejection, and the development of externalizing behavior from kindergarten to fourth grade. *Journal of Child Psychology and Psychiatry, 52*(1), 72–79.

Pisterman, S., Firestone, P., McGrath, P., Goodman, J. T., Webster, I., Mallory, R., et al. (1992). The role of parent training in treatment of preschoolers with ADHD. *American Journal of Orthopsychiatry, 62*, 397–408.

Pisterman, S., McGrath, P. J., Firestone, P., & Goodman, J. T. (1989). Outcome of parent-mediated treatment of preschoolers with attention deficit disorder with hyperactivity. *Journal of Consulting and Clinical Psychology, 57*(5), 628–635.

Shelton, T. L., Berkley, R. A., Crosswait, C., Moorehouse, M., Fletcher, K., Barrett, S., et al. (2000). Multimethod psychoeducational intervention for preschool children with disruptive behavior: Two-year post-treatment follow-up. *Journal of Abnormal Child Psychology 28*, 253–266.

Sonuga-Barke, E. J. S., Daley, D., Thompson, M., Laver-Bradbury, C., & Weeks, A. (2001). Parent-based therapies for preschool attention-deficit/hyperactivity disorder: A randomized, controlled trial with a community sample. *Journal of American Academy of Child Psychiatry, 40*, 402–408.

Sturge, C. (1982). Reading retardation and antisocial behavior. *Journal of Child Psychology and Psychiatry, 23*, 21–23.

Webster-Stratton, C. (1998). *Wally's detective book for solving problems at home.* Seattle, WA: Incredible Years.

Webster-Stratton, C. (1999). *How to promote children's social and emotional competence.* London, England: Sage Publications.

Webster-Stratton, C. (2012a). *Collaborating with parents to reduce children's behavior problems: A book for therapists using the Incredible Years programs.* Seattle, WA: Incredible Years Inc.

Webster-Stratton, C. (2012b). *Incredible Teachers.* Seattle: Incredible Years Inc.

Webster-Stratton, C., & Hammond, M. (1997). Treating children with early-onset conduct problems: A comparison of child and parent training interventions. *Journal of Consulting and Clinical Psychology, 65*(1), 93–109.

Webster-Stratton, C., & Lindsay, D. W. (1999). Social competence and early-onset conduct problems: Issues in assessment. *Journal of Child Clinical Psychology, 28*, 25–93.

Webster-Stratton, C., & Reid, M. J. (2005). *Adapting the Incredible Years Child Dinosaur Social, Emotional and Problem Solving intervention to address co-morbid diagnoses and family risk factors* Seattle, WA: Incredible Years.

Webster-Stratton, C., & Reid, M. J. (2007). Incredible Years Parents and Teachers Training Series: A Head Start partnership to promote social competence and prevent conduct problems In P. Tolin, J. Szapocznick, & S. Sambrano (Eds.), *Preventing youth substance abuse* (pp. 67–88). Washington, DC: American Psychological Association.

Webster-Stratton, C., & Reid, M. J. (2008). Adapting the Incredible Years Child Dinosaur Social, Emotional and Problem Solving intervention to address co-morbid diagnoses. *Journal of Children's Services, 3*(3), 17–30.

Webster-Stratton, C., & Reid, M. J. (2009). Parents,teachers and therapists using the child-directed play therapy and coaching skills to promote children's social and emotional competence and to build positive relatiionships. In C. E. Schaefer (Ed.), *Play therapy for preschool children* (pp. 245–273). Washington, DC: American Psychological Association.

Webster-Stratton, C., & Reid, M. J. (2010). The Incredible Years Parents, Teachers and Children Training Series: A multifaceted treatment approach for young children with conduct problems. In A. E. Kazdin & J. R. Weisz (Eds.), *Evidence-based psychotherapies for children and adolescents, 2nd edition* (pp. 194–210). New York: Guilford Publications.

Webster-Stratton, C., Reid, M. J., & Beauchaine, T. P. (2013). One-Year Follow-Up of Combined Parent and Child Intervention for Young Children with ADHD. *Journal of Clinical Child and Adolescent Psychology, 42*(2), 251–261.

Webster-Stratton, C., Reid, M. J., & Beauchaine, T. P. (2011). Combining parent and child training for young children with ADHD. *Journal of Clinical Child and Adolescent Psychology, 40*(2), 1–13.

Webster-Stratton, C., Reid, M. J., & Hammond, M. (2001a). Preventing conduct problems, promoting social competence: A parent and teacher training partnership in Head Start. *Journal of Clinical Child Psychology, 30*(3), 283–302.

Webster-Stratton, C., Reid, M. J., & Hammond, M. (2001b). Social skills and problem solving training for children with early-onset conduct problems: Who benefits? *Journal of Child Psychology and Psychiatry, 42*(7), 943–952.

Webster-Stratton, C., Reid, M. J., & Hammond, M. (2004). Treating children with early-onset conduct problems: Intervention outcomes for parent, child, and teacher training. *Journal of Clinical Child and Adolescent Psychology, 33*(1), 105–124.

Webster-Stratton, C., Reid, M. J., & Stoolmiller, M. (2008). Preventing conduct problems and improving school readiness: Evaluation of the Incredible Years Teacher and Child Training Programs in high-risk schools. *Journal of Child Psychology and Psychiatry 49*(5), 471–488.

Whitehurst, G. J., Zevenbergen, A. A., Crone, D. A., Schultz, M. D., Velting, O. N., & Fischel, J. E. (1999). Outcomes of an emergent literacy intervention from Head Start through second grade. *Journal of Educational Psychology, 91*, 261–272.

7

Psychopharmacologic Interventions in Preschool Children with ADHD

General Considerations and Evidence

JASWINDER K. GHUMAN AND

HARINDER S. GHUMAN

General Considerations

Pharmacologic agents are seen as the first-line treatment options in school-age children (Pliszka, 2007). Evidence for their indications and efficacy in preschool children with attention-deficit/hyperactivity disorder (ADHD) is less robust, and use is generally reserved for severe ADHD. Moreover, there are greater concerns about the safety of available ADHD medications in preschoolers. The rapid neuronal maturation process during preschool years is influenced by the monoamine neurotransmitters that regulate the proliferation of neural progenitor cells, neuronal migration, axonal outgrowth, synaptogenesis, and pruning (Crandall et al., 2007), and these neurotransmitters are also targets of action for many psychopharmacologic agents (Coyle, 1997). The consequences of altering the aminergic systems in the immature brain of a preschooler are not known or understood (Ghuman, Arnold, & Anthony, 2008).

Regardless, preschool children are prescribed psychopharmacologic agents to treat ADHD. From 1991 to 1995, methylphenidate (MPH) use for treatment of ADHD tripled in 2- through 4-year-old children enrolled in two state Medicaid programs and a health maintenance program (Zito et al., 2000). More recently, the Medical Expenditure Panel Survey data were analyzed from 1996 to 2008 for therapeutic stimulant use in children. The Medical Expenditure Panel Survey is a nationally representative household survey of healthcare use and costs conducted by the Agency for Healthcare Research and Quality. The study authors reported that stimulant use in children under age 6 decreased significantly ($t = 3.71$, $p < .001$) and remained low (0.1%) from 2004 to 2008 compared to the period from 1996 to 2003 (Zuvekas & Vitiello, 2012). In 2001, a stimulant use rate of 67.3% and an α-agonist use rate of 26% were reported among 2- to 4-year-old children treated with psychotropic agents (Zito, Safer, & Valluri, 2007). Of the preschool children who were enrolled in a managed care organization and were prescribed medication for ADHD in 2003, one fifth were treated with atomoxetine (Van Brunt et al., 2005). Approximately 39% of preschoolers in New England were prescribed ADHD medications in the first year following diagnosis (Emond, Ollendorf, Colby, Reed, & Pearson, 2012). The rate of initiating drug treatment in newly diagnosed German children showed a linear increase from age 3 years to 5 years but remained below 10% until age 5 years, followed by a sharper increase between ages 5 and 8 years (Lindemann et al., 2012).

Despite reports of recent decreased stimulant use in preschoolers with ADHD, some concerning trends continue. These trends include prescription of pharmacologic agents in preschool children (1) as an initial treatment strategy without a trial of psychosocial treatments first and/or concurrent administration; (2) with inadequate monitoring and follow-up; and (3) with severe long-term adverse effects or no proven efficacy in ADHD (Minde, 1998; Rappley et al., 2002). For example, analysis of the Michigan Medicaid claims data revealed that pharmacologic agents were prescribed for 57% of the 1- to 3-year-old children with ADHD treated with medications, while psychosocial treatments were prescribed for only 26% (Rappley et al., 1999); 40% of the children were prescribed medications alone, while only 9% were prescribed psychosocial treatments alone. Follow-up visits occurred every 3 months for 59% of the children and at intervals greater than 6 months for 19% of the children (Rappley et al., 2002). Antipsychotic agents were prescribed for 16% and selective serotonin reuptake inhibitors for 11% (Rappley et al., 2002). A more recent survey of insurance claims databases showed that antipsychotic use in 2- through 5-year-old children with ADHD increased from 28.5/1,000 per year in 1999–2001 to 48.4/1,000 per year in 2007. Mental health assessment, a psychotherapy visit, or a psychiatrist visit occurred for less than half (40.8%, 41.4%, and 42.6%, respectively) of the young children treated with antipsychotics (Olfson, Crystal, Huang, & Gerhard, 2010). Zito and colleagues (Zito, Burcu, Ibe, Safer, & Magder, 2013) reported a significant increase in antipsychotic use from 0.1% in 1997 to 0.5% in 2006 (p <.001) in the 2- to 4-year-old age group enrolled in a mid-Atlantic state Medicaid program; the increase in this younger age group did not differ significantly from the increase in the oldest 10- to 17-year-old age group. Antipsychotic use for children with an ADHD diagnosis increased from 7.3% in 1997 to 20.2% in 2006 (p <.01). The adjusted odds ratio of receiving antipsychotic medication increased significantly over the 10-year study period for a diagnosis of disruptive behavior or ADHD (adjusted odds ratio = 2.48; confidence interval = 2.86–4.24) compared with a diagnosis of pervasive developmental disorders and intellectual disability. The increased use of antipsychotic medications for ADHD in preschoolers is not limited to the United States. Compared to 2005, a threefold increase in the rate of recommending antipsychotic medications for ADHD was reported in 2009 in 1- to 18-year-old Canadian children and adolescents; the median duration of risperidone use was 90 days in the 1- to 6-year-old age group (Pringsheim, Lam, & Patten, 2011).

Primary healthcare and mental healthcare providers are increasingly being asked to assess and manage preschool children with ADHD. Developmental factors make treatment of preschool children with ADHD more challenging, more controversial, and in some ways riskier than treatment of older children with ADHD. The currently available evidence base for ADHD treatment modalities in preschoolers, in general, is stronger for psychosocial interventions compared to psychopharmacologic interventions and/or alternative treatments. Reports of pharmacologic treatments in preschool children formally diagnosed with ADHD are limited in number. In this chapter we discuss practice guidelines, pharmacologic treatment controversies, dilemmas and challenges, benefits of treatment, failure of the FDA Modernization Act in promoting meaningful pharmacologic research in preschoolers, and the currently available evidence for pharmacologic treatments. We also address special medication treatment considerations for preschool children with developmental disorders and preschoolers with swallowing difficulties.

CLINICAL PRACTICE GUIDELINES FOR TREATMENT OF ADHD IN PRESCHOOLERS

The most recent American Academy of Child and Adolescent Psychiatry (AACAP) practice parameters (Pliszka, 2007) do not provide clear guidelines for the treatment of ADHD in preschool children other than highlighting the results and conclusions from the Preschoolers with ADHD Treatment Study (PATS). The practice parameters do specifically note that a conservative titration strategy should be used and that the optimal MPH dose for the preschoolers in the PATS was lower than for the school-age children in the Multimodal Treatment Study of Children with ADHD (MTA) (Pliszka, 2007). The AACAP-sponsored Preschool Pharmacology Working Group (PPWG) recommended a trial of parent behavior management training or other behavioral intervention first and concurrent pharmacologic intervention only if a minimum of 5 weeks of behavioral intervention fails to provide adequate control of symptoms in preschool children with ADHD (Gleason et al., 2007).

The American Academy of Pediatrics (AAP) has more specifically incorporated the PATS protocol and results into clinical practice guidelines for the assessment and treatment of preschoolers with ADHD. The AAP recommendations specify behavior therapy as the first-line treatment for ADHD in preschool children. Pharmacologic treatment should be considered only if the preschooler's ADHD symptoms have not responded to a 10- to 14-week course of appropriate behavioral intervention (parent behavior training or other evidence-based behavioral treatments). The AAP guidelines further recommend that if evidence-based behavioral treatments are not available in certain areas, the clinicians need to weigh the risks of starting medication at an early age against the harm of delaying diagnosis and treatment. The AAP recommends considering enrolling the child in a preschool program and obtaining consultation from a mental health specialist with specific experience with preschool-age children.

The AAP guidelines specify that pharmacologic treatment can be considered in 4- to 5-year-old children with ADHD for moderate to severe continuing disturbance in a child's functioning as indicated by symptom duration of 9 months or longer (based on the PATS inclusion criteria) and clear impairment in both the home and daycare/preschool settings (AAP, 2011). Kaplan and Adesman (2011) have provided additional examples of moderate to severe impairment from ADHD symptoms in preschoolers, including history of repeated expulsions (or threatened expulsion) from preschool or nursery/daycare, accidental injury to the child, other children, or caregivers, and inability to participate in or benefit from other interventions (e.g., speech/language therapy, behavior therapy).

The United Kingdom National Institute of Clinical Excellence (NICE) guidelines do not recommend drug treatment for ADHD in children under the age of 5 years (Kendall, Taylor, Perez, & Taylor, 2008).

PHARMACOLOGIC TREATMENT CONTROVERSIES, DILEMMAS, AND CHALLENGES

The trickle-down phenomenon is common in the diagnosis and treatment of psychiatric disorders in children. Often, interventions in older children are modified for use in preschool children without adequate guidelines regarding dosages and frequency of administration in the younger age group. However, differences in development between preschool and school-age children can affect pharmacokinetics and drug disposition and may make it difficult to apply data collected in older children to preschool children. Also, preschool children may respond differently to medications used in older children (Ghuman et al., 2001, 2008; Greenhill et al., 2006) and may have specific toxicities compared to school-age children (Ghuman, Aman, Ghuman, et al., 2009; Ghuman, Aman, Lecavalier, et al., 2009; Ghuman, Byreddy, & Ghuman, 2011; Wigal et al., 2006).

Given the concerns and limited empirical information, clinicians and caregivers are often reluctant to consider pharmacologic treatments for young children. Past reports of increased rates of stimulant prescriptions in preschoolers have led to political objections that the ADHD diagnosis is "intended to facilitate behavioral control and suppression" and can result in "the psychiatric drugging of toddlers" (Breggin, 2000).

On the other hand, only a quarter of the preschoolers with a diagnosis of ADHD were referred for evaluation or treatment (Egger, Kondo, & Angold, 2006; Lavigne et al., 1998). Parents frequently complain that healthcare providers dismiss their concerns about the preschooler's problems with hyperactivity, impulsivity, and inattention. They are often told to wait to pursue an evaluation for their child *after* the child is in school. However, starting school is a major transition and a stressful time for preschoolers and their parents. Parents desire early detection and intervention (Vitiello, 2001) to enhance their child's chances for a successful transition to school. Parents' worry is further supported by several studies suggesting that preschoolers diagnosed with ADHD are at a considerable risk for school behavior problems, poor academic performance, increased conflict in teacher–child interactions, poor peer relationships, and subsequent substance abuse and poor job performance, resulting in staggering lifetime socioeconomic costs to society (Barkley, 1998; Egger et al., 2006; Kessler, Lane, Stang, & Van Brunt, 2009).

Early intervention prior to a preschooler's first major transition point to school can have an impact on the course of illness by altering a pernicious developmental trajectory in preschoolers with ADHD. A preschooler's early success or failure in adapting to school can set the stage for the child's future school behavior and his or her relationships with teachers and peers, as well as the quality of the parents' relationship with the teachers and schools. School connectedness has been shown to predict a variety of health outcomes (Thompson, Iachan, Overpeck, Ross, & Gross, 2006). Furthermore, there is evidence that the younger the child at the time of intervention, the more positive the child's behavioral adjustment at home and school and with peers (Boisjoli, Vitaro, Lacourse, Barker, & Tremblay, 2007; Strain, Steele, Ellis, & Timm, 1982).

Another treatment challenge is that even though psychosocial interventions are rec-ommended as the first-line treatment for preschool children with ADHD, psychosocial interventions may not be available to and/or preferred by many parents (Rappley et al., 1999). Parent behavior training and behavior management programs require a signifi-cant commitment of clinicians' and caregivers' time and effort. Lower compliance was reported with psychosocial intervention recommendations (58%) than for medication consultation (78%) in a study of 80 children between the ages of 5 and 13 years (Dreyer, O'Laughlin, Moore, & Milam, 2010). Only 25% of the parents attended more than four parent behavior training sessions in a study of kindergarteners (N = 158) with high rat-ings of hyperactive, impulsive, inattentive, and aggressive behavior (Barkley et al., 2000; Shelton et al., 2000). Practical and financial issues related to the availability of properly trained professionals in the community (Kaplan & Adesman, 2011) and difficulty with billing codes for parent behavior training delivered without the child being present or in a group setting (Emond et al., 2012) are other hindrances.

BENEFITS OF TREATMENT OF ADHD

Short-term benefits of treatment on ADHD symptoms have been reported and will be addressed in the section on evidence for pharmacologic treatments. Long-term benefits with pharmacologic treatment of ADHD have been reported in improving academic achievement in elementary school children (Scheffler et al., 2009), health-related qual-ity of life, and brain dysfunction in children and adolescents (Matza, Stoeckl, Shorr, & Johnston, 2006). Shaw and colleagues (2012) conducted a systematic review evaluating the treatment impact on the long-term outcome of ADHD. Untreated ADHD children followed over 2 to 9 years were reported to have significant impairment from baseline in academic outcomes (increased number of failing grades over 2 years and decline in math and reading scores over 9 years), peer rejection, and increase in tobacco use. Treatment of ADHD resulted in improved self-esteem, social function, academic out-comes, and drug use/addictive behaviors, and decreased service use (Shaw et al., 2012). There are no studies reporting on the long-term benefits of pharmacologic interven-tions in preschool children with ADHD.

Impact on brain development. There is evidence of a positive influence of therapeutic interventions on structural brain development (Luby et al., 2012), functional connectiv-ity between neural networks (Wong and Stevens, 2012), hypothalamic-pituitary-adrenal activity, and cognitive development (Nelson et al., 2007).

There are reports of neuroprotective and normalizing effects of stimulants in the treatment of ADHD in children and adolescents. Psychostimulant-treated children and adolescents with ADHD had similar rates of cortical thinning (Shaw et al., 2009) and larger right anterior cingulate volume (Semrud-Clikeman, Pliszka, Bledsoe, & Lancaster, 2012; Semrud-Clikeman, Pliszka, Lancaster, & Liotti, 2006) as age-matched healthy controls, compared to a more rapid cortical thinning and smaller right ante-rior cingulate volume (Semrud-Clikeman et al., 2006, 2012) in unmedicated ADHD children and adolescents. Strengthened connectivity of some of the frontoparietal regions on functional magnetic resonance imaging (fMRI) and improvements in a working memory performance task were seen with clinically effective doses of stimu-lants compared to placebo in children and adolescents with ADHD (Wong & Stevens,

2012). Brain activation during performance on an inhibition task was compared on a single MPH dose and placebo in 12 medication-naïve boys with ADHD, as well as in healthy age-matched controls, for potential normalization effects. During the MPH condition, ADHD boys showed significant upregulation and normalization effects in the underfunctioning inferior and ventromedial frontostriatal networks (Rubia, Halari, Mohammad, Taylor, & Brammer, 2011). MPH increased the resting theta-band activity over the left frontal region of the brain and was positively correlated with improvement in attention and decreased alpha activity in both hemispheres in a high-density magneto-encephalography (MEG) study (Wienbruch, Paul, Bauer, & Kivelitz, 2005).

Given the reports of neuroprotective benefits of pharmacologic interventions in ADHD in older children, we have had caregivers ask whether the purported improvements in brain development with pharmacologic agents can enhance the chances of normalizing their preschooler's developmental process. It is important to discuss with parents the preliminary nature of these findings in older children, as well as the fact that no specific information is available about the effects of stimulants on the brain development of preschool children or long-term safety in preschool children.

Impact on substance abuse. There are contradictory reports of the long-term impact of pharmacologic treatment of ADHD on stimulant abuse, cigarette smoking, and alcohol and substance abuse in children and adolescents. The recent 8-year follow-up of the MTA sample reported that substance use and substance use disorder were both greater in the ADHD than the non-ADHD samples. Medication for ADHD neither protected nor contributed to the risk of substance use or substance use disorder by adolescence (Molina et al., 2013). On the other hand, a reduced risk of cigarette smoking and alcohol and substance use disorders was reported with pharmacologic treatment of ADHD in other studies (Vazquez Marrufo, Vaquero, Cardoso, & Gomez, 2001; Wilson, Wetzel, White, & Knott, 2012). A recent report of neurobiologic similarities in ADHD and substance abuse-type cravings in positron emission tomography (PET) and fMRI studies suggests that treatment of ADHD may potentially reduce craving for substances and may also reduce the risk for relapse (Frodl, 2010).

IMPACT OF THE FDA MODERNIZATION ACT IN PROMOTING MEANINGFUL PHARMACOLOGIC RESEARCH IN PRESCHOOL CHILDREN

Even though pharmacologic agents are prescribed to treat ADHD in preschoolers, most ADHD medications are not approved by the U.S. Food and Drug Administration (FDA) for use in preschool children. The FDA Modernization Act was passed in 1997 to stimulate research to improve labeling of medications for children. The Modernization Act provided financial incentives to pharmaceutical firms to perform clinical trials in children by granting additional market exclusivity. Additional new regulations (the "Pediatric Rule") gave the FDA the authority to require that pediatric studies be conducted on drugs currently under development whenever a potential use in children can be anticipated (FDA, 1998). As a result, even though the number of medications with FDA-approved pediatric indication has increased, gaps still exist, especially for preschoolers. For example, a review of insurance databases for antihypertensive drug use in 2008 revealed that 29% of the drugs used in children younger than 6 years did not have an FDA indication for use in the younger age group (Welch, Yang, Taylor-Zapata, & Flynn, 2012). Analysis of the drugs granted pediatric exclusivity from 1998 to 2006 revealed that the majority of the 135 drugs granted pediatric exclusivity were rarely used in children. On the contrary, the pediatric studies to obtain market exclusivity did not include frequently used drugs in children. Market considerations, rather than the needs of patients, seem to drive the drugs selected for pediatric exclusivity studies, as suggested by the finding that many of the 135 included drugs were among the highest-selling medications in the United States in 2005 (Boots et al., 2007).

The clinical trials that led to the recent approval for indications of the transdermal, liquid, and beaded (beads can be sprinkled on food) formulations for ADHD did not include preschool children, even though these formulations are easier to administer to preschool children. Pharmaceutical companies have not been willing to fund investigations for treating ADHD in preschool children, citing the increased safety and medicolegal risks (personal communication). However, one wonders if another reason for their lack of interest stems from financial considerations, since ADHD drug utilization in preschoolers is a much smaller market share (Zuvekas & Vitiello, 2012) compared to school-age children, adolescents, and adults.

Evidence

EVIDENCE OF PHARMACOLOGIC TREATMENT OF ADHD IN PRESCHOOL CHILDREN

ADHD is characterized by frontosubcortical pathway dysfunction and dopaminergic and noradrenergic system imbalance. Stimulant and nonstimulant dopamine and norepinephrine transporter blockers are frequently used to treat ADHD and have been studied extensively in school-age children. In preschool children MPH is the most-used and most-studied pharmacologic agent for treatment of ADHD, with about 22 published reports of blinded and open-label studies. In contrast, there are one blinded and two open-label studies about the use of the nonstimulant atomoxetine, two case reports on the use of α_2-adrenergic agonists, and one case report on the use of the selective serotonin reuptake inhibitor fluoxetine in preschool children with ADHD.

STIMULANTS

In 1937, Charles Bradley first reported on the benefit of stimulants in improving the behavior of "delinquent children." Stimulants increase levels of norepinephrine and dopamine by facilitating their release in the prefrontal cortex. MPH blocks the reuptake of dopamine from the synaptic cleft by binding to the dopamine transporter. Amphetamines displace norepinephrine and dopamine from the presynaptic terminal storage sites into the synaptic cleft and block the action of a degradative enzyme, catechol-o-methyltransferase. Stimulants (with the exception of immediate-release amphetamines) are approved by the FDA to treat ADHD in children over 6 years of age. Immediate-release (IR) amphetamines are approved for children 3 years of age or older despite lack of empirical data on their efficacy and safety in such young children.

Stimulants are available in short-acting IR and long-acting delayed- or extended-release formulations and are considered first-line pharmacologic agents in the treatment of ADHD in school-age children. There are several double-blind, placebo-controlled trials providing evidence of efficacy and safety in children over 6 years of age.

Stimulant studies in preschool children. Stimulant studies in preschool children have mostly been conducted with IR formulations. The randomized controlled trials (RCTs) conducted prior to the PATS had small sample sizes, ranging from 11 to 59. Some of the studies included both preschool and older children with ADHD and did not provide specific and/or separate efficacy and safety outcome information for the preschool participants. The trial duration of the RCTs ranged from 3 to 9 weeks and stimulant dose ranged from 0.15 to 0.6 mg/kg. All but one of the RCTs evaluated the treatment response to MPH. The only study that included evaluation of amphetamine response was conducted by Short, Manos, Findling, and Schubel (2004) and compared preschool study participants' response to placebo and the best dose of either MPH (n = 22) or mixed amphetamine salts (n = 6). Most of the RCTs reported a positive response to the stimulant treatment. Response rates ranged from 80% to 93% in typically developing preschool children with ADHD (Conners, 1975; Greenhill et al., 2006; Short et al., 2004) and 71% to 73% in preschool children with developmental disorders (Ghuman, Aman, Lecavalier, et al., 2009; Ghuman et al., 2001; Handen, Feldman, Lurier, & Murray, 1999). One study by Schleifer and colleagues (1975) reported no improvement with MPH based on direct nursery school observations of the preschool participants.

Treatment emergent adverse events (TEAEs) of dysphoria, crying, whining, irritability, and solitary play were reported more frequently in the preschool participants than in older children (Ghuman et al., 2008). TEAEs reports were contradictory; Schleifer et al. (1975) reported TEAEs in 89%, whereas Conners (1975) and Barkley (1988) reported minimal or clinically negligible TEAEs in the preschool study participants. Short and colleagues (2004) cautioned that irritability, sadness, and crying may be associated with the disorder rather than resulting from medication management in the preschoolers. Rates of TEAEs ranged from 45% to 50% in preschool children with developmental disorders (Ghuman, Aman, Lecavalier, et al., 2009; Ghuman et al., 2001; Handen et al., 1999; Mayes, Crites, Bixler, Humphrey, & Mattison, 1994).

PATS. The NIMH-funded, six-center, multiphase, 70-week PATS is the largest trial and has become the landmark study for pharmacologic treatment of ADHD in preschool children. The PATS was designed to determine the short-term efficacy and safety and 10-month effectiveness and tolerability of IR MPH in preschoolers with ADHD. The PATS study sites were the Columbia University/New York State Psychiatric Institute, Duke University, Johns Hopkins University, New York University, the University of California Los Angeles, and the University of California Irvine.

The preschoolers had a DSM-IV-TR diagnosis of ADHD, combined or predominantly hyperactive subtype. The DSM-IV-TR diagnoses of ADHD and comorbid disorders were established using a multimethod and multistep approach. For screening purposes, parents completed a computer-assisted structured diagnostic interview, the Diagnostic Interview Schedule for Children Version 4.0–Parent Version (DISC-IV-P), conducted by a research assistant. The DISC-IV-P was followed by a semistructured psychiatric interview with the caregiver conducted by a child psychiatrist or a child psychologist. The PATS psychiatric interview included age-appropriate probes to systematically assess the presence of the DSM-IV-TR symptoms of ADHD and associated comorbid disorders. The ADHD symptom frequency was rated on a scale of 0 (never) to 5 (always) by the clinician; a score of 3 (often) or above was considered a clinically significant symptom (Posner et al., 2007). The ADHD symptoms were required to be present for a minimum of 9 months (Kollins et al., 2006). All areas of ADHD impairment, including home, school, peer relations, other settings, and physical risk and injury, were systematically assessed. All children were attending a preschool. The preschoolers had a hyperactive-impulsive subscale T score of 65 on both the parent and the teacher Conners Rating Scales-Revised (CRS-R) and a Children's Global Assessment scale (CGAS) impairment score of less than 55. Children with a diagnosis of adjustment disorder, pervasive developmental disorders, mental retardation, bipolar disorder, psychosis, or significant suicidality were excluded. A unanimous consensus vote of the PATS cross-site diagnostic panel was required to confirm the DSM-IV-TR diagnosis of ADHD and comorbid disorders and study eligibility.

Of the 303 eligible preschoolers, 279 entered and 261 completed 10 weeks of parent behavior training prior to MPH treatment. Following parent behavior training, 34 preschoolers discontinued the study because caregivers did not want medication for their preschooler or declined further study participation. Significant improvement (based on 30% or more reduction on the CPRS-R or CTRS-R or a Clinical Global Impression-Improvement [CGI-I] rating of less than "improved" by at least two of the three raters [parent, teacher, clinician] completing the CGI) with parent behavior training in 19 preschoolers made them ineligible to participate in the medication part of the study. Parents of 18 preschoolers were satisfied with the improvement with parent behavior training and did not want their child to take medication. Seven preschoolers were lost to follow-up.

Subsequently, 183 preschoolers were enrolled in the open-label safety lead-in phase and 11 preschoolers experienced moderate to severe TEAEs and were not eligible to enter the titration phase. An additional 21 preschoolers did not tolerate the highest IR MPH dose (7.5 mg MPH TID) and participated in a modified titration trial. A total of 165 preschoolers were randomized into a 5-week MPH titration trial and received 1 week each of MPH 1.25 mg TID, 2.5 mg TID, 5 mg TID, and 7.5 mg TID and placebo TID. Compared with placebo, significant decreases in ADHD symptoms were reported on the combined parent and teacher ratings with IR MPH doses of 2.5 mg TID ($p <.01$), 5 mg TID ($p <.001$), and 7.5 mg TID ($p <.001$), with effect sizes of 0.4 to 0.8. It is important to note that the preschoolers showed significant improvement on the 1.25-mg TID dose based on teacher ratings ($p <.02$) but not on parent ratings.

A subsequent parallel-group 4-week efficacy trial randomized 114 preschoolers to their best MPH dose (determined at the end of the titration trial) or placebo. Only 21% on the best MPH dose and 13% on placebo were rated as excellent responders and met the MTA-defined categorical criterion for remission. The mean optimal total IR MPH dose was 14 ± 8 mg/day (0.7 ± 0.4 mg/kg/day).

Fourteen PATS participants (4 to 5 years of age) and 9 school-age children (6 to 8 years of age) were enrolled in a laboratory analog classroom for a pharmacokinetic study. The preschoolers were found to metabolize MPH more slowly than school-age children after a single morning dose of IR MPH (Wigal et al., 2007). This is in contrast to the usual belief that hepatic activity is enhanced in the preschool developmental period, leading to more rapid metabolism of most medications (Cote, 2005).

The presence of comorbid disorders moderated MPH treatment response in the PATS. Preschoolers with no or one comorbid disorder (primarily oppositional defiant disorder) had a large treatment response with IR MPH 7.5 mg TID (Cohen's $d = 0.89$ and 1.00, respectively), similar to school-age children, and two comorbid disorders predicted a moderate treatment response (Cohen's $d = 0.56$), but preschoolers with three or more comorbid disorders did not benefit from IR MPH (Cohen's $d = -0.37$) (Ghuman et al., 2007). Additionally, there was a general increasing trend in family adversity with increasing numbers of comorbid disorders. Preschoolers with three or more comorbid disorders had comparatively fewer fathers who were employed, more families on welfare, fewer parents who were married, and more children living in single-caregiver homes. However, the small sample size limits the generalization of the findings, as there were only 15 preschoolers (9% of the sample) with three or more comorbid disorders compared to 150 preschoolers with two comorbid disorders (21% of the sample), one comorbid disorder (42% of the sample), or no comorbid disorders (28% of the sample).

Preschoolers were seen monthly for open-label medication follow-up visits for 10 months (n = 140). Improvement was maintained in symptom severity, general functioning, and social skills. The mean total IR MPH dose increased over the 10 months from 14 ± 8 mg/day (0.7 ± 0.4 mg/kg/day) to 20 ± 10 mg/day (0.92 ± 0.4 mg/kg/day) (Vitiello et al., 2007).

Thirty percent of the preschoolers experienced TEAEs, including reduced appetite, stomachache, difficulty falling asleep, and a reduction in growth velocity, similar to school-age children treated with MPH. Preschoolers continued to experience appetite loss, trouble sleeping, skin picking, and worried/anxious during the 10-month open-label follow-up (Vitiello et al., 2007). Additional TEAEs, especially at higher doses, were unique to preschoolers, including more irritability and mood changes and increased rates of social withdrawal and lethargy (Greenhill et al., 2006; Wigal et al., 2006), and decreased over time during the 10 months of open-label maintenance treatment. No significant differences in blood pressure and pulse rate were observed between placebo and active MPH treatment; transient, one-time elevations in blood pressure and pulse were reported in five children. No episodes of mania, hypomania, depression, or suicidality were reported.

Compared with the Centers for Disease Control and Prevention (CDC) norms, the preschool children with ADHD in the PATS were 2.0 cm taller and 1.8 kg heavier at baseline. A 20%-less-than-expected annual height gain (-1.38 cm/year) and a 55%-less-than-expected annual weight gain (-1.32 kg/year) were reported for the children who continued MPH for a year in the open-label follow-up phase (Swanson et al., 2006). Decrease in weight velocity was evident at the end of the 5-week double-blind crossover phase (Greenhill et al., 2006).

More preschoolers discontinued the study due to TEAEs with IR MPH during the open-label safety lead-in, efficacy, and maintenance phases than school-age children in the MTA. Complaints of increased crying, emotional outbursts, and irritability were the most common reasons for study discontinuation. Complaints of tics (eye blinking, mouth grimacing, and head jerking) were reported in five preschoolers, formication and nail biting and increased sucking and chewing on fingers in two preschoolers, drug withdrawal symptoms of increased emotionality and irritability in the evening while coming down from medication were reported in two preschoolers, one child had a possible seizure, and one preschooler developed rash on three separate occasions while taking MPH (Wigal et al., 2006). Other reasons for study discontinuation in the PATS included parent preference related to not wanting medications for their preschooler, satisfaction with the child's improvement in the parent training phase, and switching to long-acting stimulants in the continuation phase (Greenhill et al., 2006).

Even though the PATS is the largest RCT and was very carefully designed, several clinical questions remain unanswered. The parent behavior training program, the Community Parent Education model, used in the PATS was not validated in preschool children with ADHD and was not part of the original study design (Fanton & Gleason, 2009). Rather, it was added later as required by the ethics and safety monitoring review boards and was not designed to evaluate comparative efficacy of parent behavior training versus MPH or as a sequential or combination intervention.

The MPH doses used in the PATS were lower than used in school-age children in the MTA, with the upper limit placed at 10 mg TID. It is possible that some preschoolers may have done better at higher doses (Fanton & Gleason, 2009). On the other hand, many preschoolers may not be able to tolerate the higher doses (Ghuman, Aman, Lecavalier, et al., 2009).

Long-acting stimulants. Several long-acting stimulant formulations are available with proven efficacy in school-age children. However, there are no controlled studies of long-acting stimulant formulations in preschool children with ADHD. There are two open-label case series of using long-acting MPH formulations in preschool children with ADHD, the dl-MPH transdermal system (MTS) patch and the long-acting beaded MPH capsule (MPH LA).

The efficacy of MTS has been shown in many controlled trials in school-age children, but there are no controlled studies of MTS treatment in preschool children with ADHD. One open-label case series provides clinical support for its effectiveness (Ghuman et al., 2011). Three preschool boys (47, 53, and 67 months old) were treated openly with MTS in a naturalistic prospective manner (Ghuman et al., 2011). Due to lack of empirical guidance regarding MTS starting dose and titration schedule in preschool children, a very careful and slow MTS titration schedule was instituted. MTS was initiated with the 12.5-cm^2 patch size (with an estimated drug delivery rate of 1.1 mg/hour) with a wear time of 1 hour daily, increased by 1 hour every 2 to 3 days to a maximum of 9 hours daily. The dose was further increased to a patch size of 18.75 cm^2 (with an estimated drug delivery rate of 1.6 mg/hour) for 9 hours daily if needed and tolerated. All three children responded to MTS and tolerated a maximum daily MPH dose of 8 to 15 mg. TEAEs included poor appetite and irritability, crying, and whiny, especially when MTS was initiated, but they subsided (Ghuman et al., 2011).

MPH LA is a once-daily long-acting MPH formulation approved by the FDA for treating ADHD in children 6 years and older based on proven efficacy and safety in several RCTs (Biederman et al., 2003). There are no controlled studies of MPH LA in preschool children. Clinical effectiveness and tolerability of MPH LA was reported in 4- and 5-year-old children (N = 11) in an open-label pilot study. A once-daily dose of MPH LA was initiated at 10 mg each morning and increased to a maximum dose of 30 mg/day. If a child was not able to swallow the MPH LA capsule, parents were instructed to open the capsule and sprinkle the contents on food. The mean daily MPH LA dose was 17.73 mg; six children were treated with a dose of 20 mg/day and one child took 30 mg/day; the children on a dose of 10 mg/day were not able to tolerate the higher doses. Decreased appetite was the most common TEAE reported (it occurred in 64% of the children) and was persistent throughout the 4 weeks of the study. TEAEs of difficulty sleeping (27%) and emotional lability and stomachache (18%) abated by the end of 4 weeks. Three children discontinued the study due to TEAEs, including stomachache, vomiting, and irritability. For children who continued to take MPH LA after the open-label study was completed and were not able to tolerate titration at the lowest available dose of 10-mg increments, parents were instructed to open the capsule and administer half of the capsule contents (Maayan et al., 2009).

NONSTIMULANTS

Nonstimulants are usually considered second-line medications for ADHD in school-age children in case of an inadequate response to stimulants (Dulcan & Benson, 1997). Nonstimulant response is considered less robust than stimulant response (Shier, Reichenbacher, Ghuman, & Ghuman, 2012). Effect sizes were reported at 0.6 to 0.7 for most nonstimulants and 0.95 for stimulants in a meta-analysis of double-blind placebo-controlled ADHD treatment trials (Biederman & Faraone, 2005; Faraone, 2009). Two classes of nonstimulants, atomoxetine and α_2-adrenergic agonists, are the most common nonstimulants used in preschoolers with ADHD. Atomoxetine is the only nonstimulant medication that has a placebo-controlled RCT in 5- and 6-year-old children with ADHD; there are no controlled trials with α_2-adrenergic agonists.

Atomoxetine. Atomoxetine is a potent inhibitor of the presynaptic norepinephrine transporter with minimal affinity for other noradrenergic receptors or for other neurotransmitter transporters or receptors. It acts to increase levels of extracellular norepinephrine and dopamine in the prefrontal cortex but has a limited effect in the striatum. Atomoxetine is the first long-acting nonstimulant formulation with FDA approval for ADHD in individuals over 6 years of age. There are several double-blind, placebo-controlled trials showing its efficacy in children over 6 years of age and adults with ADHD.

The only controlled trial of atomoxetine was conducted in 5- and 6-year-old children with ADHD. One hundred one children were enrolled and 93 (mean age = 6.1 ± 0.6 years) completed an 8-week placebo and atomoxetine parallel-groups trial (Kratochvil et al., 2011). Atomoxetine was initiated at 0.5 mg/kg/day and titrated to 0.8 mg/kg/day, 1.2 mg/kg/day, 1.4 mg/kg/day, and a maximum dose of 1.8 mg/kg/day. Parent and teacher ratings on the ADHD Rating Scale showed improvement with atomoxetine, but the response was less robust, with effect sizes of 0.6 based on teacher ratings and 0.7 based on parent ratings. Many children experienced continued residual symptoms and functional impairment despite reduction in ADHD symptom ratings. The atomoxetine mean total daily dose was 1.4 mg/kg. TEAEs included mild to moderately severe gastrointestinal upset, reduced appetite, weight loss, and sedation (Kratochvil et al., 2011).

A prospective, naturalistic open-label atomoxetine treatment study was conducted in 12 preschool children with ADHD between the ages of 3 and 5 years (mean age = 5.0 ± 0.72 years). One study participant was 3½ years old, five were 4 years old, and six were 5 years old. Atomoxetine was initiated at 10 mg administered at bedtime and was titrated based on treatment response and if tolerated. Titration visits occurred at weekly intervals, and the dose was increased to 18 mg/day at week 2, 25 mg/day at week 3, 30 mg/day at week 4, 35 mg/day at week 5, and a maximum dose of 40 mg/day (1.8 mg/kg/day) at week 6. Maximum atomoxetine dose for children weighing less than 17 kg was limited to 30 mg/day. Atomoxetine was administered once daily at bedtime or in the morning or could be administered twice a day if a single daily dose resulted in adverse effects. The mean endpoint daily dose of atomoxetine was 31 ± 7.8 mg (range 20 to 40 mg/day) or 1.59 ± 0.3 mg/kg. At the completion of dose titration, children were maintained on their optimal dose for 4 weeks. About one third of the preschoolers were unable to swallow the atomoxetine capsules. Parents poured the contents of the capsules into a small amount of liquid. None of the parents reported any problem with eye irritation or refusal on their child's part to take atomoxetine due to unpleasant taste.

Atomoxetine treatment resulted in significant improvement from baseline on parent ratings of ADHD ($p < .0001$); 75% of the preschoolers were reported as positive responders. Approximately two thirds of the children experienced TEAEs. Gastrointestinal complaints of stomach upset, reduced appetite, vomiting, constipation/diarrhea, and/or increased thirst were the most common TEAEs, and complaints of irritability, defiance, and aggression were of most concern to the parents. Parents described the children as crying/whiny, grouchy/irritable, having increased frequency of tantrums, aggression, and agitation (Ghuman, Aman, Ghuman, et al., 2009).

A prospective open-label atomoxetine treatment study enrolled 5- and 6-year-old children with ADHD. Mean age of the children was 6.06 ± 0.58 years; 10 children were 5 years old and 12 were 6 years old. Improvement in hyperactive, impulsive, and inattentive symptoms was reported (Kratochvil et al., 2007). TEAEs included mood lability, reduced appetite, and weight loss; no child discontinued the study due to adverse events or lack of efficacy.

a$_2$*-Adrenergic agonists.* The α_2-adrenergic agonists guanfacine and clonidine are antihypertensive agents that act on presynaptic α_2-adrenoreceptors (α_{2A}, α_{2B}, and α_{2C}) in the prefrontal cortex to inhibit norepinephrine release and downregulate the noradrenergic system. Guanfacine is a selective α_{2A} adrenoreceptor agonist, whereas clonidine has relatively high affinity for all three α_2 adrenoreceptors. Even though the IR α_2-adrenergic agonists clonidine and guanfacine do not have FDA-approved indications for ADHD, they are often prescribed "off-label" for children with ADHD both as monotherapy and in combination with stimulants (Hazell & Stuart, 2003; Hunt, Minderaa, & Cohen, 1985). Response to α_2-adrenergic agonists is less robust, with an effect size of 0.58 for clonidine compared to an effect size of 0.82 for stimulants (Connor, Fletcher, & Swanson, 1999).

In addition to IR tablets, clonidine is also available as sustained-release capsules and a transdermal patch. Clonidine is more sedating than guanfacine and is often prescribed to treat insomnia in children with ADHD or insomnia related to stimulant side effects. Recently, long-acting clonidine and guanfacine were approved by the FDA to treat ADHD as monotherapy and as adjunctive treatment to stimulants in children over 6 years of age (Biederman et al., 2008; Connor et al., 2010; Jain, Segal, Kollins, & Khayrallah, 2011; Kollins et al., 2011; Sallee, Kollins, & Wigal, 2012; Sallee, Lyne, Wigal,

& McGough, 2009; Sallee, McGough, et al., 2009; Spencer, Greenbaum, Ginsberg, & Murphy, 2009). However, there are no controlled studies of IR or long-acting α_2-adrenergic agonists in preschool children with ADHD. There is one published case report of open-label treatment with guanfacine in four 2- and 3-year-old children with ADHD (Lee, 1997). Guanfacine improved hyperactive, impulsive, aggressive, and destructive behaviors. There is a case report of clonidine treatment in one 4-year-old child infected with human immunodeficiency virus type 1 who had a sudden onset of impulsivity, hyperactivity, aggressive behavior, and initial insomnia (Cesena, Lee, Cebollero, & Steingard, 1995). Improvement in sleep, hyperactivity, and impulsivity was reported with a clonidine dose of 0.025 mg TID (Cesena et al., 1995; Lee, 1997).

Selective serotonin reuptake inhibitors. Selective serotonin reuptake inhibitors do not have an FDA indication for treatment of ADHD. However, they have been prescribed in preschool children with ADHD (Rappley et al., 1999). There is one published case report of open-label treatment with fluoxetine in a 3-year-old boy with ADHD, defiance, anger outbursts, and aggression. Previous trials with MPH 7.5 mg TID over several weeks followed by thioridazine 12.5 mg BID and 25 mg at bedtime had not been successful. The fluoxetine trial was initiated with 5 mg in the morning and eventually increased to 10 mg as it was felt that the child had ADHD and comorbid depression. Improvement in attention span and more appropriate social interactions were observed and no significant adverse effects were reported (Campbell, Tamburrino, Evans, & Franco, 1995).

SPECIAL PHARMACOLOGIC TREATMENT CONSIDERATIONS: PRESCHOOLERS WITH DEVELOPMENTAL DISORDERS

Even though pervasive developmental disorders (PDDs) are included as exclusionary criteria for the DSM-IV-TR diagnosis of ADHD (proposed to be removed in the DSM-5 ADHD diagnostic criteria), symptoms of ADHD are very common in children with PDDs and intellectual disability (APA, 2000; Lecavalier, 2006). Stimulants are frequently prescribed to treat ADHD in school-age children with PDD and intellectual disability; however, the response rate is lower (50% to 60%) compared to typically developing children with ADHD, and the rate of TEAEs is higher (Aman, Buican, & Arnold, 2003; Elia, Borcherding, Rapoport, & Keysor, 1991; RUPP Autism Network, 2005; Spencer et al., 1996). The lower stimulant response rate in PDD and intellectual disability is compounded in preschool children since typically developing preschoolers with ADHD also have a lower and less robust response to stimulants (Greenhill et al., 2006).

Stimulant efficacy for ADHD symptoms in preschool children with PDD and intellectual disability has been studied. Fourteen preschoolers (mean age = 4.8 ± 1.0 years; age range 3.0 to 5.9 years) diagnosed with PDD (n = 12) and/or intellectual disability (n = 2) and symptoms of hyperactivity, impulsivity, and inattention participated in a placebo-controlled IR MPH short-term crossover efficacy trial (Ghuman, Aman, Lecavalier, et al., 2009). Parent-rated ADHD symptoms improved with IR MPH administered BID compared to placebo ($p = .002$). Positive response to IR MPH was reported in 50% of the preschoolers (effect size of 0.5), similar to school-age children with PDDs (RUPP Autism Network, 2005) and typically developing ADHD preschoolers with two or more comorbid disorders (Ghuman et al., 2007). The lower stimulant response in preschool children with PDD and intellectual disability is not surprising given the reports of a lower ADHD treatment response in children with higher comorbidity (Ghuman et al., 2007; Owens et al., 2003). PDD and/or intellectual disability and associated communication disorder, in addition to "ADHD," in preschoolers with PDD and/or intellectual disability could be akin to having two or more "comorbid disorders" as in typically developing ADHD preschoolers in the PATS.

Similar to older children with PDD and/or intellectual disability (Aman et al., 2003; RUPP Autism Network, 2005), TEAEs with MPH were reported more frequently occurring in 50% of the preschoolers; one child discontinued the study due to dysphoria, crying, and whining. The MPH TEAEs included increased stereotypic and repetitive behavior, upset stomach, sleep-related difficulties, and emotional lability, similar to typically developing preschoolers treated with MPH (Greenhill et al., 2006).

TEAEs limited upward dose adjustments in the preschoolers with PDD and/or intellectual disability. The average IR MPH dose was 15 mg/day (0.76 ± 0.3 mg/kg/day), and many children had residual symptoms and impairment. Even then, parents and teachers were happy with the modest improvement in the children's behavior. They felt that the children's behavior was more manageable and the children were better able to participate in educational settings and various recommended therapies.

A placebo-controlled MPH study in preschoolers with intellectual disability (preschoolers with PDD were excluded) reported improvement in ADHD symptoms in 8 of the 11 preschoolers (Handen et al., 1999). Adverse effects included social withdrawal, increased crying, and irritability, especially at the higher dose (0.6 mg/kg BID).

PRESCHOOLERS WITH PILL-SWALLOWING DIFFICULTIES

Preschool children often have difficulty swallowing pills and may have difficulty taking the commonly available ADHD medication formulations in the form of tablets or capsules (Beck, Cataldo, Slifer, Pulbrook, & Ghuman, 2005; Ghuman, Cataldo, Beck, & Slifer, 2004). We have published step-by-step instructions to teach preschool children how to swallow pills (Beck et al., 2005; Ghuman et al., 2004). This is a brief behavioral instruction by practicing swallowing increasing sizes of cake decorations (Beck et al., 2005; Ghuman et al., 2004). The available transdermal (MTS and clonidine patch), liquid (methylin), and beaded formulations (e.g., MPH LA, MPH CD, d-MPH ER, dextroamphetamine Spansules, and extended-release mixed amphetamine salts capsules can be opened and sprinkled on food) may provide alternative treatment options for preschool children with pill-swallowing difficulties.

Clinical Recommendations

1. The available evidence base for ADHD treatment modalities in preschoolers is stronger for psychosocial interventions than for psychopharmacologic interventions and/or alternative treatments.
2. Professional guidelines for treatment of ADHD in preschool children (AACAP-PPWG and AAP) call for a trial of appropriate psychosocial treatment (parent behavior management training or other evidence-based behavioral intervention) first.

2.1. Psychosocial treatment should be of adequate duration (AACAP-PPWG recommends a minimum of 5 weeks and AAP recommends a 10- to 14-week course).

2.2. If the child is not attending a preschool, consider recommending enrolling the child in a preschool program to provide opportunities for appropriate peer interaction and learning socially accepted behavioral norms.

3. Psychopharmacologic intervention may be considered if evidence-based behavioral treatments are not available and/or preferred by parents.

4. In most circumstances, psychopharmacologic intervention should be considered only if adequate control of symptoms is not achieved despite a trial of psychosocial treatment.

5. Pharmacologic intervention should always be provided concurrently with psychosocial treatments.

5.1. The AAP guidelines recommend that pharmacologic treatment should be considered only in children 4 years of age or older. The UK-NICE guidelines recommend pharmacologic treatment only in children 5 years of age or older.

6. Psychopharmacologic intervention may be considered if the preschooler experiences moderate to severe disturbance in functioning, as indicated by:

6.1. ADHD symptom duration of 9 months or longer

6.2. Clear impairment in both the home and the daycare/preschool settings

6.3. History of repeated expulsions (or threatened expulsion) from preschool or nursery/daycare

6.4. Accidental injury to the child, other children, or caregivers

6.5. Inability to participate in or benefit from other interventions

7. Keep in mind that for pharmacologic treatment:

7.1. A conservative titration strategy is recommended with treatment initiation at a low dose and titration at a relatively slower pace.

7.2. Preschoolers have more frequent TEAEs, especially at higher doses, and have a unique adverse event profile.

7.2.1. Lower optimal dose may limit robustness of response in preschoolers.

7.3. The presence of comorbid disorders moderates clinical response.

7.4. In preschool children with PDD and intellectual disability, the pharmacologic treatment response is less robust and TEAEs are more frequent.

7.5. Many preschoolers have difficulty swallowing pills and may need treatment with alternative formulations.

Summary

The PATS has provided evidence for the short-term efficacy and safety of IR MPH in preschool children with ADHD. A less robust response and lower response rates are reported compared to school-age children. Preschoolers have difficulty tolerating higher doses and have a unique adverse effect profile, including more irritability and mood changes. There are no controlled trials of long-acting stimulant formulations. There are two open-label case reports, one each for MTS and MPH LA, showing clinical effectiveness and tolerability in preschool children with ADHD.

One controlled and two open-label studies are available regarding the effectiveness and tolerability of one nonstimulant, atomoxetine, in preschool children with ADHD indicating benefit. The response is reported to be less robust, and gastrointestinal complaints are the most common TEAEs reported. Only two case reports of the use of IR α_2-adrenergic agonists for the treatment of ADHD in preschoolers are available; no information is available on the use of long-acting α_2-adrenergic agonists. In the community, α_2-adrenergic agonists are commonly prescribed in preschoolers with ADHD, as monotherapy or more frequently concomitantly with stimulants, especially if there are complaints about aggressive behavior, tics, or sleep difficulties.

Despite improvements in core ADHD symptoms with pharmacologic agents, improvements in long-term interpersonal relationships, which are important in predicting outcomes for children with disruptive behaviors, have not been shown (Coie & Dodge, 1998; Pelham, Wheeler, & Chronis, 1998; Rubin et al., 2006). Moreover, information is not available about long-term safety and the effects of psychopharmacologic agents on brain development in preschool children. Hence, caution is needed when considering pharmacologic treatments in preschool children with ADHD (Ghuman et al., 2008).

Psychosocial interventions should always be implemented as first-line treatment in preschoolers with ADHD. Pharmacologic treatments, if indicated, should always be administered concomitantly with psychosocial interventions. However, there are times when parents may have difficulty in implementing psychosocial interventions and/ or the severity of the ADHD symptoms may require immediate attention. In such circumstances, pharmacologic interventions may be prescribed first. With the resulting improvements in the child's attention, compliance, and disruptive behaviors, it may be easier to implement psychosocial interventions, and the parents may, in turn, become more amenable and accepting of psychosocial interventions.

More research is needed to find the best possible treatments matched with parent preferences. Given the safety concerns with pharmacologic treatments and the lack of information regarding the short- and long-term impact of pharmacologic agents on the developing brains of preschool children, there is an urgent need for comparative, sequential and/or combined efficacy and safety of pharmacologic, psychosocial, and alternative treatments in well-characterized samples of preschool children with ADHD.

Disclosures

Jaswinder K. Ghuman, M.D., has received past funding from the NIMH for a K-23 career development grant, the Arizona Institute for Mental Health Research, and from Bristol-Myers Squibb for a clinical trial in autistic disorder. She received funding from the Health Resources and Services Administration–Maternal and Child Health (HRSA-MCH) for a training grant for the University of Arizona Leadership Education in Neurodevelopmental Disabilities Training Program (AZLEND).

Harinder S. Ghuman, M.D., has no conflicts of interest.

References

AAP. (2011). ADHD: clinical practice guideline for the diagnosis, evaluation, and treatment of attention-deficit/hyperactivity disorder in children and adolescents. *Pediatrics, 128*(5), 1007–1022.

Aman, M. G., Buican, B., & Arnold, L. E. (2003). Methylphenidate treatment in children with borderline IQ and mental retardation: analysis of three aggregated studies. *Journal of Child & Adolescent Psychopharmacology, 13*(1), 29–40.

APA. (2000). *Diagnostic and statistical manual of mental disorders, text revision* (DSM-IV-TR).Washington, DC: American Psychiatric Association.

Barkley, R. A. (1988). The effects of methylphenidate on the interactions of preschool ADHD children with their mothers. *Journal of the American Academy of Child & Adolescent Psychiatry, 27*(3), 336–341.

Barkley, R. A. (1998). Attention-deficit hyperactivity disorder. *Scientific American, 279*(3), 66–71.

Barkley, R. A., Shelton, T. L., Crosswait, C., Moorehouse, M., Fletcher, K., Barrett, S., et al. (2000). Multi-method psycho-educational intervention for preschool children with disruptive behavior: preliminary results at post-treatment. *Journal of Child Psychology & Psychiatry, 41*(3), 319–332.

Beck, M. H., Cataldo, M., Slifer, K. J., Pulbrook, V., & Ghuman, J. K. (2005). Teaching children with attention deficit hyperactivity disorder (ADHD) and autistic disorder (AD) how to swallow pills. *Clinical Pediatrics, 44*(6), 515.

Biederman, J., & Faraone, S. V. (2005). Attention-deficit hyperactivity disorder. *Lancet, 366*(9481), 237–248.

Biederman, J., Melmed, R., Patel, A., McBurnett, K., Konow, J., Lyne, A., et al. (2008). A randomized, double-blind, placebo-controlled study of guanfacine extended release in children and adolescents with attention-deficit/hyperactivity disorder. *Pediatrics, 121*(1), e73–84.

Biederman, J., Quinn, D., Weiss, M., Markabi, S., Weidenman, M., Edson, K., et al. (2003). Efficacy and safety of Ritalin LA, a new, once daily, extended-release dosage form of methylphenidate, in children with attention deficit hyperactivity disorder. *Paediatric Drugs, 5*(12), 833–841.

Boisjoli, R., Vitaro, F., Lacourse, E., Barker, E. D., & Tremblay, R. E. (2007). Impact and clinical significance of a preventive intervention for disruptive boys: 15-year follow-up. *British Journal of Psychiatry, 191*, 415–419.

Boots, I., Sukhai, R. N., Klein, R. H., Holl, R. A., Wit, J. M., Cohen, A. F., et al. (2007). Stimulation programs for pediatric drug research—do children really benefit? *European Journal of Pediatrics, 166*(8), 849–855.

Breggin, P. R. (2000). The psychiatric drugging of toddlers. *Ethical Human Sciences and Services, 2*(2), 83–86.

Campbell, N. B., Tamburrino, M. B., Evans, C. L., & Franco, K. N. (1995). Fluoxetine for ADHD in a young child. *Journal of the American Academy of Child & Adolescent Psychiatry, 34*(10), 1259–1260.

Cesena, M., Lee, D. O., Cebollero, A. M., & Steingard, R. J. (1995). Case study: behavioral symptoms of pediatric HIV-1 encephalopathy successfully treated with clonidine. *Journal of the American Academy of Child & Adolescent Psychiatry, 34*(3), 302–306.

Coie, J. D., & Dodge, K. A. (1998). Aggression and antisocial behavior. In W. D. N. Eisenberg (Ed.), *Handbook of child psychology* (5th ed., Vol. 3, pp. 779–862). New York: Wiley.

Conners, C. K. (1975). Controlled trial of methylphenidate in preschool children with minimal brain dysfunction. *International Journal of Mental Health, 4*(1-2), 61–74.

Connor, D., Findling, R., Kollins, S., Sallee, F., Lopez, F., Lyne, A., et al. (2010). Effects of guanfacine extended release on oppositional symptoms in children aged 6-12 years with attention-deficit hyperactivity disorder and oppositional symptoms: a randomized, double-blind, placebo-controlled trial. *CNS, 24*(9), 755–768.

Connor, D., Fletcher, K., & Swanson, J. (1999). A meta-analysis of clonidine for symptoms of attention-deficit hyperactivity disorder. *Journal of the American Academy of Child & Adolescent Psychiatry, 38*(12), 1551–1559.

Cote, C. J. (2005) Pediatric anesthesia. In: R. D. Miller (Ed.), *Miller's anesthesia*, 6th ed. Philadelphia: Elsevier.

Coyle, J. (1997). Biochemical development of the brain: neurotransmitters and child psychiatry. In C. Popper (Ed.), *Psychiatric pharmacosciences of children and adolescents* (pp. 3–25). Washington, DC.

Crandall, J. E., McCarthy, D. M., Araki, K. Y., Sims, J. R., Ren, J. Q., & Bhide, P. G. (2007). Dopamine receptor activation modulates GABA neuron migration from the basal forebrain to the cerebral cortex. *Journal of Neuroscience, 27*(14), 3813–3822.

Dreyer, A. S., O'Laughlin, L., Moore, J., & Milam, Z. (2010). Parental adherence to clinical recommendations in an ADHD evaluation clinic. *Journal of Clinical Psychology, 66*(10), 1101–1120.

Dulcan, M. K., & Benson, R. S. (1997). AACAP Official Action. Summary of the practice parameters for the assessment and treatment of children, adolescents, and adults with ADHD. *Journal of the American Academy of Child & Adolescent Psychiatry, 36*(9), 1311–1317.

Egger, H. L., Kondo, D., & Angold, A. (2006). The epidemiology and diagnostic issues in preschool attention-deficit/ hyperactivity disorder: A review. *Infants & Young Children, 19*(2), 109–122.

Elia, J., Borcherding, B. G., Rapoport, J. L., & Keysor, C. S. (1991). Methylphenidate and dextroamphetamine treatments of hyperactivity: are there true nonresponders? *Psychiatry Research, 36*(2), 141–155.

Emond, S. K., Ollendorf, D. A., Colby, J. A., Reed, S. J., & Pearson, S. D. (2012). Management strategies for attention-deficit/hyperactivity disorder: a regional deliberation on the evidence. *Postgraduate Medicine, 124*(5), 58–68.

Fanton, J., & Gleason, M. M. (2009). Psychopharmacology and preschoolers: a critical review of current conditions. *Child & Adolescent Psychiatric Clinics of North America, 18*(3), 753–771.

Faraone, S. V. (2009). Using meta-analysis to compare the efficacy of medications for attention-deficit/hyperactivity disorder in youths. *Pharmacy & Therapeutics, 34*(12), 678–694.

FDA. (1998). Regulations requiring manufacturers to assess the safety and effectiveness of new drugs and biological products in pediatric patients: final rule. *Federal Register* (63), 66631–66672.

Frodl, T. (2010). Comorbidity of ADHD and substance use disorder (SUD): a neuroimaging perspective. *Journal of Attention Disorders, 14*, 109–120.

Ghuman, J. K., Aman, M. G., Ghuman, H. S., Reichenbacher, T., Gelenberg, A., Wright, R., et al. (2009). Prospective, naturalistic, pilot study of open-label atomoxetine treatment in preschool children with attention-deficit/hyperactivity disorder. *Journal of Child & Adolescent Psychopharmacology, 19*(2), 155–166.

Ghuman, J. K., Aman, M. G., Lecavalier, L., Riddle, M. A., Gelenberg, A., Wright, R., et al. (2009). Randomized, placebo-controlled, crossover study of methylphenidate for attention-deficit/ hyperactivity disorder symptoms in preschoolers with developmental disorders. *Journal of Child & Adolescent Psychopharmacology, 19*(4), 329–339.

Ghuman, J. K., Arnold, L. E., & Anthony, B. J. (2008). Psychopharmacological and other treatments in preschool children with attention-deficit/hyperactivity disorder: current evidence and practice. *Journal of Child & Adolescent Psychopharmacology, 18*(5), 413–447.

Ghuman, J. K., Byreddy, S., & Ghuman, H. S. (2011). Methylphenidate transdermal system in preschool children with attention-deficit/hyperactivity disorder. *Journal of Child & Adolescent Psychopharmacology, 21*(5), 495–498.

Ghuman, J. K., Cataldo, M. D., Beck, M. H., & Slifer, K. J. (2004). Behavioral training for pill-swallowing difficulties in young children with autistic disorder. *Journal of Child and Adolescent Psychopharmacology, 14*(4), 601–611.

Ghuman, J. K., Ginsburg, G. S., Subramaniam, G., Ghuman, H. S., Kau, A. S., & Riddle, M. A. (2001). Psychostimulants in preschool children with attention-deficit/hyperactivity disorder: clinical evidence from a developmental disorders institution. *Journal of the American Academy of Child & Adolescent Psychiatry, 40*(5), 516–524.

Ghuman, J. K., Riddle, M. A., Vitiello, B., Greenhill, L. L., Chuang, S. Z., Wigal, S. B., et al. (2007). Comorbidity moderates response to methylphenidate in the Preschoolers with

Attention-deficit/Hyperactivity Disorder Treatment Study (PATS). *Journal of Child and Adolescent Psychopharmacology, 17*(5), 563–580.

Gleason, M. M., Egger, H. L., Emslie, G. J., Greenhill, L. L., Kowatch, R. A., Lieberman, A. F., et al. (2007). Psychopharmacological treatment for very young children: contexts and guidelines. *Journal of the American Academy of Child & Adolescent Psychiatry, 46*(12), 1532–1572.

Greenhill, L., Kollins, S., Abikoff, H., McCracken, J., Riddle, M., Swanson, J., et al. (2006). Efficacy and safety of immediate-release methylphenidate treatment for preschoolers with ADHD. *Journal of the American Academy of Child & Adolescent Psychiatry, 45*(11), 1284–1293.

Handen, B. L., Feldman, H. M., Lurier, A., & Murray, P. J. (1999). Efficacy of methylphenidate among preschool children with developmental disabilities and ADHD. *Journal of the American Academy of Child & Adolescent Psychiatry, 38*(7), 805–812.

Hazell, P. L., & Stuart, J. E. (2003). A randomized controlled trial of clonidine added to psychostimulant medication for hyperactive and aggressive children. *Journal of the American Academy of Child & Adolescent Psychiatry, 42*(8), 886–894.

Hunt, R. D., Minderaa, R. B., & Cohen, D. J. (1985). Clonidine benefits children with attention deficit disorder and hyperactivity: report of a double-blind placebo-crossover therapeutic trial. *Journal of the American Academy of Child & Adolescent Psychiatry, 24*(5), 617–629.

Jain, R., Segal, S., Kollins, S. H., & Khayrallah, M. (2011). Clonidine extended-release tablets for pediatric patients with attention-deficit/hyperactivity disorder. *Journal of the American Academy of Child & Adolescent Psychiatry, 50*(2), 171–179.

Kaplan, A., & Adesman, A. (2011). Clinical diagnosis and management of attention deficit hyperactivity disorder in preschool children. *Current Opinion Pediatrics, 23*(6), 684–692.

Kendall, T., Taylor, E., Perez, A., & Taylor, C. (2008). Diagnosis and management of attention-deficit/hyperactivity disorder in children, young people, and adults: summary of NICE guidance. *BMJ, 337*, a1239.

Kessler, R. C., Lane, M., Stang, P. E., & Van Brunt, D. L. (2009). The prevalence and workplace costs of adult attention deficit hyperactivity disorder in a large manufacturing firm. *Psychological Medicine, 39*(1), 137–147.

Kollins, S. H., Jain, R., Brams, M., Segal, S., Findling, R. L., Wigal, S. B., et al. (2011). Clonidine extended-release tablets as add-on therapy to psychostimulants in children and adolescents with ADHD. *Pediatrics, 127*(6), e1406–1413.

Kollins, S., Greenhill, L., Swanson, J., Wigal, S., Abikoff, H., McCracken, J., et al. (2006). Rationale, design, and methods of the Preschool ADHD Treatment Study (PATS). *Journal of the American Academy of Child & Adolescent Psychiatry, 45*(11), 1275–1283.

Kratochvil, C. J., Vaughan, B. S., Mayfield-Jorgensen, M. L., March, J. S., Kollins, S. H., Murray, D. W., et al. (2007). A pilot study of atomoxetine in young children with attention-deficit/hyperactivity disorder. *Journal of Child & Adolescent Psychopharmacology, 17*(2), 175–186.

Kratochvil, C. J., Vaughan, B. S., Stoner, J. A., Daughton, J. M., Lubberstedt, B. D., Murray, D. W., et al. (2011). A double-blind, placebo-controlled study of atomoxetine in young children with ADHD. *Pediatrics, 127*(4), e862–868.

Lavigne, J. V., Arend, R., Rosenbaum, D., Binns, H. J., Christoffel, K. K., Burns, A., et al. (1998). Mental health service use among young children receiving pediatric primary care. *Journal of the American Academy of Child & Adolescent Psychiatry, 37*(11), 1175–1183.

Lecavalier, L. (2006). Behavioral and emotional problems in young people with pervasive developmental disorders: relative prevalence, effects of subject characteristics, and empirical classification. *Journal of Autism & Development Disorders, 36*(8), 1101–1114.

Lee, B. J. (1997). Clinical experience with guanfacine in 2- and 3-year-old children with attention deficit hyperactivity disorder. *Infant Mental Health, 18*, 300–305.

Lindemann, C., Langner, I., Kraut, A. A., Banaschewski, T., Schad-Hansjosten, T., Petermann, U., et al. (2012). Age-specific prevalence, incidence of new diagnoses, and drug treatment of attention-deficit/hyperactivity disorder in Germany. *Journal of Child & Adolescent Psychopharmacology, 22*(4), 307–314.

Luby, J. L., Barch, D. M., Belden, A., Gaffrey, M. S., Tillman, R., Babb, C., et al. (2012). Maternal support in early childhood predicts larger hippocampal volumes at school age. *Proceedings of the National Academy of Science USA, 109*(8), 2854–2859.

Maayan, L., Paykina, N., Fried, J., Strauss, T., Gugga, S. S., & Greenhill, L. (2009). The open-label treatment of attention-deficit/hyperactivity disorder in 4- and 5-year-old children with beaded methylphenidate. *Journal of Child & Adolescent Psychopharmacology, 19*(2), 147–153.

Matza, L. S., Stoeckl, M. N., Shorr, J. M., & Johnston, J. A. (2006). Impact of atomoxetine on health-related quality of life and functional status in patients with ADHD. *Expert Review of Pharmacoeconomics & Outcomes Research, 6*(4), 379–390.

Mayes, S. D., Crites, D. L., Bixler, E. O., Humphrey, F. J., 2nd, & Mattison, R. E. (1994). Methylphenidate and ADHD: influence of age, IQ and neurodevelopmental status. *Developmental Medicine & Child Neurology, 36*(12), 1099–1107.

Minde, K. (1998). The use of psychotropic medication in preschoolers: Some recent developments. *Canadian Journal of Psychiatry-Revue Canadienne de Psychiatrie, 43*(6), 571–575.

Molina, B. S., Hinshaw, S. P., Eugene Arnold, L., Swanson, J. M., Pelham, W. E., Hechtman, L., et al. (2013). Adolescent substance use in the multimodal treatment study of Attention-Deficit/Hyperactivity Disorder (ADHD) (MTA) as a function of childhood ADHD, random assignment to childhood treatments, and subsequent medication. *Journal of the American Academy of Child & Adolescent Psychiatry, 52*(3), 250–263.

Nelson, C. A., 3rd, Zeanah, C. H., Fox, N. A., Marshall, P. J., Smyke, A. T., & Guthrie, D. (2007). Cognitive recovery in socially deprived young children: the Bucharest Early Intervention Project. *Science, 318*(5858), 1937–1940.

Olfson, M., Crystal, S., Huang, C., & Gerhard, T. (2010). Trends in antipsychotic drug use by very young, privately insured children. *Journal of the American Academy of Child & Adolescent Psychiatry, 49*(1), 13–23.

Owens, E. B., Hinshaw, S. P., Kraemer, H. C., Arnold, L. E., Abikoff, H. B., Cantwell, D. P., et al. (2003). Which treatment for whom for ADHD? Moderators of treatment response in the MTA. *Journal of Consulting Clinical Psychology, 71*(3), 540–552.

Pelham, W. E., Jr., Wheeler, T., & Chronis, A. (1998). Empirically supported psychosocial treatments for attention deficit hyperactivity disorder. *Journal of Clinical Child Psychology, 27*(2), 190–205.

Pliszka, S. (2007). Practice parameter for the assessment and treatment of children and adolescents with attention-deficit/hyperactivity disorder. *Journal of the American Academy of Child & Adolescent Psychiatry, 46*(7), 894–921.

Posner, K., Melvin, G. A., Murray, D. W., Gugga, S. S., Fisher, P., Skrobala, A., et al. (2007). Clinical presentation of attention-deficit/hyperactivity disorder in preschool children: the Preschoolers with Attention-Deficit/Hyperactivity Disorder Treatment Study (PATS). *Journal of Child & Adolescent Psychopharmacology, 17*(5), 547–562.

Pringsheim, T., Lam, D., & Patten, S. B. (2011). The pharmacoepidemiology of antipsychotic medications for Canadian children and adolescents: 2005–2009. *Journal of Child & Adolescent Psychopharmacology, 21*(6), 537–543.

Rappley, M. D., Eneli, I. U., Mullan, P. B., Alvarez, F. J., Wang, J., Luo, Z., et al. (2002). Patterns of psychotropic medication use in very young children with attention-deficit hyperactivity disorder. *Journal of Developmental & Behavioral Pediatrics, 23*(1), 23–30.

Rappley, M. D., Mullan, P. B., Alvarez, F. J., Eneli, I. U., Wang, J., & Gardiner, J. C. (1999). Diagnosis of attention-deficit/hyperactivity disorder and use of psychotropic medication in very young children. *Archives of Pediatric & Adolescent Medicine, 153*(10), 1039–1045.

Rubia, K., Halari, R., Mohammad, A. M., Taylor, E., & Brammer, M. (2011). Methylphenidate normalizes frontocingulate underactivation during error processing in attention-deficit/hyperactivity disorder. *Biological Psychiatry, 70*(3), 255–262.

Rubin, K. H., Bukowski, W. M., Parker, J. G., Eisenberg, N., Damon, W., & Lerner, R. M. (2006). Peer interactions, relationships, and groups. In *Handbook of child psychology: Vol. 3, Social, emotional, and personality development* (6th ed., pp. 571–645). John Wiley & Sons Inc.

RUPP Autism Network. (2005). Randomized, controlled, crossover trial of methylphenidate in pervasive developmental disorders with hyperactivity. *Archives of General Psychiatry, 62*(11), 1266–1274.

Sallee, F. R., Kollins, S. H., & Wigal, T. L. (2012). Efficacy of guanfacine extended release in the treatment of combined and inattentive only subtypes of attention-deficit/hyperactivity disorder. *Journal of Child and Adolescent Psychopharmacology, 22*(3), 206–214.

Sallee, F., Lyne, A., Wigal, T., & McGough, J. (2009). Long-term safety and efficacy of guanfacine extended release in children and adolescents with attention-deficit/hyperactivity disorder. *Journal of Child & Adolescent Psychopharmacology, 19*(3), 215–226.

Sallee, F., McGough, J., Wigal, T., Donahue, J., Lyne, A., & Biederman, J. (2009). Guanfacine extended release in children and adolescents with attention-deficit/hyperactivity disorder: a placebo-controlled trial. *Journal of the American Academy of Child & Adolescent Psychiatry, 48*(2), 155–165.

Scheffler, R. M., Brown, T. T., Fulton, B. D., Hinshaw, S. P., Levine, P., & Stone, S. (2009). Positive association between attention-deficit/hyperactivity disorder medication use and academic achievement during elementary school. *Pediatrics, 123*(5), 1273–1279.

Schleifer, M., Weiss, G., Cohen, N., Elman, M., Cvejic, H., & Kruger, E. (1975). Hyperactivity in pre-schoolers and effect of methylphenidate. *American Journal of Orthopsychiatry, 45*(1), 38–50.

Semrud-Clikeman, M., Pliszka, S. R., Lancaster, J., & Liotti, M. (2006). Volumetric MRI differences in treatment-naive vs. chronically treated children with ADHD. *Neurology, 67*(6), 1023–1027.

Semrud-Clikeman, M., Pliszka, S., Bledsoe, J., & Lancaster, J. (2012). Volumetric MRI differences in treatment-naive and chronically treated adolescents with ADHD-combined type. *Journal of Attention Disorders* [epub May 31, 2012].

Shaw, M., Hodgkins, P., Caci, H., Young, S., Kahle, J., Woods, A. G., et al. (2012). A systematic review and analysis of long-term outcomes in attention deficit hyperactivity disorder: effects of treatment and non-treatment. *BMC Medicine, 10*, 99.

Shaw, P., Sharp, W., Morrison, M., Eckstrand, K., Greenstein, D. K., Clasen, L. S., et al. (2009). Psychostimulant treatment and the developing cortex in attention deficit hyperactivity disorder. *American Journal of Psychiatry, 166*(1), 58–63.

Shelton, T. L., Barkley, R. A., Crosswait, C., Moorehouse, M., Fletcher, K., Barrett, S., et al. (2000). Multimethod psychoeducational intervention for preschool children with disruptive behavior: two-year post-treatment follow-up. *Journal of Abnormal Child Psychology, 28*(3), 253–266.

Shier, A. C., Reichenbacher, T., Ghuman, H. S., & Ghuman, J. K. (2012). Pharmacological treatment of attention deficit hyperactivity disorder in children and adolescents: clinical strategies. *Journal of Central Nervous System Diseases, 5*, 1–17.

Short, E. J., Manos, M. J., Findling, R. L., & Schubel, E. A. (2004). A prospective study of stimulant response in preschool children: insights from ROC analyses. *Journal of the American Academy of Child & Adolescent Psychiatry, 43*(3), 251–259.

Spencer, T., Biederman, J., Wilens, T., Harding, M., O'Donnell, D., & Griffin, S. (1996). Pharmacotherapy of attention-deficit hyperactivity disorder across the life cycle. *Journal of the American Academy of Child & Adolescent Psychiatry, 35*(4), 409.

Spencer, T., Greenbaum, M., Ginsberg, L., & Murphy, W. (2009). Safety and effectiveness of coadministration of guanfacine extended release and psychostimulants in children and adolescents with attention-deficit/hyperactivity disorder. *Journal of Child & Adolescent Psychopharmacology, 19*(5), 501–510.

Strain, P. S., Steele, P., Ellis, T., & Timm, M. A. (1982). Long-term effects of oppositional child treatment with mothers as therapists and therapist trainers. *Journal of Applied Behavioral Analys, 15*(1), 163–169.

Swanson, J., Greenhill, L., Wigal, T., Kollins, S., Stehli, A., Davies, M., et al. (2006). Stimulant-related reductions of growth rates in the PATS. *Journal of the American Academy of Child & Adolescent Psychiatry, 45*(11), 1304–1313.

Thompson, D. R., Iachan, R., Overpeck, M., Ross, J. G., & Gross, L. A. (2006). School connectedness in the health behavior in school-aged children study: the role of student, school, and school neighborhood characteristics. *Journal of School Health, 76*(7), 379–386.

Van Brunt, D. L., Johnston, J. A., Ye, W., Pohl, G. M., Sun, P. J., Sterling, K. L., et al. (2005). Predictors of selecting atomoxetine therapy for children with attention-deficit-hyperactivity disorder. *Pharmacotherapy, 25*(11), 1541–1549.

Vazquez Marrufo, M., Vaquero, E., Cardoso, M. J., & Gomez, C. M. (2001). Temporal evolution of alpha and beta bands during visual spatial attention. *Brain Research & Cognitive Brain Research, 12*(2), 315–320.

Vitiello, B. (2001). Psychopharmacology for young children: clinical needs and research opportunities. *Pediatrics, 108*(4), 983–989.

Vitiello, B., Abikoff, H. B., Chuang, S. Z., Kollins, S. H., McCracken, J. T., Riddle, M. A., et al. (2007). Effectiveness of methylphenidate in the 10-month continuation phase of the Preschoolers with Attention-Deficit/Hyperactivity Disorder Treatment Study (PATS). *Journal of Child & Adolescent Psychopharmacology, 17*(5), 593–604.

Welch, W. P., Yang, W., Taylor-Zapata, P., & Flynn, J. T. (2012). Antihypertensive drug use by children: are the drugs labeled and indicated? *Journal of Clinical Hypertension (Greenwich), 14*(6), 388–395.

Wienbruch, C., Paul, I., Bauer, S., & Kivelitz, H. (2005). The influence of methylphenidate on the power spectrum of ADHD children—an MEG study. *BMC Psychiatry, 5*, 29.

Wigal, S. B., Gupta, S., Greenhill, L., Posner, K., Lerner, M., Steinhoff, K., et al. (2007). Pharmacokinetics of methylphenidate in preschoolers with attention-deficit/hyperactivity disorder. *Journal of Child & Adolescent Psychopharmacology, 17*(2), 153–164.

Wigal, T., Greenhill, L., Chuang, S., McGough, J., Vitiello, B., Skrobala, A., et al. (2006). Safety and tolerability of methylphenidate in preschool children with ADHD. *Journal of the American Academy of Child & Adolescent Psychiatry, 45*(11), 1294–1303.

Wilson, T. W., Wetzel, M. W., White, M. L., & Knott, N. L. (2012). Gamma-frequency neuronal activity is diminished in adults with attention-deficit/hyperactivity disorder: a pharmaco-MEG study. *Journal of Psychopharmacology, 26*(6), 771–777.

Wong, C. G., & Stevens, M. (2012). The effects of stimulant medication on working memory functional connectivity in attention-deficit/hyperactivity disorder. *Biological Psychiatry, 71*(5), 458–466.

Zito, J. M., Burcu, M., Ibe, A., Safer, D. J., & Magder, L. S. (2013). Antipsychotic use by Medicaid-insured youths: impact of eligibility and psychiatric diagnosis across a decade. *Psychiatric Services, 64*(3), 223–229.

Zito, J. M., Safer, D. J., dosReis, S., Gardner, J. F., Boles, M., & Lynch, F. (2000). Trends in the prescribing of psychotropic medications to preschoolers. *Journal of the American Medical Association, 283*(8), 1025–1030.

Zito, J. M., Safer, D. J., & Valluri, S. (2007). Psychotherapeutic medication prevalence in Medicaid-insured preschoolers. *Journal of Child and Adolescent Psychopharmacology, 17*(2), 195.

Zuvekas, S. H., & Vitiello, B. (2012). Stimulant medication use in children: a 12-year perspective. *American Journal of Psychiatry, 169*(2), 160–166.

8

Psychopharmacologic Interventions

Clinical Practice in Preschool Children with ADHD

JASWINDER K. GHUMAN AND

HARINDER S. GHUMAN

Psychosocial interventions are the first line of treatment for preschoolers with attention-deficit/hyperactivity disorder (ADHD), as emphasized in Chapters 2, 7, and 8 (Dulcan, 1997; Gleason et al., 2007). If the preschooler continues to have severe impairing symptoms that cause significant interference in daily functioning even after psychosocial interventions have been in place, pharmacologic intervention can be considered. There are exceptional circumstances when pharmacologic treatment may be considered in preschoolers without first implementing psychosocial interventions due to the severity of the impairment resulting from presenting symptoms. However, pharmacologic treatment should always be prescribed concurrently with psychosocial interventions. In this chapter, we will address the baseline workup prior to starting pharmacologic agents, psychoeducation, and informed consent. We discuss clinical strategies for titration, monitoring for and dealing with treatment emergent adverse events (TEAEs) of stimulants and nonstimulants, and dealing with comorbid disorders.

Baseline Workup

PSYCHIATRIC ASSESSMENT

A thorough psychiatric assessment should be conducted in preschool children with presenting complaints related to ADHD symptoms following the guidelines presented in Chapter 2. The assessment should not only determine whether a diagnosis of ADHD is confirmed or ruled out, but should also evaluate if there are any comorbid disorders present in the preschool-age child (described in detail in Chapter 4). Rating scales should be obtained from caregivers and preschool "teachers" and/or daycare providers for baseline behavioral status (described in detail in Chapter 3) and subsequently on a regular basis to monitor the preschooler's progress during treatment. Performance-based measures as described in Chapter 3 on neuropsychological assessment can be helpful to determine the baseline status of a wide range of cognitive functions (e.g., attention span, working memory). A preschooler with obvious or suspected speech, language, hearing, or cognitive concerns should be referred for the pertinent assessments to determine the contribution of communication, cognitive, and learning disorders to the child's ADHD symptoms, and vice versa. A developmental/educational assessment may also be indicated if a child shows evidence of developmental delays and the parents are worried that the child is not able to learn and keep up with his or her peers. These assessments are usually obtained either through the educational (Child Find program) or clinical settings. Child Find programs identify and serve 0- to 5-year-old children with disabilities and their families who are in need of the federally mandated Early Intervention (Part C) or Preschool Special Education (Part B) services of the Individuals with Disabilities Education Act (IDEA). An interdisciplinary team of professionals should be established for integrated delivery of care with the child's primary healthcare and mental healthcare providers, school psychologists, educators, therapists, and the parents (Taylor et al., 2004).

MEDICAL ASSESSMENT

It is recommended that parents schedule an appointment with the child's primary healthcare provider for a careful physical examination and assessment of any medical conditions contributing to the preschooler's ADHD symptoms or confounding the diagnosis; see Chapter 4 for details. It is important to communicate with the primary healthcare provider for any underlying medical illness or if the child is taking any medications.

Prior to prescribing medication for ADHD, a detailed history of child's appetite and eating and sleep habits and/or problems should be obtained. Detailed information should be obtained regarding sleep arrangements, bedtime and bedtime routine, what time the child wakes up in the morning, whether the child gets up in the middle of the night, and any difficulty going back to sleep when up at night. Clinicians should ask about any history of preexisting motor and/or vocal tics in the child or family.

A careful targeted cardiac history should be obtained to determine any cardiovascular risks in the child, including a previous history of cardiac problems, heart murmur, palpitations, shortness of breath, fainting or dizziness (particularly with exercise), syncope, seizures, and a family history of cardiac arrhythmia and/or sudden death in children or young adults (Ghuman & Ghuman, 2012; Perrin, Friedman, & Knilans, 2008; Vetter et al., 2008). The U.S. Food and Drug Administration (FDA) issued a safety announcement on November 1, 2011, for healthcare professionals to take special note that stimulant products and atomoxetine should generally not be used in patients with serious heart problems, or in those for whom an increase in blood pressure or heart rate would be problematic. Patients treated with ADHD medications should be periodically monitored for changes in heart rate or blood pressure.

The physical examination should be specifically focused on any abnormal heart murmurs, hypertension, irregular or rapid heart rhythm, and physical findings suggestive of Marfan syndrome (Vetter et al., 2008). The need for an electrocardiogram (ECG) prior to starting ADHD medications has been debated. The American Heart Association recommends that it is reasonable to obtain an ECG to identify cardiovascular abnormalities (e.g., hypertrophic cardiomyopathy, long-QT syndrome, and Wolff-Parkinson-White syndrome) (Vetter et al., 2008). An ECG may not identify all individuals with cardiac conditions, but it can increase the sensitivity of the evaluation, especially if there are suspicions of high-risk conditions. Even though there are no practice guidelines that require it, we routinely obtain an ECG along with a complete blood count, a comprehensive metabolic screen, a thyroid screen, and a lead level prior to starting psychiatric medications in preschoolers in our Infant and Preschool Psychiatry Clinic.

ASSESSMENT OF THE FAMILY'S ABILITY TO SAFELY ADMINISTER AND STORE MEDICATIONS

When considering prescribing pharmacotherapy for a preschool child with ADHD, it is important to assess the caregivers' ability to understand the importance of personally administering the medication to the preschooler as prescribed and safely storing the medication out of reach of young children, and to ensure and monitor against drug diversion by the child's siblings, other family members, and/or friends or other people visiting the house. Clinicians should enquire if caregivers or other household members have a history of drug use and/or abuse.

Psychoeducation

Misperceptions about ADHD are common among caregivers, providers, and the public regarding whether ADHD is a legitimate diagnosis, what causes ADHD (Bussing, Zima, et al., 2012), and how it should be treated. Caregivers and teachers may attribute the cause of ADHD to the child's preferential interest in play and fun and exciting activities and relatively low effort and disinterest in academic tasks and learning new skills. We often hear from parents, "He does not like learning activities," "only wants to do what he likes," "doesn't want to do what I ask him to do," "only wants to play." Caregivers may have difficulty accepting their child's ADHD diagnosis and look for alternative explanations for the child's behavior—for example, "He is just bad," "needs more discipline," "just wants attention," "His mother is too soft and gives in to him easily." In a study designed to understand how caregivers experience their children's ADHD symptoms, about one third of the caregivers expressed alternative explanation for the child's behavior (Larson, Yoon, Stewart, & dosReis, 2011).

Parents may be ambivalent about potential ADHD interventions (Larson et al., 2011) and may receive misleading, skewed, and contradictory information and/or advice from family, friends, social networks, and media. Parents may feel pressured to consider or reject the ADHD diagnosis and certain interventions and feel distressed from the mixed advice and pressure. For example, 1,393 adults were interviewed regarding their attitudes and beliefs about treatment and psychiatric medications in children with mental health problems in the National Stigma Study-Children. Many participants believed that children are overmedicated for behavior problems (Larson et al., 2011; Pescosolido, Perry, Martin, McLeod, & Jensen, 2007), giving psychiatric medications to young children interferes with families' motivation to work out behavior problems themselves (Pescosolido et al., 2007), and psychiatric medications change children's personality to "zombie"-like and "drugged" (DosReis, Barksdale, Sherman, Maloney, & Charach, 2010). These beliefs can likely lead parents to have adversarial interactions with schools and clinicians (Larson et al., 2011), have difficulty accepting treatment recommendations, and delay treatment initiation or become inconsistent with follow-through (Bussing, Zima, et al., 2012; Lebowitz, 2013).

Psychoeducation has been shown to improve treatment acceptance and promote maintenance of treatment gains and treatment adherence (Chacko et al., 2009; Nock & Kazdin, 2005). Further, psychoeducation was associated with improvement in the family's knowledge of ADHD, opinion of the use of medication, treatment satisfaction, and adherence to medical recommendations (Montoya, Colom, & Ferrin, 2011). Psychoeducation can clarify misperceptions and explore caregivers' concerns and expectations for treatment. Encouraging parents to actively participate in the decision-making process is important in formulating an acceptable treatment plan in line with the parents' personal values.

It is important to provide psychoeducation early on in the evaluation and treatment process to address areas identified as high risk for treatment attrition (Bussing, Koro-Ljungberg, et al., 2012) and to maximize treatment engagement. As part of the initial psychiatric evaluation and treatment planning, parents' expectations, perceptions, and treatment preferences should be assessed. Clinicians should enquire about personal values and health beliefs regarding the disease mechanism, etiology, and treatment response mechanism and attribution. Parents should be asked about their beliefs regarding what they think contributed to their child developing ADHD. It is important to explore if the parents think the problem lies in the child only, the parents only, both the parents and the child, teachers only, and/or disruptive peers at school. What would they like to see change in their child, in themselves, and/or at school? What do they think will be helpful to improve their child's behavior? What specific treatment interventions are they interested in for their child? Medication? Therapy for the child? Both medication and therapy? Therapy for themselves? What if any interventions are they not interested in considering? Clinicians should also enquire about parents' perceived sense of stress and burden related to the child's behaviors (Larson et al., 2011).

Clinicians should present well-balanced information about all the available treatment options and expected outcomes (both benefits and adverse effects) for each option so parents can be more confident participants in the shared decision-making process. The information should be presented as a choice and the parents should know sufficient details about each option to help them make a well-informed decision. Treatment recommendations should take into account parent preferences and personal and family values in order to increase compliance and acceptability of the treatment, and thus improve outcome. At the same time, clinicians need to ensure that parent preferences are based on well-balanced and current information.

According to the Health Beliefs model, whether treatment is sought depends on knowledge and awareness of a health condition and its treatments (Bussing, Koro-Ljungberg, et al., 2012). Three fifths of the adults participating in the National Stigma Study-Children were not able to identify ADHD symptoms correctly (Pescosolido et al., 2008). Parents should be provided with information regarding ADHD symptom presentation, associated health problems such as accident proneness, learning and academic difficulties, and risk for substance abuse and conduct problems, and comorbid psychiatric disorders.

Parents should be educated about ADHD's etiology, the life course of the disorder, developmental differences at different ages, and the consequences of failing to treat the disorder.

Instructions for medication dose and time of administration should be explained to the parents in clear and simple language. Written instructions should be given clearly specifying the times of medication administration. One mother told us at the time of the initial evaluation that her child had been taking stimulant medication in the morning and at bedtime per the instructions on the bottle for twice-a-day administration. It is also important to emphasize to the parents that they should personally administer the medication to the child. We have had occasional instances of parents delegating the responsibility for the preschooler's medication administration to an adolescent sibling.

Parents should be educated regarding the reasons for the recommended dose and the timing of administration and why the medication dose should not be increased suddenly. For example, a high dose of a stimulant could lead to agitation, hallucinations, and appetite reduction; a high dose of a a_2-adrenergic agonist could lead to hypotension. Similarly, the reasons for not stopping some medications suddenly should also be explained to the parents—for example, stopping a_2-adrenergic agonists can lead to rebound hypertension. It is important to discuss with caregivers situations for which the treatment contract could be terminated—for example, noncompliance with the specified dose and time of medication administration in case of a_2-adrenergic agonists and frequent requests for stimulant refills before the prescription should have run out.

Informed Consent

Pros and cons of treating the preschooler with medication should be thoroughly discussed without pressuring the parents to start medication. Parents should have ample time to ask questions and consult among themselves and with other family members and the child's primary healthcare provider. Parents should be given written information about the medication that is written in simple and straightforward language without professional jargon. There is an excellent simple pamphlet on Tufts University's website with information on stimulants for parents: https://research.tufts-nemc.org/help4kids/docs/SANDAP%20HANDOUTS/ParentInfoMeds.pdf

Parents should be informed at the outset that most ADHD medications (with the exception of immediate-release amphetamines) do not have FDA approval to treat ADHD in preschool children and are used "off-label." There should be a thorough discussion with the parents regarding the known side effects of the medication. Parents should be informed about the sensitivity of preschoolers to ADHD medications and the unique adverse effects that are more common in preschool children compared to older children. The discussion of adverse effects and the option of not medicating should be presented in a well-balanced manner. It is important to inform parents about the findings of suppression of growth velocity in preschool children treated with stimulants (Greenhill et al., 2006; Swanson et al., 2006). Parents who are short-statured themselves may be reluctant to consider stimulant medication if their preschooler is also short-statured compared to parents who are tall themselves and have a tall preschooler.

Parents should be informed about the FDA "black-box" warning for Adderall due to the very preliminary reports of sudden death associated with the use of stimulants (Ghuman & Ghuman, 2012; Gould et al., 2009; Nissen, 2006). The FDA Pediatric Advisory Committee recommended highlighting for all stimulant medications that "children with structural heart defects, cardiomyopathy, or heart-rhythm disturbances may be at risk for adverse cardiac events, including sudden death." Parents should also be informed about the FDA warning that stimulants have a high potential for abuse, chronic abuse can lead to drug intolerance, and frank psychotic episodes can occur, especially with parenteral abuse.

Parents should be informed in detail about the requirements for baseline workup, frequency of appointments, and regular monitoring for height, weight, blood pressure, and pulse. Given the reports of increased and unique sensitivity to side effects of ADHD medications, preschoolers should be monitored closely.

Questions Parents Ask

Parents may be ambivalent about giving medication to their preschooler at such a young age. They often worry about the adverse effects of the medication and how the medication may affect the child in the long run. Sometimes there is disagreement between the preschooler's father and mother and/or other family members about medicating the child. A joint appointment should be scheduled with both parents and/or other family members, as indicated, to discuss the assessment findings and treatment recommendations and to answer questions and address their reservations. Parents should be informed that the child will be seen regularly for medication monitoring and that medication will be started at a very low dose and titrated slowly as indicated and tolerated by the child. The monitoring process should be described for any TEAEs. Parents should be informed how they can contact the clinician in case of TEAEs. Clinicians should inform the parents about steps to minimize TEAEs and what will be done if the child develops TEAEs. For example, parents are advised to give the stimulant medication to the child with or after meals to manage the appetite-suppressant effect. Parents worry, "Will the medication change my child's personality? I don't want my child to look like a zombie." Parents can be reassured that the medication dose will be decreased if the dose proves to be too high for the child or stopped if the child is not able to tolerate the medication.

Parents frequently ask, "How long will my child need to take medication?" Parents should be informed about the recommendation of the American Academy of Child and Adolescent Psychiatry (AACAP) Preschool Pharmacology Working Group (PPWG) to discontinue the medication after 6 months to reassess if the child needs to continue taking it and/or is still deriving benefit from it (Gleason et al., 2007). Regarding the parents' worry, "Will my child become dependent on the medication?", parents should be informed about the need to periodically increase/adjust the medication dose during follow-up. Parents often worry, "Will my child become addicted to the medication?" The clinician should discuss with the parents the current knowledge base about the high prevalence of substance use disorders associated with a diagnosis of ADHD and the evidence base supporting a protective role or a neutral and/or no impact of ADHD medications in the development of substance use disorders (Barkley, Fischer, Smallish, & Fletcher, 2003; Biederman et al., 2008; Faraone, Biederman, Wilens, & Adamson, 2007; Mannuzza et al., 2008; Molina et al., 2013; Wilens and Fusillo, 2007).

ADHD Medications

In the following sections, we present information regarding the clinical practice of stimulants and nonstimulants for the treatment of ADHD in preschool children.

STIMULANTS

Stimulants, particularly methylphenidate (MPH), are the most common medications used in preschool children with ADHD. There are no guidelines to help decide whether MPH or amphetamine should be started first, which children will respond better to one stimulant over the other, or which stimulant is better for predominantly hyperactive or inattentive symptoms. Some school-age children may respond better to one stimulant over the other and may experience TEAEs with one stimulant and not with the other (Elia, Borcherding, Rapoport, & Keysor, 1991). Both dextroamphetamine and MPH were equally efficacious relative to placebo in a double-blind crossover treatment study of dextroamphetamine, MPH, and placebo in a group of 48 school-age boys (mean age = 8.6 ± 1.7 years) with ADHD (Elia, Borcherding, Rapoport, & Keysor, 1991). Arnold (2000) conducted a review of the controlled crossover comparison studies of MPH and amphetamine in school-age children with ADHD and reported an overall stimulant response rate of 87%. Furthermore, 41% of the children participating in the reviewed studies responded both to amphetamine and MPH, 69% responded to amphetamine, and 57% to MPH (Arnold, 2000; Elia et al., 1991). There are no comparative studies of MPH and amphetamine efficacy in preschoolers with ADHD; hence, clinical decisions are frequently made in collaboration with caregivers regarding their preference (Shier, Reichenbacher, Ghuman, & Ghuman, 2012).

Because stimulants are controlled substances, a written prescription is needed and the prescription can't be called in to the pharmacy. The FDA limits the stimulant prescription duration to a maximum of 30 days, and no refills are allowed.

MPH. MPH products are generally based on racemic dextro and levo isomers (dl-MPH), available in immediate-release (IR) form as Ritalin and Methylin, and dextro threo enantiomer (d-MPH), available in IR form as Focalin. Both Ritalin and Methylin reach peak levels in 1 to 1½ hours, have a 3- to 4-hour duration of action, and are frequently prescribed BID or TID in preschoolers with ADHD. Available dosage strengths of Ritalin and Methylin are 5-mg, 10-mg, and 20-mg tablets. Methylin is also available as a chewable tablet with dosage strengths of 2.5 mg, 5 mg, and 10 mg and as a grape-flavored oral solution in strengths of 5 mg/5 mL and 10 mg/5 mL. Methylin chewable tablets can swell and may not be appropriate for preschool children due to the risk of choking if the tablets are not chewed thoroughly before swallowing and taken with at least 8 ounces of liquid.

Focalin contains only the active dextro threo enantiomer and hence requires half of racemic MPH to be effective. Available dosage forms include 2.5-mg, 5-mg, and 10-mg tablets. Focalin has a longer duration of action, for 6 hours, and can be given BID. Ritalin and Focalin can be crushed and given in soft food such as applesauce or ice cream (Chavez et al., 2009) for preschoolers with pill-swallowing difficulties.

In preschool children, treatment is usually initiated with IR short-acting formulations. Medication is started at a half-tablet (and occasionally a quarter-tablet) of the smallest dosage strength available, as in the PATS and Ghuman studies (Ghuman et al., 2001; 2009; Greenhill et al., 2006). Following the PATS titration schedule, IR MPH is initiated with once-daily dosing in the morning (usually dl-MPH 2.5 mg in the morning, or d-MPH 1.25 mg in the morning) for the first 3 to 7 days. Parents are asked to call the clinician in 3 to 7 days; if there are no TEAEs, the dose can be increased to BID dosing (dl-MPH 2.5 mg in the morning and 2.5 mg at noon) for the next 3 to 7 days, followed by dl-MPH 5 mg in the morning and 2.5 mg at noon. At this point, parents should be scheduled for a follow-up visit and all subsequent dose adjustments should be done after an in-person clinic visit usually every 2 weeks. Dose adjustments are based on the child's response, the parent and "teacher" ratings on ADHD rating scales. and any medication TEAEs. Based on the child's response and if tolerated, the dl-MPH dose can be further titrated in a stepwise fashion to 5 mg in the morning and 5 mg at noon, 7.5 mg in the morning and 5 mg at noon, 10 mg in the morning and 5 mg or 7.5 mg at noon, and 10 mg in the morning and 10 mg at noon. Sometimes the upward titration may be done at a slower pace if the preschooler experiences moderate TEAEs. If TID dosing is desired, a 5-mg dose can be added around 4 p.m. On rare occasions, a QID dosing may be of use—for example adding a very small dose of 2.5 mg around 6 or 6:30 p.m. if the parents complain that the child is not able to settle down for sleep (Brown & McMullen, 2001). In a retrospective chart review of 3- to 5-year-old children treated with stimulants for ADHD, stimulants were prescribed QID for approximately one fifth of the children and QD for approximately one tenth of the children (Ghuman et al., 2001).

An optimal dose is one that produces the maximal effect with minimal side effects. Initially, the child should be seen every 2 weeks for the first 1 to 2 months; once the medication dose is stabilized, follow-up visits can be scheduled once a month. Response to medication should be monitored with regularly administered ADHD rating scales completed by the parents and the preschooler's "teacher."

Many parents desire coverage only while their child is at preschool and occasionally as needed for organized afternoon activities. Similarly, some parents desire medication for their preschooler only during weekdays and only occasionally during the weekend as needed for structured activities (e.g., church or Sunday school). This may be particularly important for the preschoolers if they experience a moderate decrease in appetite with the stimulant. On the other hand, some parents have difficulty managing their child's behavior and elect for TID dosing throughout the week including weekends, especially if the child does not have any untoward TEAEs.

Several long-acting stimulant formulations are available for use in school-age children. Long-acting formulations allow single daily dosing and have become the standard of care in older children. Long-acting stimulant formulations provide increased convenience, all-day coverage, and smoother action without the peaks and valleys seen with short-acting formulations. Once a preschooler's IR stimulant dose is stabilized, some parents may prefer to switch to a long-acting formulation to avoid the need to give the medication multiple times.

However, there are several concerns regarding long-acting formulations in preschool children with ADHD. First, preschoolers may have trouble swallowing bigger tablet of many long-acting formulations. Second, given the heightened sensitivity of preschoolers to stimulant TEAEs, such as more irritability and proneness to crying (Ghuman, Aman, Lecavalier, et al., 2009; Ghuman, Arnold, & Anthony, 2008; Ghuman, Byreddy, & Ghuman, 2011; Ghuman & Ghuman, 2012; Ghuman et al., 2001; Greenhill et al., 2006), especially at higher doses, the available dosage strengths of the long-acting formulations may prove to be too high and may not permit small incremental titration desired for preschoolers. Third, some caregivers do not want their preschooler to be under the effect of medication for most of the day. Thus, when treating ADHD in preschool children, IR short-acting agents have an advantage as lower doses can be given, more precise dosing is possible, and TEAEs can be minimized (e.g., poor appetite throughout the day and sleep disturbance). Appetite suppression is especially important for preschool children because they are in an active growing developmental period. Sleep disturbance is important not just because it affects the child's behavior and functioning, but also because it interferes with the parents' sleep and day-to-day functioning.

On the other hand, certain long-acting formulations may bypass swallowing difficulties and allow tailored intermediate dosing strengths and duration of medication effect. For example, The racemic dl-MPH transdermal system (MTS) patch (Daytrana) is a long-acting transdermal patch that does not require oral administration, can be cut for dispensing the desired amount of the drug (Arnold et al., 2007), and can be removed to allow the desired duration of the medication effect. Ritalin-LA, Metadate-CD, and Focalin-XR capsules are long-acting formulations that can be opened and the beaded contents divided to give smaller doses, and the contents can be sprinkled on food.

The MTS patch is a long-acting formulation that uses a diffusion-based transdermal drug delivery route. Daytrana is available in a 12.5-cm^2 patch size (10 mg MPH dose equivalent per 9-hour daily MTS wear-time at an estimated drug delivery rate of 1.1 mg/hour), an 18.75-cm^2 patch size (15 mg MPH dose equivalent per 9-hour daily MTS wear-time at an estimated drug delivery rate of 1.6 mg/hour), a 25-cm^2 patch size (20 mg MPH dose equivalent per 9-hour daily MTS wear-time at an estimated drug delivery rate of 2.2 mg/hour), and a 37.5-cm^2 patch size (30 mg MPH dose equivalent per 9-hour daily MTS wear-time at an estimated drug delivery rate of 3.3 mg/hour). The MTS patch may be applied while a child is still sleeping to overcome the delayed onset of MTS action (usually seen 2 hours after application). MTS effect usually lasts 3 hours after patch removal.

MTS is not affected by meals or the first-pass effect of the enteric and hepatic de-esterification. Consistent MPH absorption from MTS administration results in a smoother action. MTS offers a retrievable form of drug delivery (in milligrams per hour) rather than a fixed non-retrievable dose (in milligrams per dose) (Arnold et al., 2007). It offers flexibility to determine the optimal dose by controlling the patch size (influencing milligrams delivered/hour) and patch wear-time (influencing total milligrams delivered/day). It allows the flexibility to control the optimal duration of the medication effect and specific hours of the day when the drug effect is required or needs to be terminated; the patch can be applied and removed at the desired times to manage a child's behavior and TEAEs. The MethyPatch (the MTS's predecessor) could be cut to the desired size, thus allowing intermediate doses for custom titration. However, with MethyPatch's sale to Shire/Noven, the premarketing study protocols did not allow the patch to be cut; thus, the package insert instructs not to cut the patch. However, since MPH is dispersed uniformly throughout the MTS patch adhesive, Arnold and colleagues (2007) concluded that the MTS patch can be cut to individualize the dose. If the patch is cut, the corners should be rounded to prevent catching on clothes. The MTS patch can be worn while swimming. Clinicians should educate parents regarding management of wear-time to optimize the daily time course of clinical benefits.

Parents should be informed about how to properly apply the patch and should be given skin hygiene instructions for good patch adhesion and management of any resulting irritation. The MTS patch should be applied to clean skin (after bathing) without using lotion, oil, or powder and making sure there are no cuts, abrasions, or irritation on the skin. It is preferable to apply the patch to a child's lateral hip for consistent absorption; the site should be rotated every day. To promote good patch adhesion, the patch should be cool (10 to 15 minutes in the refrigerator might help in hot weather) and applied soon after removing the protective liner from the patch. The patch should be pressed firmly for 30 to 60 seconds to ensure adhesion. The patch should be removed gently; there may be a residual adhesive outline, which can be removed by gently swabbing with mineral/vegetable oil or petroleum jelly. Minimal to moderate localized transient contact dermatitis (erythema) resulting from the mild irritant qualities of MPH (Arnold et al., 2007) has been reported and usually resolves within 24 to 36 hours after removing the patch. If redness persists for 2 days or longer or the skin surface is raised and/or feels rough due to papules, parents should call the prescriber. The patch application site should be rotated every day to minimize erythema and allow skin recovery in between applications. In some cases, if the child is unable to tolerate the transdermal application, patch use may need to be stopped.

Heat, including fever, generally increases the absorption rate of drugs with transdermal delivery systems (Hull, 2002); this can increase up to twice the normal MPH delivery rate in case of the MTS (Noven/Shire, 2005). Hence, a heating pad, heated waterbed, or electric blanket should never be used while wearing an MTS. If a preschooler spends considerable time outdoors in hot weather, the MTS dose may need to be decreased. The child must be monitored closely and/or may need to discontinue the MTS temporarily. There is a risk for overdose if the patch is not removed after the recommended wear-time. Additionally, there is a risk for diversion and abuse potential and/or accidental poisoning, especially since a substantial amount of MPH remains in the MTS patch after removal.

Beaded formulations of MPH can be opened and the contents divided to achieve intermediate doses to allow small incremental titration desired for preschoolers. For preschoolers with swallowing difficulties, the contents can be sprinkled on soft food. The contents should be mixed evenly with the food; the food should not be heated and should be consumed right away in its entirety and not stored for later use.

Ritalin-LA (MPH LA) is a beaded formulation capsule that uses Spheriodal Oral Drug Absorption System (SODAS) to deliver dl-MPH. It has 50% IR beads and 50% enteric-coated (pH-dependent polymer) delayed-release beads, resulting in a biphasic drug release. MPH LA has an 8- to 10-hour duration of action and is taken once daily in the morning. MPH LA is available in 10-mg, 20-mg, 30-mg, and 40-mg dosage strengths. Alteration of the gastrointestinal tract pH with co-administration of antacids can affect release of the pH-dependent MPH LA delayed-release beads.

Metadate-CD (MPH CD) uses a beaded drug-delivery system; different layers applied over the drug core determine the rate of drug release (Chavez et al., 2009). MPH CD has 30% IR beads and 70% beaded drug delivery system release beads with time to peak concentration of 1 to 3 hours and a biphasic/extended drug release. MPH CD has an 8-hour duration of action and is taken once daily in the morning. Available capsule dose strengths are 10 mg, 20 mg, 30 mg, 40 mg, 50 mg, and 60 mg. A high-fat meal can potentially delay time to peak concentration.

Focalin-XR (d-MPH ER) is a beaded formulation capsule that contains 50% d-MPH IR beads and 50% d-MPH enteric-coated delayed-release SODAS beads, resulting in a biphasic drug release with peak concentrations at 1.5 and 6.5 hours following oral administration. Focalin-XR has a 10- to 12-hour duration of action and is taken once daily in the morning. It is available in 5-mg, 10-mg, 15-mg, and 20-mg dosage strengths.

Amphetamines. If a preschooler with ADHD does not respond to MPH, the AACAP-PPWG recommended switching to dextroamphetamine or mixed amphetamine salts (Gleason et al., 2007). IR amphetamine formulations are available as dextroamphetamine (Dexedrine and Dextrostat tablets and Liquadd as liquid oral suspension) and mixed amphetamine salts (Adderall tablets) and have FDA approval for treating ADHD in children 3 years and older.

Dextroamphetamine reaches peak levels in 1 to 1½ hours, has a 4- to 5-hour duration of action, and is usually prescribed two or three times daily. Dexedrine is available as 5-mg tablet, Dextrostat as 5-mg and 10-mg tablets, and Liquadd as mg/5 mL oral suspension.

Adderall (dextroamphetamine salts) has a 3:1 ratio of d-amphetamine to l-amphetamine. Adderall (dl-AMP) has a slightly longer duration of action (4 to 6 hours) and is usually taken twice daily. It is available in 5-mg, 7.5-mg, 10-mg, 12.5-mg, 15-mg, 20-mg, and 30-mg IR tablets.

Amphetamine titration and monitoring guidelines are similar to those described for MPH. Medications are initiated at a half- or quarter-strength of the smallest dose available, and a slow dose titration schedule is followed to aim for an optimal dose with maximal effect and minimal TEAEs. Preschoolers should be monitored closely with more frequent visits during titration and monthly follow-up maintenance visits. Like MPH, amphetamines are controlled by the FDA, so written prescriptions are needed, prescription duration is limited to a maximum of 30 days, and no refills are allowed.

Dextroamphetamine is available in long-acting capsule (Dexedrine Spansules) and pro-drug (Vyvanse) forms; dextroamphetamine salts are available as a long-acting (Adderall-XR) beaded formulation. The long-acting amphetamine formulations are approved for children 6 years and older. The beaded amphetamine formulations (Dexedrine Spansules and Adderall-XR) can be opened and the contents divided to achieve intermediate doses to allow small incremental titration desired for preschoolers. For preschoolers with swallowing difficulties, the contents can be sprinkled on soft food. Instructions for administering the amphetamine beaded formulations mixed with food are similar to those given for stimulant beaded formulations.

Dexedrine Spansules contain 50% d-AMP IR beads and 50% d-AMP delayed-absorption beads, resulting in a biphasic drug release. The duration of action is 8 hours. Spansules are taken once daily in the morning and are available as 5-mg, 10-mg, and 15-mg capsules.

Vyvanse (lisdexamphetamine) is an inactive pro-drug that contains l-lysine and d-AMP. It undergoes rate-limited hydrolysis to release d-AMP in the gut. It has a 12-hour duration of action and should be taken once daily in the morning. Vyvanse is available in 20-mg, 30-mg, 40-mg, 50-mg, and 60-mg capsules. The capsule contents can be dissolved in water and smaller doses can be given (Fanton & Gleason, 2009). When dissolved in water, it should be consumed right away and not stored for later use.

Adderall-XR contains a two-pulsed, microbead delivery system with 50% IR and 50% delayed-release beads, resulting in a biphasic dl-AMP release. Time to maximum plasma concentration is 7 hours, with a 10- to 12-hour duration of action. Adderall-XR is taken once daily in the morning. It is available in 5-mg, 10-mg, 15-mg, 20-mg, and 30-mg capsules.

HANDLING STIMULANT SIDE EFFECTS

Appetite suppression. Caregivers should administer stimulant medications with or after a meal so the child can eat before the stimulant's appetite-suppressant effect sets in. Caregivers should be flexible with meal schedules and allow the preschooler to eat between meals or on demand if he or she gets hungry later than the scheduled mealtimes. Preschoolers should be offered large, nutritious meals in the morning and evening and extra after-dinner high-energy nutritious snacks (e.g., cheese, protein shakes, peanut butter, trail mix, nuts, granola, energy bars) to prevent weight loss. The child's appetite, weight, height, and BMI should be regularly monitored and graphed on a growth chart at 3- to 6-month intervals. "Drug holidays" should be considered to improve appetite and promote growth rebound (Graham et al., 2011) if the child is losing weight or not maintaining the age-expected growth trajectory. Consultation with a pediatric endocrinologist may be sought if the child is short-statured to begin with or if there are ongoing serious concerns regarding the child's growth.

Sleep problems. Stimulants increase wakefulness, most likely via their sympathomimetic action. A sleep diary is helpful to monitor any sleep problems arising during stimulant treatment. Sleep hygiene and behavior therapy techniques should be discussed with parents. Parents should establish a regular bedtime and bedtime routine, a quiet and calming activity prior to bedtime, and a firm structure. The afternoon dose of IR stimulant should not be administered later than 4:30 p.m. to minimize sleep difficulties. If the child has sleep difficulties, the stimulant dose may be lowered and/or administered earlier. Occasionally, a small dose of stimulant taken late in the evening can help the child settle down for sleep (Ghuman et al., 2001), especially in case of restlessness related to the rebound effect of stimulants (Brown & McMullen, 2001). Melatonin and clonidine are commonly used by community practitioners to treat stimulant-induced insomnia. In case of a history of significant sleep problems, stimulants may need to be stopped and a nonstimulant trial with α_2-adrenergic agonists or atomoxetine may be advisable.

Cardiac adverse effects. Blood pressure and pulse should be checked prior to starting stimulants and at each subsequent visit thereafter. If there are concerns about elevated blood pressure (above 110/72 for 3-year-olds and 115/74 for 6-year-olds) or tachycardia above 120 beats/min (Bernstein, 2000), a referral to the primary healthcare provider and/or to a pediatric cardiologist may be needed for further evaluation and recommendations. Parents should be asked to call the prescriber if the preschooler complains of palpitations, chest ache, dizziness, or fainting.

Reports of sudden deaths in individuals taking stimulants led to the recommendation by the FDA Advisory Committee of a "black-box warning" for stimulants (FDA, 2006; Nissen, 2006). A subsequent FDA review of the Adverse Events Reporting System data for marketed safety experience with therapeutic use of stimulants did not reveal the base rate of sudden death in children treated for ADHD to be above the rate of sudden death in the general population (Schelleman et al., 2011; Villalaba, 2006). A careful targeted cardiac history, including a history of cardiac problems and a family history of sudden death in children or young adults, should be obtained prior to starting stimulants (Ghuman & Ghuman, 2012). If preschool children with known serious structural cardiac abnormalities, cardiomyopathy, serious heart rhythm abnormalities, hypertension, or other serious cardiac problems, or at risk for cardiac problems (e.g., children with Marfan syndrome), are being considered for pharmacologic treatment due to severe impairment from ADHD symptoms, a referral to a pediatric cardiologist should be made. Pharmacologic treatment should be prescribed only in consultation with and with ongoing monitoring by the pediatric cardiologist.

Tics. Preschoolers should be monitored closely for the development of new tics or exacerbation of preexisting tics as part of medication follow-up. If a child develops new tics or preexisting tics worsen, the stimulant dose should be reduced to see if they improve. Observation for at least 3 months is recommended (Graham et al., 2011) due to the natural history of waxing and waning of tics. If tics are persistent, a switch to atomoxetine or α_2-adrenergic agonists may be indicated, although there has been at least one report of exacerbation of tics with atomoxetine treatment in school-age children.

Abuse potential and diversion. Given the risk of abuse potential and diversion of stimulants, some clinicians consider stimulant prescription to be relatively contraindicated if there is a current or past history of substance abuse in the family; instead, they will recommend treatment with a nonstimulant. If stimulants are prescribed due to severity of the preschooler's ADHD symptoms, extremely close and careful monitoring and accurate documentation should be maintained regarding the number of tablets authorized to be dispensed each time a prescription is written and the duration between each prescription renewal.

Stimulants should not be prescribed to a child if there is a history of cocaine abuse in the family members due to the potentially lethal hazards of combining the shared neurochemical effects of cocaine and dopaminergic drugs like stimulants.

Seizures. ADHD medications have the potential to lower seizure threshold. MPH can prolong the duration of kindled seizures in rats (Babington & Wedeking, 1973), and amphetamine has been found to both increase and decrease seizure risk in animals (Greer & Alpern, 1980; King & Burnham, 1980). On the other hand, there was no difference in the incidence of seizures between ADHD medication and placebo in prospective trials, retrospective cohort studies, and postmarketing surveillance in ADHD patients without epilepsy (Graham et al., 2011).

Because of their young age, preschool children with ADHD may not have yet developed or been identified with seizures and may develop seizures for the first time during stimulant treatment. Hence, a careful history of seizures should be obtained in preschool children and potential risks of lowered seizure threshold with stimulants should be discussed with the parents. Preschoolers should be closely monitored while taking the medication.

Psychotic symptoms. Reported psychotic adverse events with stimulants are rare. A FDA review of RCTs of ADHD drug treatment in children (Mosholder, Gelperin, Hammad, Phelan, & Johann-Liang, 2009) found a total of 11 psychosis/mania events during 743 person-years of exposure with ADHD drug treatment compared to no psychosis events reported with placebo. The postmarketing surveillance reported rate of psychosis events is 1 in 2,500 cases of ADHD treated with dexamphetamine, MPH, and atomoxetine. A report of "hearing voices and seeing adults when no one was there" in an 8-year-old boy treated with 40 mg/day MPH was reported; the psychotic symptoms resolved with a dosage decrease (Ross, 2006). No information is available about psychotic symptoms in preschool children treated with stimulants. Caution should be used when prescribing stimulants to children with a family history of psychosis or a past history suggestive of psychotic symptoms.

Mutagenic adverse effects. An alarming report of increased cytogenetic anomalies in the peripheral blood cultured from 12 children (mean age = 8.5 ± 3.5 years) treated with therapeutic doses of MPH for 3 months (El-Zein et al., 2005) spurred a wave of investigations into the mutagenic risk of stimulants. No increased frequencies of cytogenetic anomalies were found in peripheral blood lymphocytes cultured after 3 months of prospective MPH treatment and behavior therapy compared to behavior therapy alone in 109 children aged 6 to 12 years (Tucker et al., 2009; Walitza et al., 2009). Several further cytogenetic evaluations that included a healthy control group, a chronically MPH-treated (>12 months) group, and a drug-naïve ADHD group and examination of buccal mucosa cells in addition to the peripheral lymphocytes did not demonstrate elevated cytogenetic damage (Walitza et al., 2010). Furthermore, peripheral blood of mice treated with high doses of MPH (30, 60, or 125 mg/kg) did not show any evidence of increased micronucleated erythrocytes and micronucleated polychromatic erythrocytes, nor was there a decline in polychromatic erythrocytes (Zamora-Perez et al., 2011).

Drug holidays. In our clinical experience, ADHD drug holidays during the summer months are often requested, preferred, and implemented by parents of preschoolers. Parents reason that since the child does not have many structured activities and demands during the summer, drug holidays can help the preschooler "catch up" with the reduced appetite and growth and reduce the long-term effects of ADHD medications. Drug holidays can also be used to assess whether the child still needs the medication after a period of treatment and behavior stability.

In the only double-blind RCT to address drug holidays and ADHD drug effects, 6- to 14-year-old children and adolescents were randomized to receive BID methylphenidate either 7 days a week, or 5 days a week and placebo over the weekend (Martins et al., 2004). No reduction in therapeutic effects on weekends (as rated by parents) or on the following day of school (as rated by teachers) was found.

However, drug holidays can be problematic for the child and the family because the ADHD symptoms will often re-emerge or worsen during the period that medication is withheld. Higher health costs per year due to accidents and emergency room visits were reported for children with ADHD not receiving their normal ADHD medication (Leibson et al., 2006).

NONSTIMULANTS: ATOMOXETINE AND α_2-ADRENERGIC AGONISTS

The AACAP-PPWG algorithm for pharmacotherapy of ADHD recommends a trial of α_2-adrenergic agonists or atomoxetine in preschoolers who do not respond to an adequate trial of either of the stimulant classes or experience intolerable or unacceptable TEAEs. Nonstimulant agents may be considered without a stimulant trial first if there are comorbid tic, anxiety, and depressive disorders, aggressive behavior, or a family history of substance abuse, and/or if parents are adamantly opposed to their child taking a stimulant.

Based on more common use of α_2-adrenergic agonists in preschoolers, a higher level of evidence for α_2-adrenergic agonists than for atomoxetine was cited by the AACAP-PPWG. However, in our discussions with community practitioners, monotherapy with atomoxetine is usually considered more efficacious than monotherapy with α_2-adrenergic agonists, and α_2-adrenergic agonists are frequently used as adjunct treatments for ADHD. Moreover, there are no controlled empirical data for the use of α_2-adrenergic agonists in preschoolers with ADHD other than two case reports of open-label treatment in five preschool children with ADHD (Cesena, Lee, Cebollero, & Steingard, 1995; Lee, 1997). On the other hand, efficacy of atomoxetine versus placebo was reported in 101 preschoolers aged 5 and 6 years treated for ADHD (Kratochvil et al., 2011).

Atomoxetine. Atomoxetine is longer-acting, with a half-life of about 5 hours, and time to maximum concentration is 1 to 2 hours. It is available in capsule form; available doses are 10 mg, 18 mg, 25 mg, 40 mg, 60 mg, 80 mg, and 100 mg. Unlike stimulants, atomoxetine dosing is weight-based. In school-age children, atomoxetine is usually initiated at 0.5 mg/kg/daily for 3 to 5 days and subsequently increased to 1.2 to 1.4 mg/kg/day. The FDA-recommended maximum dose is 1.8 mg/kg/day.

Atomoxetine is usually started at bedtime due to its sedating effect, especially initially. In preschoolers, we initiate atomoxetine at 10 mg at bedtime. The dosage can be titrated at 1- to 2-week intervals to 18 mg, 25 mg, 30 mg, and 35 mg based on the child's weight, response, and TEAEs; we usually don't exceed 40 mg/day. If there are moderate TEAEs, a slower titration schedule may be needed. Atomoxetine can be prescribed QD or BID (in divided doses), usually determined by TEAEs to decrease sedation and gastrointestinal side effects (Greenhill, Newcorn, Gao, & Feldman, 2007) and/or parent preference. Similar to the follow-up schedule for stimulant prescription, we see the children every 2 weeks for the first 1 to 2 months and then monthly once the dose is stabilized. Unlike stimulants, it takes 3 to 4 weeks for improvement in symptoms and may take over 3 months for remission of symptoms (Dickson et al., 2011). Some preschoolers may not be able to swallow atomoxetine capsules. Parents may open the capsule and pour the contents of the capsules in small amounts of liquid (Ghuman, Aman, Ghuman, et al., 2009). Since atomoxetine powder is an eye irritant, parents should be advised to wash their hands right away.

Abdominal pain, vomiting, decreased appetite, somnolence, dizziness, fatigue, and irritability are common TEAEs with atomoxetine. Both weight loss and a decrease in expected height and no significant growth impairment have been reported in children treated with atomoxetine (Spencer et al., 2007). Atomoxetine can increase heart rate and blood pressure due to its noradrenergic effects. Atomoxetine should not be used in children with known serious structural cardiac abnormalities, cardiomyopathy, and serious heart rhythm abnormalities (Lilly, 2008).

Atomoxetine has been shown to lead to rare hepatic injury (Bangs et al., 2008). Parents should be advised to watch for symptoms of hepatotoxicity, including itching, yellow conjunctiva, skin and urine, nausea and vomiting, and abdominal tenderness. Combining atomoxetine with antiepileptic agents might increase the risk for liver toxicity. Epileptic patients treated with atomoxetine and antiepileptic medications should be carefully monitored. Elevation of liver enzymes, however, is a poor predictor of impending hepatotoxicity.

Atomoxetine is metabolized by the hepatic cytochrome P450 2D6 enzyme, and caution should be exercised with concomitant use of fluoxetine and paroxetine due to an increase in the atomoxetine blood level. A slow and cautious titration schedule should be followed if atomoxetine is prescribed concomitantly with fluoxetine or paroxetine; atomoxetine should be initiated at a lower dose of 0.5 mg/kg/day for the first month and the target dose should be limited to 1.2 mg/kg/day. Additionally, 7% of Caucasian and 2% of African-American youths are slow metabolizers, and lower doses of 0.5 mg/kg/day should be used to prevent cardiac and gastrointestinal side effects, which can become severe when the blood level reaches steady state (Kasi, Mounzer, & Gleeson, 2011).

Apparently due to its molecular similarity to fluoxetine, atomoxetine has been associated with suicidal ideation (FDA, 2005). Analysis of adverse-event data from the atomoxetine clinical trials database identified a small but statistically significant increase in risk of suicidal thoughts among atomoxetine-treated children and adolescents compared with placebo. This resulted in a FDA "black-box" warning to the product labeling of atomoxetine in September 2005.

Families and caregivers should be educated regarding the need to recognize any emergence of mood change or self-injurious behavior in the child and to inform the prescriber. Preschoolers being treated with ADHD drugs should be observed for mood changes, increased crying, irritability, and talk of self-harm. If mood symptoms emerge during treatment, dose reduction or discontinuation is recommended, especially if these symptoms are severe or abrupt in onset or were not part of the presenting symptoms (Shier et al., 2012).

a$_2$-adrenergic agonists. Since the popularity of IR guanfacine has increased, clonidine has fallen out of favor due to its sedating effect and comparatively shorter duration of action than IR guanfacine. In community practice, IR clonidine is more commonly used for treatment of sleep difficulties in children with ADHD with or without stimulant treatment. Prior to initiating treatment with a$_2$-adrenergic agonists, the AACAP-PPWG algorithm guidelines recommend an assessment of the caregivers' ability to administer and store the medication safely (Gleason et al., 2007) because of their antihypertensive properties and the risk of precipitating a hypertensive crisis with abrupt discontinuation.

α_2-adrenergic agonists may be contraindicated if the family is not able to do so (Gleason et al., 2007).

IR clonidine is usually initiated at a half-tablet of the smallest dosage strength available at a dose of 0.025 mg at night to minimize adverse effects, especially sedation. A morning dose of 0.025 mg can then be added a week later, followed by a midday dose of 0.025 mg 3 to 7 days later. The dosage can be titrated in this manner in increments of 0.025 mg BID or TID (may also be given QID). We recommend that any single dose should not exceed 0.1 mg and the total daily dose should not exceed 0.3 mg.

ER clonidine can be initiated at a dose of 0.1 mg at bedtime and increased, as needed to obtain an optimal response, by 0.1 mg at weekly intervals. ER clonidine should be administered twice daily with an equal or higher dose at bedtime. We prefer to limit the maximum total daily dose to 0.3 mg.

IR guanfacine is usually initiated at a dose of 0.25 mg at night to minimize sedation (Strange, 2008). The dosage can be titrated every 7 days in increments of 0.25 mg, first by adding a morning dose of 0.25 mg, followed by an after-school dose of 0.25 mg 7 days later. The dose can be titrated in this manner; we recommend that any single dose should not exceed 0.5 mg and the maximum total daily dose should not exceed 1.5 mg to 2 mg. Somnolence and fatigue are the most common TEAEs, especially during early titration, and can be managed by a slower titration or by lowering the dose.

ER guanfacine is taken once daily, either in the morning or evening. However, sedation with ER guanfacine may be a problem in preschool children, so it may need to be taken in the evening. It should not be taken with a high-fat meal as it can increase exposure. ER guanfacine is usually started at 1 mg once daily and can be titrated at 1- to 2-week intervals; we prefer to limit the maximum total daily dose to 3 mg. It may take 2 to 3 weeks to see a response (Sallee, Kollins, & Wigal, 2012).

TEAEs with clonidine and guanfacine have usually been mild and include sedation, fatigue, headache, dry mouth, constipation, upper abdominal pain, mid-sleep awakening, vivid dreams, irritability, dizziness, bradycardia, orthostatic hypotension, and withdrawal hypertension. Somnolence can be significant and may require a slower rate of titration. Guanfacine is generally less sedating than clonidine.

Because α_2-adrenergic agonists are antihypertensive agents, parents should be warned to monitor the preschooler closely for complaints of dizziness, syncope, and postural hypotension. Blood pressure and heart rate should be monitored at every visit. α_2-adrenergic agonists should not be discontinued abruptly due to the risk of precipitating a hypertensive crisis, making compliance with alpha agonists especially important. A slow taper is recommended when stopping α_2-adrenergic agonists. IR clonidine should be tapered by 0.05 mg, ER clonidine by 0.1 mg, IR guanfacine by 0.5 mg, and ER guanfacine by 1 mg every 3 to 7 days.

There were several case reports of sudden death in 8- to 10-year-old children taking a combination of clonidine and MPH (Cantwell, Swanson, & Connor, 1997). However, later reports failed to establish a definite causal link between combination treatment with clonidine and MPH and sudden death (Wilens, Spencer, Swanson, Connor, & Cantwell, 1999). Nevertheless, in children with a history of preexisting myocardial or structural heart disease or renal disease that can increase a child's risk for developing hypertension, cardiac consultation should be obtained prior to considering treatment with α_2-adrenergic agonists alone or in combination with stimulants.

Clonidine is often used for sleep problems associated with ADHD and/or stimulant treatment. However, its use can be problematic in some children due to the TEAEs of mid-sleep awakening and vivid dreams. We know of anecdotal reports of repeated increases in the bedtime dose of clonidine due to parents' repeated complaints of the child waking up in the middle of the night. Parents complain that there is initial improvement in the preschooler's sleep with each instance of clonidine dose increase, but it is short-lived, with return of mid-sleep awakening. We also know of anecdotal reports of parents giving an additional dose of clonidine when the child wakes up in the middle of the night. Clinicians should educate parents regarding the importance of giving only the prescribed dose, not to increase the child's clonidine dose without the prescriber's recommendation, and not to stop the child's clonidine abruptly. If the parents are not able to follow these guidelines, we recommend that the preschooler's clonidine be stopped following a slow taper.

Clinical Strategies for Management of Comorbid Disorders

It is important to assess for and incorporate treatment of comorbid disorders in the overall treatment plan since they are very common (as detailed in Chapter 4) and comorbidity has been shown to moderate treatment response in ADHD (Ghuman et al., 2007; MTA, 1999; Owens et al., 2003).

Developmental, communication, and learning disorders can confound the diagnosis of ADHD and vice versa. Appropriate referrals should be sought if developmental, communication, and learning disorders are suspected. The preschooler may need to be referred to a special education preschool, and specific classroom interventions should be implemented to address learning issues. Parent behavior training, behavior management, and classroom interventions (as detailed in Chapters 5 and 6) help address issues related to oppositional defiant disorder and disruptive behavior disorders. Depending on the severity of the oppositional defiant disorder symptoms and disruptive behaviors and psychosocial needs, additional individual, group, and family therapies may be indicated.

Children with ADHD and comorbid anxiety and tic disorders have been treated with stimulants without exacerbation of anxiety or tic symptoms (Abikoff et al., 2005; Erenberg, 2005). Nonstimulant agents, atomoxetine, or α_2-adrenergic agonists should be considered in case of severe anxiety or tic symptoms or worsening with stimulants. Clinical improvement in both ADHD and anxiety ratings was seen on parent report with open-label atomoxetine treatment in 3-to 5-year-old children with ADHD (Ghuman, Aman, Ghuman, et al., 2009). Improvement in anxiety and ADHD symptoms with atomoxetine versus placebo was reported in 8- to 17-year-old children with ADHD and comorbid anxiety disorders (Geller et al., 2007). If a preschooler presents with both ADHD and anxiety symptoms, atomoxetine can be instituted as a first-line treatment.

α_2-adrenergic agonists alone or as adjunct treatment to stimulants have been shown to improve tic and ADHD symptoms (Scahill et al., 2001; Tourette's Syndrome Study Group, 2002) and may be preferred agents for the treatment of children with moderate to severe comorbid tic disorders. Atomoxetine was also reported to improve both ADHD and tic symptoms in children and adolescents with ADHD and comorbid Tourette's disorder or chronic motor tic disorder (Allen et al., 2005; Spencer et al., 2008). On the other hand, open-label atomoxetine treatment resulted in onset of motor and/or vocal tics and worsening of tics in 9- to 15-year old boys with ADHD (Ledbetter, 2005; Lee, Lee, Lombroso, & King, 2004).

For preschoolers with comorbid mood disorders and self-harm issues, treatment is determined by whether it is ADHD or the comorbid disorder that is causing the greatest impairment. If self-harm issues and mood symptoms are paramount, appropriate safety precautions should be implemented and mood symptoms should be addressed first. Caution should be exercised if pharmacologic agents are prescribed to treat impairing ADHD symptoms in children with comorbid mood disorders since stimulants have been associated with induction of psychosis and manic symptoms in young children (Ross, 2006).

Clinical Recommendations

1. Psychosocial interventions are the first line of treatment for preschoolers with ADHD.
2. When considering treating preschoolers for ADHD, first a thorough psychiatric assessment should be conducted that includes a psychiatric history to address presenting complaints related to ADHD symptoms, comorbid disorders, medical/neurological conditions, medications, mental status examination of the preschooler, and collateral information from multiple sources and settings.
   2.1. Appropriate referrals for the pertinent assessments should be made for any obvious or suspected speech, language, and hearing, cognitive or medical\neurological concerns.
3. Caregivers should be provided psychoeducation to clarify misconceptions about ADHD and its treatment.
   3.1. The decision to treat ADHD in preschoolers should be a shared decision-making process with the child's caregivers and should take into account their values and beliefs.
   3.2. If there is disagreement between the parents and other family members about treating the child, a joint appointment should be scheduled to answer any questions and address their reservations.
4. Prior to prescribing psychopharmacological agents, the caregivers' ability to understand the importance of personally administering the medication as prescribed, to safely store the medication out of reach of young children, and to prevent and monitor for drug diversion should be assessed.
5. Prior to prescribing medication for ADHD, a detailed history should be obtained regarding the child's appetite, eating and sleep habits and/or problems, and tics, along with a careful targeted history about any cardiovascular, seizures, and psychosis risks in the child.
6. Parents should be informed at the outset that most ADHD medications (with the exception of immediate-release amphetamines) do not have FDA approval to treat ADHD in preschool children and are used "off-label."

7. Instructions for medication dose and time of administration should be explained to the parents in simple language, and written instructions should be provided clearly specifying the times of medication administration.

    7.1. Preschoolers should be seen regularly for medication monitoring.

    7.2. Rating scales should be obtained before starting treatment and then regularly throughout treatment to monitor response to medication and TEAEs.

    7.3. Parents should be informed of TEAEs associated with the prescribed medication and how to deal with the TEAEs, along with a discussion regarding the need for and/or appropriateness of drug holidays.

8. Treatment is usually initiated with IR short-acting stimulant formulations.

    8.1. Medication is started at a half-tablet (occasionally a quarter-tablet) of the smallest dosage strength available.

    8.2. Follow the rule: start low, go slow.

    8.3. Be cautious, don't prescribe very high doses, but at the same time be careful not to undertreat.

    8.4. Once a preschooler's IR medication dose is stabilized, some parents may prefer to switch to a long-acting formulation.

    8.5. If there is no response or a subthreshold response to one stimulant class:

        8.5.1. Switch to another stimulant class.

        8.5.2. If the response is still inadequate, switch to a nonstimulant formulation.

    8.6. Be sure to address comorbid disorders.

Summary

Thorough psychiatric and medical assessment is essential before instituting pharmacologic treatment for ADHD in preschoolers. Psychoeducation and informed consent should be provided early in the assessment and treatment process. Parents should be informed about the "off-label" status of the use of most of the ADHD pharmacologic agents in preschoolers. There should be thorough discussion of possible adverse effects of pharmacologic agents, including the FDA "black-box" warnings and the very preliminary reports of death associated with ADHD medications. There should be ample time for parents to ask questions and consult with family members and/or the preschooler's primary healthcare provider while considering treatment options for the preschooler. The decision to treat the preschooler with pharmacologic agents should be made jointly with the parents.

Prescription of pharmacologic agents should follow the rule of "start low, go slow." Close monitoring for treatment response, dose adjustments, and TEAEs, with sufficient time on each dosage, should be instituted. Monitoring visits should occur every 2 weeks for the first 1 to 2 months until the preschooler is on an optimal dose and then once a month for follow-up. Parent and "teacher" rating scales should be obtained prior to starting medication and repeated regularly to monitor treatment response during follow-up visits. Weight, height, blood pressure, and pulse should be monitored on a regular basis. The AACAP-PPWG recommends discontinuing medication after 6 months to assess the need for ongoing pharmacologic intervention in preschoolers (Gleason et al., 2007).

Disclosures

Jaswinder K. Ghuman, M.D., has received past funding from the NIMH for a K-23 career development grant, the Arizona Institute for Mental Health Research, and from Bristol-Myers Squibb for a clinical trial in autistic disorder. She received funding from the Health Resources and Services Administration–Maternal and Child Health (HRSA-MCH) for a training grant for the University of Arizona Leadership Education in Neurodevelopmental Disabilities Training Program (AZLEND).

Harinder S. Ghuman, M.D., has no conflicts of interest.

References

Abikoff, H., McGough, J., Vitiello, B., McCracken, J., Davies, M., Walkup, J., et al. (2005). Sequential pharmacotherapy for children with comorbid attention-deficit/hyperactivity and anxiety disorders. *Journal of the American Academy of Child & Adolescent Psychiatry, 44*(5), 418–427.

Allen, A. J., Kurlan, R. M., Gilbert, D. L., Coffey, B. J., Linder, S. L., Lewis, D. W., et al. (2005). Atomoxetine treatment in children and adolescents with ADHD and comorbid tic disorders. *Neurology, 65*(12), 1941–1949.

Arnold, L. E. (2000). Methylphenidate vs. amphetamine: Comparative review. *Journal of Attention Disorders, 3*(4), 200–211.

Arnold, L. E., Lindsay, R. L., Lopez, F. A., Jacob, S. E., Biederman, J., Findling, R. L., et al. (2007). Treating attention-deficit/hyperactivity disorder with a stimulant transdermal patch: the clinical art. *Pediatrics, 120*(5), 1100–1106.

Babington, R. G., & Wedeking, P. W. (1973). The pharmacology of seizures induced by sensitization with low intensity brain stimulation. *Pharmacology Biochemistry & Behavior, 1*(4), 461–467.

Bangs, M., Jin, L., Zhang, S., Desaiah, D., Allen, A., Read, H., et al. (2008). Hepatic events associated with atomoxetine treatment for attention-deficit hyperactivity disorder. *Drug Safety, 31*(4), 345–354.

Barkley, R. A., Fischer, M., Smallish, L., & Fletcher, K. (2003). Does the treatment of attention-deficit/hyperactivity disorder with stimulants contribute to drug use/abuse? A 13-year prospective study. *Pediatrics, 111*(1), 97–109.

Bernstein, D. (2000). *Evaluation of the cardiovascular system* (16th ed.). Philadelphia: W.B. Saunders.

Biederman, J., Monuteaux, M. C., Spencer, T., Wilens, T. E., Macpherson, H. A., & Faraone, S. V. (2008). Stimulant therapy and risk for subsequent substance use disorders in male adults with ADHD: a naturalistic controlled 10-year follow-up study. *American Journal of Psychiatry, 165*(5), 597–603.

Brown, T. E., & McMullen, W. J., Jr. (2001). Attention deficit disorders and sleep/arousal disturbance. *Annals of the New York Academy of Science, 931,* 271–286.

Bussing, R., Koro-Ljungberg, M., Noguchi, K., Mason, D., Mayerson, G., & Garvan, C. W. (2012). Willingness to use ADHD treatments: a mixed methods study of perceptions by adolescents, parents, health professionals and teachers. *Social Science & Medicine, 74*(1), 92–100.

Bussing, R., Zima, B. T., Mason, D. M., Meyer, J. M., White, K., & Garvan, C. W. (2012). ADHD knowledge, perceptions, and information sources: perspectives from a community sample of adolescents and their parents. *Journal of Adolescent Health, 51*(6), 593–600.

Cantwell, D., Swanson, J., & Connor, D. (1997). Case study: adverse response to clonidine. *Journal of the American Academy of Child & Adolescent Psychiatry, 36*(4), 539–544.

Cesena, M., Lee, D. O., Cebollero, A. M., & Steingard, R. J. (1995). Case study: behavioral symptoms of pediatric HIV-1 encephalopathy successfully treated with clonidine. *Journal of the American Academy of Child & Adolescent Psychiatry, 34*(3), 302–306.

Chacko, A., Wymbs, B. T., Wymbs, F. A., Pelham, W. E., Swanger-Gagne, M. S., Girio, E., et al. (2009). Enhancing traditional behavioral parent training for single mothers of children with ADHD. *Journal of Clinical Child & Adolescent Psychology*, 38(2), 206–218.

Chavez, B., Sopko, M. A., Jr., Ehret, M. J., Paulino, R. E., Goldberg, K. R., Angstadt, K., et al. (2009). An update on central nervous system stimulant formulations in children and adolescents with attention-deficit/hyperactivity disorder. *Annals of Pharmacotherapy*, 43(6), 1084–1095.

Dickson, R., Maki, E., Gibbins, C., Gutkin, S., Turgay, A., & Weiss, M. (2011). Time courses of improvement and symptom remission in children treated with atomoxetine for attention-deficit/hyperactivity disorder: analysis of Canadian open-label studies. *Child Psychiatry & Mental Health*, 5, 14.

DosReis, S., Barksdale, C. L., Sherman, A., Maloney, K., & Charach, A. (2010). Stigmatizing experiences of parents of children with a new diagnosis of ADHD. *Psychiatric Services*, 61(8), 811–816.

Dulcan, M. (1997). Practice parameters for the assessment and treatment of children, adolescents, and adults with attention-deficit/hyperactivity disorder. *Journal of the American Academy of Child & Adolescent Psychiatry*, 36(10 Suppl), 85S–121S.

Elia, J., Borcherding, B. G., Rapoport, J. L., & Keysor, C. S. (1991). Methylphenidate and dextro-amphetamine treatments of hyperactivity: are there true nonresponders? *Psychiatry Research*, 36(2), 141–155.

El-Zein, R. A., Abdel-Rahman, S. Z., Hay, M. J., Lopez, M. S., Bondy, M. L., Morris, D. L., et al. (2005). Cytogenetic effects in children treated with methylphenidate. *Cancer Letters*, 230(2), 284–291.

Erenberg, G. (2005). The relationship between Tourette syndrome, attention deficit hyperactivity disorder, and stimulant medication: a critical review. *Seminars in Pediatric Neurology*, 12(4), 217–221.

Fanton, J., & Gleason, M. M. (2009). Psychopharmacology and preschoolers: a critical review of current conditions. *Child & Adolescent Psychiatric Clinics of North America*, 18(3), 753–771.

Faraone, S. V., Biederman, J., Wilens, T. E., & Adamson, J. (2007). A naturalistic study of the effects of pharmacotherapy on substance use disorders among ADHD adults. *Psychological Medicine*, 37(12), 1743–1752.

FDA. (2005). FDA issues public health advisory on Strattera (atomoxetine) for attention deficit disorder, September 29, 2005. Accessed 6/30/2012 at: http://www.fda.gov/NewsEvents/Newsroom/PressAnnouncements/2005/ucm108493.htm.

FDA. (2006). Drug Safety and Risk Management Advisory Committee Meeting, February 9, 2006: Briefing January 12, 2006. Accessed January 27, 2012, at http://www.fda.gov/ohrms/dockets/ac/06/briefing/2006-4202B1_05_FDA-Tab05.pdf.

Geller, D., Donnelly, C., Lopez, F., Rubin, R., Newcorn, J., Sutton, V., et al. (2007). Atomoxetine treatment for pediatric patients with attention-deficit/hyperactivity disorder with comorbid anxiety disorder. *Journal of the American Academy of Child & Adolescent Psychiatry*, 46(9), 1119–1127.

Ghuman, J. K., & Ghuman, H. S. (2012). Pharmacologic intervention for attention-deficit hyperactivity disorder in preschoolers: is it justified? *Paediatric Drugs*, 15(1), 1–8.

Ghuman, J. K., Aman, M. G., Ghuman, H. S., Reichenbacher, T., Gelenberg, A., Wright, R., et al. (2009). Prospective, naturalistic, pilot study of open-label atomoxetine treatment in preschool children with attention-deficit/hyperactivity disorder. *Journal of Child & Adolescent Psychopharmacology*, 19(2), 155–166.

Ghuman, J. K., Aman, M. G., Lecavalier, L., Riddle, M. A., Gelenberg, A., Wright, R., et al. (2009). Randomized, placebo-controlled, crossover study of methylphenidate for attention-deficit/hyperactivity disorder symptoms in preschoolers with developmental disorders. *Journal of Child and Adolescent Psychopharmacology*, 19(4), 329–339.

Ghuman, J. K., Arnold, L. E., & Anthony, B. J. (2008). Psychopharmacological and other treatments in preschool children with attention-deficit/hyperactivity disorder: current evidence and practice. *Journal of Child and Adolescent Psychopharmacology*, 18(5), 413–447.

Ghuman, J. K., Ginsburg, G. S., Subramaniam, G., Ghuman, H. S., Kau, A. S., & Riddle, M. A. (2001). Psychostimulants in preschool children with attention-deficit/hyperactivity disorder: clinical evidence from a developmental disorders institution. *Journal of the American Academy of Child & Adolescent Psychiatry, 40*(5), 516–524.

Ghuman, J., Byreddy, S., & Ghuman, H. (2011). Methylphenidate transdermal system in preschool children with attention-deficit/hyperactivity disorder. *Journal of Adolescent Psychopharmacology, 21*(5), 495–498.

Ghuman, J., Riddle, M., Vitiello, B., Greenhill, L., Chuang, S., Wigal, S., et al. (2007). Comorbidity moderates response to methylphenidate in the Preschoolers with Attention-Deficit/Hyperactivity Disorder Treatment Study (PATS). *Journal of Child & Adolescent Psychopharmacology, 17*(5), 563–580.

Gleason, M. M., Egger, H. L., Emslie, G. J., Greenhill, L. L., Kowatch, R. A., Lieberman, A. F., et al. (2007). Psychopharmacological treatment for very young children: contexts and guidelines. *Journal of the American Academy of Child & Adolescent Psychiatry, 46*(12), 1532–1572.

Gould, M. S., Walsh, B. T., Munfakh, J. L., Kleinman, M., Duan, N., Olfson, M., et al. (2009). Sudden death and use of stimulant medications in youths. *American Journal of Psychiatry, 166*(9), 992–1001.

Graham, J., Banaschewski, T., Buitelaar, J., Coghill, D., Danckaerts, M., Dittmann, R. W., et al. (2011). European guidelines on managing adverse effects of medication for ADHD. *European Child & Adolescent Psychiatry, 20*(1), 17–37.

Greenhill, L. L., Newcorn, J. H., Gao, H., & Feldman, P. D. (2007). Effect of two different methods of initiating atomoxetine on the adverse event profile of atomoxetine. *Journal of the American Academy of Child and Adolescent Psychiatry, 46*(5), 566–572.

Greenhill, L., Kollins, S., Abikoff, H., McCracken, J., Riddle, M., Swanson, J., et al. (2006). Efficacy and safety of immediate-release methylphenidate treatment for preschoolers with ADHD. *Journal of the American Academy of Child & Adolescent Psychiatry, 45*(11), 1284–1293.

Greer, C. A., & Alpern, H. P. (1980). Paradoxical effects of d-amphetamine upon seizure susceptibility in 2 selectively bred lines of mice. *Developmental Psychobiology, 13*(1), 7–15.

Hull, W. (2002). Heat-enhanced drug delivery: a survey paper. *Journal of Applied Research in Clinical and Experimental Therapeutics, 2*, 69–76.

Kasi, P. M., Mounzer, R., & Gleeson, G. H. (2011). Cardiovascular side effects of atomoxetine and its interactions with inhibitors of the cytochrome p450 system. *Case Report Medicine, 952584*.

King, G. A., & Burnham, W. M. (1980). Effects of d-amphetamine and apomorphine in a new animal model of petit mal epilepsy. *Psychopharmacology (Berlin), 69*(3), 281–285.

Kratochvil, C. J., Vaughan, B. S., Stoner, J. A., Daughton, J. M., Lubberstedt, B. D., Murray, D. W., et al. (2011). A double-blind, placebo-controlled study of atomoxetine in young children with ADHD. *Pediatrics, 127*(4), e862–868.

Larson, J. J., Yoon, Y., Stewart, M., & dosReis, S. (2011). Influence of caregivers' experiences on service use among children with attention-deficit hyperactivity disorder. *Psychiatric Services, 62*(7), 734–739.

Lebowitz, M. S. L. (2013). Stigmatization of ADHD: a developmental review. *Journal of Attention Disorders,* Epub February 13, 2013.

Ledbetter, M. (2005). Atomoxetine use associated with onset of a motor tic. *Journal of Child & Adolescent Psychopharmacology, 15*(2), 331–333.

Lee, B. J. (1997). Clinical experience with guanfacine in 2- and 3-year-old children with attention deficit hyperactivity disorder. *Infant Mental Health, 18*, 300–305.

Lee, T. S., Lee, T. D., Lombroso, P. J., & King, R. A. (2004). Atomoxetine and tics in ADHD. *Journal of the American Academy of Child & Adolescent Psychiatry, 43*(9), 1068–1069.

Leibson, C. L., Barbaresi, W. J., Ransom, J., Colligan, R. C., Kemner, J., Weaver, A. L., et al. (2006). Emergency department use and costs for youth with attention-deficit/hyperactivity disorder: associations with stimulant treatment. *Ambulatory Pediatrics, 6*(1), 45–53.

Lilly. (2008). FDA approves Strattera(R) for maintenance of ADHD in children and adolescents, May 8, 2008. Accessed 6/30/2012 at: http://newsroom.lilly.com/ReleaseDetail.cfm?releaseid=309001.

Mannuzza, S., Klein, R. G., Truong, N. L., Moulton, J. L., 3rd, Roizen, E. R., Howell, K. H., et al. (2008). Age of methylphenidate treatment initiation in children with ADHD and later substance abuse: prospective follow-up into adulthood. *American Journal of Psychiatry, 165*(5), 604–609.

Martins, S., Tramontina, S., Polanczyk, G., Eizirik, M., Swanson, J. M., & Rohde, L. A. (2004). Weekend holidays during methylphenidate use in ADHD children: a randomized clinical trial. *Journal of Child & Adolescent Psychopharmacology, 14*(2), 195–206.

Molina, B. S., Hinshaw, S. P., Eugene Arnold, L., Swanson, J. M., Pelham, W. E., Hechtman, L., et al. (2013). Adolescent substance use in the Multimodal Treatment Study of Attention-Deficit/ Hyperactivity Disorder (ADHD) (MTA) as a function of childhood ADHD, random assignment to childhood treatments, and subsequent medication. *Journal of the American Academy of Child & Adolescent Psychiatry, 52*(3), 250–263.

Montoya, A., Colom, F., & Ferrin, M. (2011). Is psychoeducation for parents and teachers of children and adolescents with ADHD efficacious? A systematic literature review. *European Psychiatry, 26*(3), 166–175.

Mosholder, A. D., Gelperin, K., Hammad, T. A., Phelan, K., & Johann-Liang, R. (2009). Hallucinations and other psychotic symptoms associated with the use of attention-deficit/ hyperactivity disorder drugs in children. *Pediatrics, 123*(2), 611–616.

MTA. (1999). Moderators and mediators of treatment response for children with attention-deficit/ hyperactivity disorder: the Multimodal Treatment Study of Children with Attention-deficit/ hyperactivity disorder. *Archives of General Psychiatry, 56*(12), 1088–1096.

Nissen, S. E. (2006). ADHD drugs and cardiovascular risk. *N Engl J Med, 354*(14), 1445–1448.

Nock, M. K., & Kazdin, A. E. (2005). Randomized controlled trial of a brief intervention for increasing participation in parent management training. *Journal of Consulting Clinical Psychology, 73*(5), 872–879.

Noven/Shire. (2005). Pharmacokinetics/pharmacodynamics summary NDA 21-514.24, October, pp. 1–43. http://www.fda.gov/ohrms/dockets/ac/05/briefing/2005-4195B1_01_02-Noven-Appendix-1.pdf. Retrieved March 26, 2011, 2011

Owens, E. B., Hinshaw, S. P., Kraemer, H. C., Arnold, L. E., Abikoff, H. B., Cantwell, D. P., et al. (2003). Which treatment for whom for ADHD? Moderators of treatment response in the MTA. *Journal of Consulting Clinical Psychology, 71*(3), 540–552.

Perrin, J. M., Friedman, R. A., & Knilans, T. K. (2008). Cardiovascular monitoring and stimulant drugs for attention-deficit/hyperactivity disorder. *Pediatrics, 122*(2), 451–453.

Pescosolido, B. A., Jensen, P. S., Martin, J. K., Perry, B. L., Olafsdottir, S., & Fettes, D. (2008). Public knowledge and assessment of child mental health problems: findings from the National Stigma Study-Children. *Journal of the American Academy of Child & Adolescent Psychiatry, 47*(3), 339–349.

Pescosolido, B. A., Perry, B. L., Martin, J. K., McLeod, J. D., & Jensen, P. S. (2007). Stigmatizing attitudes and beliefs about treatment and psychiatric medications for children with mental illness. *Psychiatric Services, 58*(5), 613–618.

Ross, R. G. (2006). Psychotic and manic-like symptoms during stimulant treatment of attention deficit hyperactivity disorder. *American Journal of Psychiatry, 163*(7), 1149–1152.

Sallee, F. R., Kollins, S. H., & Wigal, T. L. (2012). Efficacy of guanfacine extended release in the treatment of combined and inattentive only subtypes of attention-deficit/hyperactivity disorder. *Journal of Child and Adolescent Psychopharmacology, 22*(3), 206–214.

Scahill, L., Chappell, P. B., Kim, Y. S., Schultz, R. T., Katsovich, L., Shepherd, E., et al. (2001). A placebo-controlled study of guanfacine in the treatment of children with tic disorders and attention deficit hyperactivity disorder. *American Journal of Psychiatry, 158*(7), 1067–1074.

Schelleman, H., Bilker, W. B., Strom, B. L., Kimmel, S. E., Newcomb, C., Guevara, J. P., et al. (2011). Cardiovascular events and death in children exposed and unexposed to ADHD agents. *Pediatrics, 127*(6), 1102–1110.

Shier, A. C., Reichenbacher, T., Ghuman, H. S., & Ghuman, J. K. (2012). Pharmacological treatment of attention deficit hyperactivity disorder in children and adolescents: clinical strategies. *Journal of Central Nervous System Diseases, 5*, 1–17.

Spencer, T. J., Sallee, F. R., Gilbert, D. L., Dunn, D. W., McCracken, J. T., Coffey, B. J., et al. (2008). Atomoxetine treatment of ADHD in children with comorbid Tourette syndrome. *Journal of Attention Disorders, 11*(4), 470–481.

Spencer, T., Kratochvil, C., Sangal, R., Saylor, K., Bailey, C., Dunn, D., et al. (2007). Effects of atomoxetine on growth in children with attention-deficit/hyperactivity disorder following up to five years of treatment. *Journal of Child & Adolescent Psychopharmacology, 17*(5), 689–700.

Strange, B. (2008). Once-daily treatment of ADHD with guanfacine: patient implications. *Neuropsychiatric Diseases & Treatment, 4*(3), 499–506.

Swanson, J., Greenhill, L., Wigal, T., Kollins, S., Stehli, A., Davies, M., et al. (2006). Stimulant-related reductions of growth rates in the PATS. *Journal of the American Academy of Child & Adolescent Psychiatry, 45*(11), 1304–1313.

Taylor, E., Dopfner, M., Sergeant, J., Asherson, P., Banaschewski, T., Buitelaar, J., et al. (2004). European clinical guidelines for hyperkinetic disorder—first upgrade. *European Child & Adolescent Psychiatry, 13*(Suppl 1), I7–30.

Tourette's Syndrome Study Group. (2002). Treatment of ADHD in children with tics: a randomized controlled trial. *Neurology, 58*(4), 527–536.

Tucker, J., Suter, W., Petibone, D., Thomas, R., Bailey, N., Zhou, Y., et al. (2009). Cytogenetic assessment of methylphenidate treatment in pediatric patients treated for attention deficit hyperactivity disorder. *Mutation Research, 677*(1–2), 53–58.

Vetter, V., Elia, J., Erickson, C., Berger, S., Blum, N., Uzark, K., et al. (2008). Cardiovascular monitoring of children and adolescents with heart disease receiving medications for attention deficit/hyperactivity disorder [corrected]: a scientific statement from the American Heart Association Council on Cardiovascular Disease in the Young Congenital Cardiac Defects Committee and the Council on Cardiovascular Nursing. *Circulation, 117*(8), 2407–2423.

Villalaba, L. (2006). Follow-up review of AERS search identifying cases of sudden death occurring with drugs used for the treatment of attention deficit hyperactivity disorder (ADHD). Available at: http://www.fda.gov/ohrms/dockets/ac/06/briefing/2006-4210b_07_01_safetyreview.pdf. Accessed: 7/4/12.

Walitza, S., Kampf, K., Artamonov, N., Romanos, M., Gnana Oli, R., Wirth, S., et al. (2009). No elevated genomic damage in children and adolescents with attention deficit/hyperactivity disorder after methylphenidate therapy. *Toxicology Letters, 184*(1), 38–43.

Walitza, S., Kampf, K., Oli, R., Warnke, A., Gerlach, M., & Stopper, H. (2010). Prospective follow-up studies found no chromosomal mutagenicity of methylphenidate therapy in ADHD affected children. *Toxicology Letters, 193*(1), 4–8.

Wilens, T. E., & Fusillo, S. (2007). When ADHD and substance use disorders intersect: relationship and treatment implications. *Current Psychiatry Reports, 9*(5), 408–414.

Wilens, T., Spencer, T., Swanson, J., Connor, D., & Cantwell, D. (1999). Combining methylphenidate and clonidine: a clinically sound medication option. *Journal of the American Academy of Child & Adolescent Psychiatry, 38*(5), 614–619; discussion 619–622.

Zamora-Perez, A., Lazalde-Ramos, B., Sosa-Maclas, M., Gomez-Meda, B., Torres-Bugarin, O., & Zuniga-Gonzalez, G. (2011). Methylphenidate lacks genotoxic effects in mouse peripheral blood erythrocytes. *Drug & Chemical Toxicology, 34*(3), 294–299.

9

Complementary and Alternative Treatments for Preschool Children with ADHD

NICHOLAS LOFTHOUSE AND ELIZABETH HURT

Complementary and alternative medicine (CAM) is defined by the National Center for Complementary and Alternative Medicine (NCCAM) as "a group of diverse medical and health care systems, practices, and products that are not generally considered to be part of conventional medicine" (NCCAM, 2011). As these interventions can include both noningestible (i.e., externally administered) and ingestible (i.e., orally administered) treatments, we refer to them collectively as complementary and alternative treatments (CATs). They are "complementary" when used "together with conventional medicine" and alternative when used "in place of conventional medicine" (NCCAM, 2011). Technically a complimentary or alternative treatment should be designated as such only if incremental effects when added or similar effects when compared to established treatments, respectively, are demonstrated by research. As few CATs actually fulfill these requirements, the majority of CATs should be more accurately considered as experimental treatments with the potential to become CATs. Typically, most patients and families who try CATs do so because they find conventional treatments (e.g., medication) ineffective, intolerable because of side effects, and/or practically or philosophically unacceptable. CAT use for children and adolescents with attention-deficit/hyperactivity disorder (ADHD) has been reported to range between 12% and 68% worldwide (Bussing, Zima, Gary, & Garvan, 2002; Cala, Crismon, & Baumgartner, 2003; Chan, Rappaport, & Kemper, 2003; Sinha & Efron 2005; Stubberfield, Wray, & Parry 1999), with 93% of pediatricians reporting being asked about CATs by their patients with ADHD (Sinha & Efron, 2005). Unfortunately none of these studies reported CAT use for 2- to 5-year-olds with ADHD.

Similarly, although an October 2012 PsycINFO/Medline title search (ADHD/attention-deficit, inattentive, inattention, hyperactive, hyperactivity, impulsive or impulsivity, limited to age 2 to 5 years) identified more than 1,215 citations, only 6 included randomized controlled trials (RCTs) for CATs specific to this age range (Bateman et al., 2004; Kaplan, McNicol, Conte, & Moghadam, 1989; McCann et al.,

2007; Pelsser et al., 2009, 2011 [all 5 involved elimination diets]; Li, Yu, Lin, et al., 2010 [electro-acupuncture]) and 2 included open-label evaluations of CATs for preschoolers (Halperin et al., 2012; Tamm et al., 2012 [both involved executive functioning training]), or if they involved CATs, they did not include any within-study analyses for 2- to 5-year-olds. Therefore, few published data currently exist on CATs for preschool ADHD. However, parents may not wait for science to catch up with their children's needs and may experiment with CATs on their own, especially if they sense practitioners are reluctant or lack knowledge about such interventions. Therefore, it is imperative for practitioners to have the knowledge to discuss and guide individual trials for younger patients. To assist practitioners we will discuss these six studies and the downward extension of other CAT research conducted on 5- to 18-year-olds with ADHD, which we have previously reviewed (Arnold, Hurt, Mayes, & Lofthouse, 2011; Arnold, Lofthouse, & Hurt, 2012; Hurt, Lofthouse, & Arnold, 2011a,b,c; Lofthouse, Arnold, Hersch, Hurt, & deBeus, 2012; Lofthouse, Arnold, & Hurt, 2012, in press; Lofthouse, McBurnett, Hurt, & Arnold, 2011).

For each of the following CATs, we define the intervention, describe its rationale for use, summarize the published research, and discuss its strengths and limitations and future research directions. We apply the Sensible, Easy, Cheap, and Safe (SECS) criteria and discuss whether, at this current time, an individual trial is recommended, acceptable, or not recommended for preschoolers with ADHD. Unfortunately, there is limited scientific evidence for CATs for preschoolers with ADHD. We are only aware of two reviews of nonpharmacologic treatments (i.e., CATs and behavior modification) for preschoolers with ADHD (Ghuman, Arnold, & Anthony, 2008; Rajwan, Chacko, & Moeller, 2012). In the former, the reviewed studies included children with a diagnosis or symptoms of ADHD and at least some children were less than 6 years of age. Three nonpharmacologic treatments had midlevel evidence for efficacy (based on significant differences on ADHD outcomes in one RCT, mixed results in at least two RCTs or one series of random single case design experiments): parent behavior training (N = 15 studies), child training (N = 6), and additive-free elimination diet (N = 9). Evidence for efficacy of other nonpharmacologic treatments was at a lower level (based on uncontrolled trials, case reports, retrospective chart reviews, or informed clinical opinion): vitamin/mineral and other dietary supplementation (N = 10), vestibular stimulation (N = 3), and massage (N = 3).

Rajwan and colleagues (2012) reviewed nonpharmacologic interventions for 3- to 6-year-old children with an ADHD diagnosis or symptoms and concluded that parent-based (N = 10 studies) and teacher-based (N = 3 studies) behavior modification, and to a lesser extent multimodal behavior treatment (parent-, teacher-, and child-based, N = 4 studies), changed oppositional, noncompliant, aggressive, and disruptive behaviors and also improved attention and hyperactivity. In contrast, they concluded that self-instructional/self-regulation training for children (N = 4), dietary interventions (N = 2), nutritional supplements (N = 1), and acupuncture (N = 1) needed substantially more research before being clinically used.

In a recent meta-analysis of 54 RCTs of dietary and psychological treatments for 3- to 18-year-olds with an ADHD diagnosis or symptoms, Sonuga-Barke and colleagues (2013) found that when nonblinded assessment data were used, all dietary and psychological treatments showed statistically significant effects on ADHD assessments, with standardized mean differences (i.e., effect sizes) between 0.21 to 0.48 and 0.40 to 0.64, respectively. However, when only the best "probably blinded" assessment data were used, only essential-fatty-acid supplementation (0.16) and artificial food color exclusion (0.42) remained significant, with results for behavioral interventions, neurofeedback, cognitive training, and restricted elimination diets reduced to nonsignificant levels.

There is more research on CATs for school-aged children, albeit still relatively sparse and limited by methodological flaws (see reviews by Arnold, Hurt, Mayes, & Lofthouse, 2011; Hurt, Arnold, & Lofthouse, 2011a,b,c). However, some of these CATs may be particularly palatable for parents of preschool children who do not wish to begin medication with a young child. Given this state of affairs, we will make recommendations based on available evidence for preschool children and school-age children with ADHD. Where means and standard deviations are available, we report effect sizes (ESs, Cohen's d; Cohen, 1988). For reference, d values between 0.2 and 0.4 are considered small ESs, 0.5 to 0.8 medium, and above 0.8 large. Conventional ADHD treatments have ES of 0.8 to 1.2 for stimulant medications, 0.4 to 1.0 for atomoxetine, and 0.5 to 1.0 for behavior modification in school-age children (Arnold, 2004). We include four categories of ingestible CATs (elimination diets, dietary supplementation, herbs, and homeopathic remedies) and seven categories of noningestible CATs (electro-acupuncture, executive functioning/attention/working memory training, yoga, meditation, vestibular stimulation, massage therapy, and biofeedback/neurofeedback).

Ingestible CATs

ELIMINATION DIETS

Elimination (few foods, defined, or oligoantigenic) diets involve the avoidance of foods or components to which the child might be sensitive for 1 to 3 weeks followed by their reintroduction, one at a time, while watching for any reaction. This CAT is based on the hypothesis, introduced by Feingold (1975), that many children are sensitive to dietary salicylates, artificially added food colors, flavors, and preservatives, and possibly natural food proteins. Hence, eliminating these substances may ameliorate ADHD and learning and behavioral problems. A basic elimination diet involves removing dairy products (instead, use soy milk, soy cheese, rice milk, rice-based ice cream); food products containing gluten, such as wheat and wheat-based products (including pasta), and barley, oat, or rye grains (alternative foods could include brown rice, buckwheat, spelt, millet, potatoes or sweet potatoes); citrus fruits; corn and corn-containing products; and all processed foods, including caffeine (e.g., chocolate and soda; withdrawal symptoms should last only a few days). Three RCTs and six placebo challenges (N = 704) have reported significant (p = .05 to .001) improvements in ADHD symptoms, with effect sizes of 0.5 to 2.0. All of the studies included preschoolers, but most also included school-age children (range 2 to 15 years), often selected for suspected food sensitivity and for syndromes (minimal brain dysfunction, hyperactivity) that were later gathered under the rubric of ADHD. Reviews of double-blind placebo-controlled studies of artificial food colorings suggest a small but significant negative effect on children's behavior, regardless of whether or not they have ADHD, which may be associated with a genetic vulnerability to the substances (Bateman et al., 2004; McCann et al., 2007; Stevenson et al., 2010).

Five of the studies reviewed are of particular interest for this chapter as they were done with preschool children. Three studies included only preschoolers diagnosed with ADHD (Kaplan et al., 1989; Pelsser et al., 2009, 2011) and two studies included preschool-aged children with and without ADHD symptoms (Bateman et al., 2004; McCann et al., 2007). In 1989, Kaplan and colleagues reported a within-subject, placebo-controlled double-blind crossover study of an additive-free versus placebo diet in a sample of 24 3.5- to 6-year-olds with a DSM-III diagnosis of ADHD. During the elimination diet stage and compared to baseline and placebo, parents reported significantly (p <.01) fewer ADHD symptoms, with 58% of children demonstrating behavioral and sleep improvements. In 2009, Pelsser and colleagues randomized 27 3- to 8-year-olds diagnosed with ADHD to an elimination diet or waitlist control group; after 5 weeks, there were significant improvements on nonblinded parent and teacher ratings of ADHD symptoms in the intervention group relative to the control group (p <.001). More recently, Pelsser and colleagues (2011) randomized 100 4- to 8-year-old children to an elimination diet group or a control group who received nutritional advice. After 5 weeks on the diet, the intervention group improved significantly more on blinded physician and nonblinded parent and teacher ratings of ADHD symptoms (p <.0001). Thirty-two of the 41 diet completers were considered to be clinical responders (>40% improvement on ADHD symptoms), and 30 participated in a double-blind placebo-controlled food challenge phase; 19 of the 30 relapsed to at least one food challenge.

The so-called Southampton studies involved two studies on preschoolers (Bateman et al., 2004 [N = 277]; McCann et al., 2007 [N = 153]); the latter also included 8- and 9-year-olds (N = 144). The samples were nonclinical but designated as hyperactive or not based on parent ratings and atopic or not based on a skin prick test. All children were given an elimination diet free of artificial food colorings and preservatives for 1 week and then challenged with 1 week each of a mix of artificial food colorings and sodium benzoate or placebo mixed with fruit juice. Blinding for all studies was excellent, as shown by blind adult taste panels and asking parents in the first study which order they thought the children were assigned. The first preschool study (Bateman et al., 2004) reported a greater significant increase in parent-rated hyperactivity on active challenge than on placebo in all the enrolled preschoolers, with a small to medium ES, and the second preschool study (McCann et al., 2007) replicated these results in a different sample and found dose effects. Importantly, there was no association with ADHD (defined by rating scale score) or atopy (defined by skin prick) indicating this deleterious effect applied to all children. These results led to some marked changes in Europe, with the United Kingdom government requesting that food manufacturers exchange these artificial food colorings for natural food colors/flavors and the European Union asking companies to voluntarily eliminate several artificial food colorings from foods and beverages or add a warning label. However, a 2011 U.S. Food and Drug Administration (FDA) Food Advisory Committee hearing on the behavioral effects of artificial food colorings voted not to recommend banning them or requiring a warning label (FDA Food Advisory Committee, 2011; Arnold, Lofthouse, & Hurt, 2012).

Even though dietary management, particularly restriction of artificial food colorings, does not meet specific criterion to be considered a CAT for ADHD, due to the small proven deleterious effect on hyperactivity ratings of all preschoolers (not just those with ADHD) from artificial food colorings and sodium benzoate, restriction of artificial food colorings and preservatives appears sensible and relatively safe. Restriction of other dietary components known to affect a given individual child appears sensible and relatively safe on one hand, but the potential risks of an oligoantigenic ("few foods") diet should be considered, including family stress associated with the time, effort, and expense in maintaining this type of diet and nutritional imbalance in the preschooler. Given these concerns, the "few foods" diet may be acceptable for preschoolers with ADHD who have a documented history of reactions to certain food substances. A 1- to 3-week trial could be tried, if there is benefit, foods should be added back one at a time to find the problem foods. But if there is no benefit, the diet should be abandoned. Due to the high level of organization needed for elimination diets, families may require consultation from clinicians to develop behavioral plans to assist with adherence to the diet and from dietitians to ensure nutritional adequacy of the diet. As few of the studies used subjects with a DSM diagnosis of ADHD, future research needs to include specific diagnostic assessments to better characterize the samples.

A related dietary strategy, elimination of sugar alone, despite widespread public belief, has not garnered convincing scientific support from 12 well-designed double-blind, placebo-controlled challenge studies (N = 296) and a meta-analysis (Wolraich, Wilson, & White, 1995) of 23 double-blind, placebo-controlled studies (N = 531). One study (Wender & Salanto, 1991) in the meta-analysis included young children (ages 5-7) with and without ADHD; there were no significant effects of sugar relative to placebo on observed aggressive behavior or on overall performance on a continuous performance task for either group. However, a classroom study of school-age children not selected for ADHD (N = 29) found that there was an increase in classroom inattentiveness during the course of a morning after no breakfast. The decline in inattentiveness was lessened by a whole-grain cereal breakfast with milk and was worsened by a same-calorie glucose-drink breakfast (p <.0025) (Wesnes, Pincock, Richardson, Helm, & Hails, 2003). Elimination of sugar by itself is not recommended as a CAT specific for ADHD. However, sugar is frequently accompanied by artificial flavors and dyes and in excess can have other known health implications. Because reasonable restriction of sugar has general health benefits (i.e., is sensible) and is safe and cheap, we recommend it for all children, even if it is not always easy due to the potential parent–child conflict and time needed to monitor a preschooler's eating habits. It can have an additional benefit of helping the preschooler develop healthy eating habits early on.

DIETARY SUPPLEMENTATION

Dietary supplementation involves enhancing a child's diet with various nutrients thought to be lacking in children with ADHD. Nutritional supplements can be classified into three categories: macronutrients (polyunsaturated fatty acids, glyconutritional saccharides, amino acids, and protein), micronutrients (vitamins and minerals, especially iron, zinc, and magnesium), and metabolites (melatonin, L-carnitine, and dimethylaminoethanol [DMAE]).

Macronutrient Supplementation
Polyunsaturated fatty acids (PUFAs) include alpha-linolenic acid (ALA, an omega-3 [ω-3]) and its longer-chain metabolites and linoleic acid (LA, an omega-6 [ω-6]) and its

longer-chain metabolites. Omega-3 and ω-6 are the only two essential fatty acid series known for humans—"essential" because we cannot synthesize them and they are vital in our diets for normal growth, metabolism, and functioning. Normal metabolism, which may be disrupted in some cases of ADHD (Brookes, Chen, Xu, Taylor, & Asherson., 2006), changes ALA and LA into the more desaturated and longer-chain PUFAs: eicosapentaenoic acid (EPA, ω-3) and docosahexaenoic acid (DHA, ω-3), gamma-linolenic acid (GLA, ω-6), dihomo-gamma-linolenic acid (DGLA, ω-6), and arachidonic acid (AA, ω-6). PUFAs have been used in the treatment of ADHD because of associated fatty acid deficiency symptoms and lower blood PUFA levels; DHA is especially associated with more severe ADHD symptoms (see Milte, Sinn, & Howe, 2009; Milte et al., 2011 for review).

To date, there have been 16 published double-blind, placebo-controlled RCTs, one meta-analysis (Bloch & Qawasmi, 2011), and one Cochrane review (Gillies et al., 2012) on PUFAs for children with ADHD diagnosis or symptoms. The meta-analysis, which included 10 of these 16 RCTs, reported a significant ($p < .0001$) but small effect size (0.31) for ω-3 in improving ADHD symptoms, especially for higher doses of EPA ($p < .04$, $R^2 = 0.37$). In contrast, the Cochrane review, which included 13 of the 16 RCTs, reported that the majority of the data showed no benefit for PUFA, although a minority of the data demonstrated improvement with combined ω-3 and ω-6 (GLA). As previously noted, Sonuga-Barke et al. (2013) a meta-analysis of "probably blinded" RCTs of essential fatty-acid supplementation showed a small but significant benefit (ES = 0.16). These disparate conclusions may be due to the wide variability of PUFAs and PUFA mixes used, treatment durations, doses, study designs, samples, and/or methodological limitations across these RCTs. In our own detailed examination of these 16 RCTs (N = 1,069), four used one PUFA, seven used two, and five used at least three. Where means and standard deviations were available (9/16 studies), we found the following ESs favoring PUFAs over placebo based on parent ratings ($d = 0.63$), teacher ratings ($d = 1.04$; range 0.28 to 2.56), clinician ratings ($d = 0.63$), neuropsychological tests ($d = 0.85$), and PUFA blood composition changes ($d = 1.56$). Trials with the highest ESs tended to use a combination of PUFAs. Unfortunately, many of the trials were limited by design flaws.

Even though no controlled trials are available in preschoolers with ADHD, due to brain development and cardiovascular health benefits, PUFAs appear sensible and are easy, inexpensive, and safe to use as long as mercury-free oils are used (indicated on the label or by USP seal). Based on the reported studies in school-age children, a 3- to 6-month trial of EPA/DHA (500 to 750 mg/day) may be considered in preschoolers with ADHD, especially if they do not eat oily wild ocean fish at least three times a week.

Glyconutritional supplements are derived from vegetables and contain seven basic saccharides essential for cell communication and glycoprotein and glycolipid production. In an open-label trial in 17 children between 6 and 14 years of age diagnosed with ADHD (Dykman & Dykman, 1998), a 2-week trial with glyconutritional supplements significantly reduced parent-rated inattention and hyperactivity/impulsivity ratings on a DSM-IV–based scale that was specifically constructed for the study. The improvement was sustained for 6 weeks. Similar results were reported in another open-label trial in 19 ADHD children (Dykman & McKinley, 1997). Glyconutritional supplements have little evidence but, depending on expense, may be acceptable for a trial, especially for children who do not eat vegetables.

Amino acid supplementation has been suggested as a treatment because of reports of low levels of amino acids (Baker et al., 1991; Bernstein, 1990) and nitrogen wasting in children with ADHD (Stein & Sammaritano, 1984). Several open and controlled trials have reported a short-term benefit for tryptophan, tyrosine, phenylalanine, and S-adenosyl-methionine (SAMe) for ADHD symptoms in school-age children and adults (Nemzer, Arnold, Votolato, & McConnell, 1986; Reimherr, Wender, Wood, & Ward, 1987; Shekim, Antun, Hanna, & McCracken, 1990; Wood, Reimherr, & Wender, 1985a). However, this short-term benefit of amino acids usually dissipates by 2 to 3 months (Wood, Reimherr, & Wender, 1985b). There is also some risk from toxic catabolic products from increased neurotransmitter turnover from the "supply-side metabolism." Because of metabolic risk and the lack of long-term benefits, amino acids are not recommended for preschool children. Eating adequate protein in the diet to maintain adequate substrate and to compensate for nitrogen wasting is safer and is the recommended approach for preschoolers with ADHD.

Breakfast containing protein and complex carbohydrate. Wesnes and colleagues (2003) found that children (without ADHD) who were given a whole-grain cereal and milk breakfast deteriorated less (by about half) in their attention over the course of the morning classroom session than when given no breakfast or a same-calorie glucose breakfast. A protein-containing low-sugar breakfast is sensible, easy, cheap, and safe and therefore is recommended for preschoolers with ADHD. Further, although we do not know of supporting data, attention to the protein content of lunch, dinner, and snacks may also be sensible.

Micronutrient Supplementation

Recommended daily allowance/dietary intake (RDA/RDI) multivitamins have not been systematically evaluated in ADHD, but in two double-blind placebo-controlled RCTs (Benton & Cook, 1991; Benton & Roberts, 1988), of 47 typically developing 6-year-olds and 90 school-age children, relative to a placebo, participants significantly improved in nonverbal intelligence, concentration, sustained attention, and excess motor behavior with RDI multivitamin and mineral supplementation. However, the effect may be specific to a subgroup with poor diets (Benton & Buts, 1990). Crombie and colleagues (1990) reported no significant differences on tests of reasoning in 86 typically developing 11- to 13-year-old children with 7-month RDI multivitamin and mineral supplementation versus placebo. In addition to being sensible, especially in light of the poor dietary habits of children with ADHD (Howard, Robinson, Smith, et al., 2011), this approach is inexpensive, easy, and, unless the patient has a rare genetic disorder, safe. Thus, even if there is lack of empirical evidence for improving ADHD symptoms in preschoolers, RDA/RDI multivitamin/mineral supplementation is acceptable for all preschoolers with ADHD and is recommended for picky eaters and/or those with stimulant-suppressed appetites at risk for vitamin deficiency.

Megadoses of single or multiple vitamins included some early and promising pilot data for specific single megavitamins in school-age children with hyperactivity (Brenner, 1982; Coleman et al., 1979), whereas three placebo-controlled studies of multiple megavitamins found no benefit for ADHD symptoms (Arnold, Christopher, Huestis, & Smeltzer, 1978; Haslam, Dalby, & Rademaker, 1984; Kershner & Hawke, 1979). Due to the lack of evidence and concerns about toxicity (e.g., hepatotoxicity, peripheral neuropathy), megadoses of single or multiple vitamins do not appear sensible or safe and are therefore not recommended for preschool children with ADHD.

Mineral supplementation, such as iron, magnesium, and zinc, has been suggested because of reported deficiencies in children with ADHD compared to controls (Kozielec, Starobrat-Hermelin, & Kotokowiak, 1994). Iron is a necessary co-enzyme to make catecholamines, often found to be deficient in ADHD. It has been reported to be deficient in two samples of 5- to 14-year-old children with ADHD (Cortese, Konofal, Bernadina, Mouren, & Lecendreux, 2009; Konofal et al., 2007), although the deficiency may be restricted to those with ADHD and comorbid disorders (Oner & Oner, 2008). Currently, there are only two small pilot trials of iron supplementation for ADHD symptoms. An open-label trial of 17 non-anemic 7- to 11-year-old boys with ADHD showed significantly improved parent ratings with 5 mg/kg/day of iron for 30 days (Sever, Ashkenazi, Tyano, & Weizman, 1997). A more recent placebo-controlled randomized pilot trial of 23 non-anemic 5- to 8-year-olds with ADHD and borderline-deficient iron levels reported a significant decrease in parent-reported ADHD symptoms with 12 weeks of 80 mg/day of iron sulfate (Konofal et al., 2008).

Magnesium deficiency can cause a wide variety of neurologic and psychiatric problems and can stem from multiple causes, including inadequate intake and malabsorption (Flink, 1981). Kozielec and Starobrat-Hermelin (1997) reported that 95% of 9- to 12-year-old Polish children with ADHD had deficient magnesium levels based on red cell and hair levels and 34% by serum levels. Four open-label trials in school-age European children with ADHD (total N = 173) reported significant decreases in inattention and hyperactivity after 1 to 6 months of treatment with magnesium (Mousain-Bose et al., 2006; Mousain-Bose, Roche, Rapin, & Bali, 2004; Nogovitsina & Levinia, 2007; Starobrat-Hermelin & Kozielec, 1997).

Zinc is a co-factor for more than 100 enzymes, many in the brain, and is necessary for melatonin production and regulating dopamine production; when deficient it causes hyperactivity in both animals and humans (Arnold & DiSilvestro, 2005). Compared to normal controls, 6- to 12-year-old children with ADHD had lower zinc levels (d = 2.4, p <.001, Bekaroglu et al., 1996), and serum zinc level has been found to correlate (r = −0.45) with inattention ratings (Arnold et al., 2005). Two Turkish RCTs of zinc monotherapy in a total of 626 school-age children (Bilici et al., 2004; Uckardes, Ozmert, Unal, & Yurdakok, 2009) reported more benefit for ADHD with zinc than placebo, but the benefit in the latter study was limited to children of mothers with primary school or less education. An Iranian RCT found adjunctive benefit when added to standard methylphenidate dosage in school-age children with ADHD (Akhondzadeh, Mohammadi, & Khademi, 2004). However, an American pilot RCT (Arnold, DiSilvestro, et al., 2011) in school-age children with ADHD reported that 8 weeks of zinc monotherapy was no more effective than placebo. On the other hand, there was a 37% decrease in the amphetamine dose that was added openly for 5 weeks for all the participants while they continued in their assigned treatment group (zinc or placebo) in a blinded manner. Possible reasons for the different results with zinc monotherapy between the Middle Eastern and the American trials include geographic dietary differences, genetic differences, dose and type of zinc used (zinc sulfate in the Middle East trials and glycinate in the American trial), and participants' socioeconomic status. Furthermore, zinc may also interact with food dye, as some children with hyperactivity and food dye intolerance had lower serum, urine, and nail zinc levels than normal controls. When challenged with tartrazine, their serum zinc levels declined and urine zinc levels increased, suggesting zinc wasting from the dye (Ward, 1997; Ward et al., 1990).

There are no controlled trials of safety and efficacy of iron, magnesium, and zinc supplementation in preschool children with ADHD. Although easy to administer, an excess of these minerals can cause hemochromatosis (iron), aplasia and interference with iron/copper absorption (zinc), and aggression or diarrhea (magnesium) (Arnold, Hurt, Mayes, & Lofthouse, 2011). Therefore, as controlled research has not supported their use for school-age children with ADHD, iron, magnesium, and zinc supplements beyond the RDA/RDI are acceptable only for preschoolers with ADHD who have a documented deficiency/insufficiency.

Metabolite Supplementation

Melatonin supplementation has been proposed because it is a natural hormone involved in the regulation of circadian rhythm and ADHD is often associated with sleep problems. Three studies of melatonin in 159 schoolchildren with ADHD, one open-label (Tjon Pian Gi, Broeren, Starreveld, & Versteegh, 2003), one crossover (van der Heijden, Smits, Someren, Ridderinkhof, & Gunnings, 2007), and one double-blind, placebo-controlled RCT (Weiss, Wasdell, Bomben, Rea, & Freeman, 2006) did not find any significant decreases in ADHD symptoms but did find significant improvements in sleep (d = 0.59 to 1.02). Although there are no RCTs in preschoolers with ADHD, melatonin meets the SECS criteria and is acceptable for sleep-onset delay in preschoolers with ADHD. Melatonin should be used if the usual behavioral/environmental sleep hygiene interventions are not sufficient.

Carnitine is a metabolite necessary for energy production, fatty acid metabolism, lipid transportation, and EFA elongation. Because most of us do not make enough of our own, it is considered a semi-essential nutrient, available in fish and meat. Three double-blind RCTs of carnitine supplementation of school-age children with ADHD have been reported. Significant improvements in parent- and teacher-rated attention problems and aggressive behavior were reported in 13 of 24 Dutch school-age boys (age range = 6 to 13 years) with ADHD for acetyl-L-carnitine (ALC) compared to placebo (Van Oudheusen & Scholte, 2002). Arnold and colleagues (2005, 2007) reported significantly better scores at 4 months, but not at 2 months, on a timed math test of attention for L-carnitine compared to placebo (p =.02, d = 0.67) in 112 children (age range = 5 to 12 years) diagnosed with ADHD, even though there was no benefit on the primary outcome measure, parent- and teacher-rated Conners Rating Scale-Revised. Although Arnold and colleagues (2007) found no significant differences in ADHD symptoms between carnitine and placebo in the primary analysis, a moderator effect of ADHD subtype was identified (children with inattentive type did better on carnitine). Additionally, a geographic effect was reported in this 10-site pilot study; children recruited from the three sites northwest of the Allegheny Mountains (n = 44) showed superiority of ALC, and children from the other sites (n = 68) showed a tendency in the opposite direction. Future RCTs will be helpful to examine efficacy and safety of ALC specifically on the ADHD inattentive type. Because of the documented general cardiovascular benefits, L-carnitine appears sensible, safe, easy, and inexpensive. Therefore, a 4-month trial is acceptable for preschoolers with the inattentive type of ADHD and a sluggish cognitive tempo—for example, low initiative, easily bored, fluctuating attention, slow thinking (Lee, Burns, Snell, & McBurnett, 2013) but not for those with the combined or hyperactive/impulsive type.

DiMethylAminoEthanol (DMAE, also called deanol and dimethylethanolamine) is a precursor of choline involved in acetylcholine synthesis, an important neurotransmitter (Re, 1974). A review by Arnold and colleagues (2011) reported that despite several placebo-controlled and open-label trials, there were methodologic flaws in many of the studies, and outcomes were varied, with some studies showing no effect or placebo superiority (Arnold, Hurt, Mayes, & Lofthouse, 2011). The best study was probably the three-arm RCT, in 74 school-age children with learning problems, including many with hyperactivity, comparing 500 mg DMAE to 40 mg methylphenidate and placebo. Significant effects compared to placebo were reported for DMAE (d = 0.1 to 0.6) and methylphenidate (d = 0.8 to 1.3). No serious side effects were reported with DMAE (Lewis & Young, 1975). Although significantly less effective than stimulants, DMAE appears sensible, easy, cheap, and safe, so it may be acceptable for preschoolers with very mild ADHD symptoms or if parents are specifically seeking alternative treatments.

Herbs are plant extracts with pharmacologic activity. Pycnogenol (French maritime pine bark extract) produced significant improvements in hyperactivity, inattention, and visual–motor coordination in a double-blind placebo-controlled RCT in school-age children with ADHD (N = 61). Similar findings were not found in the placebo group, and children taking Pycnogenol experienced relapse of symptoms a month after discontinuation (Trebaticka et al., 2006). *Ginkgo biloba* (gingko tree leaf) promotes brain blood flow and inhibits platelet activation. A comparative study with methylphenidate was conducted in a 6-week double-blind RCT of 6- to 14-year-olds with ADHD (N = 50). Significantly (p <.001) less improvement was seen with *Ginkgo biloba* (d = 0.02 to 0.55) on parent- and teacher-rated ADHD symptoms than methylphenidate (d = 1.36 to 1.62) (Salehi, 2010). St. John's wort, a serotonergic herb with antidepressant activity, has been examined in one double-blind, placebo-controlled RCT of 54 unmedicated 6- to 17-year-olds with ADHD, but it did not demonstrate benefit relative to placebo treatment (Weber et al., 2008). Most recently, Ningdong granules (a traditional Chinese medicine preparation of four different plant species, three animal substances, and human placenta) was examined in a methylphenidate-controlled 8-week double-blind RCT of 72 school-aged children with ADHD (Li, Li, et al., 2011). Ningdong granules led to significant (p < 0.01) decreases in teacher-reported and a downward trend in parent-reported ADHD symptoms, both comparable to the methylphenidate group. Unlike the latter, Ningdong granules also produced a significant (p <.05) pre- to post-treatment rise in homovanillic acid (thought to reflect dopamine metabolism) and significantly (p <.05) fewer side effects than MPH. Unfortunately, the safety of the ingredients is not known, and lead contamination has been reported for some Chinese and Indian herbs.

Future research on herbal approaches requires more double-blind, placebo-controlled RCTs in larger samples with longer-term follow-up. Despite being easy to use and relatively inexpensive, some herbs can cause side effects such as strokes and bleeding (*Ginkgo biloba*) and convulsions in children with epilepsy and other neurologic problems. Therefore, given minimal but promising empirical support and the involved risks, Pycnogenol and Ningdong granules may be acceptable for preschoolers with ADHD only if other safer treatments have failed. As parents may assume that herbal remedies are safer than prescription medication because they are "natural," practitioners need to educate parents that herbs are essentially "crude drugs" not regulated by the FDA, their overall quality/safety may vary across manufacturers, and they may have significant side effects, be contaminated by heavy metals (Harris, Cao, Littlefield, et al., 2011), and interact with prescription drugs (e.g., St. John's wort with serotonin reuptake inhibitors). For example, the following herbs are commonly used by patients with ADHD (Arnold, Hurt, Mays, & Lofhouse, 2011), without evidence but with associated risks: valerian (headache, mydriasis, restlessness, cardiac problems), kava kava (weakness, rash, weight loss, hematuria, increased cholesterol levels and liver problems, and chamomile (interaction with benzodiazepine receptors).

Homeopathic remedies are based on Hahnemann's Law of Similars, which states that if a substance causes sickness in a healthy person, then a lower concentration of that substance (remedy) can cure a sick person (National Center for Homeopathy, 2012). Unlike herbal medicine, homeopathy uses ultradiluted plant, mineral, or other natural substances. Of the five studies (one open-label and four double-blind RCTs, N = 283), significant (p <.05) improvement in ADHD symptoms was reported in three studies, while no significant differences were found in one placebo-controlled trial and one comparative RCT with methylphenidate (Frei & Thurneysen, 2001; Frei et al., 2005; Jacobs, Williams, Girard, Nijike, & Katz, 2005; Lamont, 1997; Strauss, 2002). A 2009 Cochrane review concluded, "There is currently little evidence for the efficacy of homeopathy for the treatment of ADHD" (Heirs & Dean, 2007, p. 4). This area needs better-controlled studies, use of standard treatment outcome measures, and the examination of specific patient factors affecting response. Despite being safe and relatively easy, homeopathy can be expensive, as it is lengthy (average response time 3.5 months) and may involve repeated doctor visits. However, short (3 to 6 months) trials may be acceptable for preschoolers with ADHD who are unresponsive to or have parents unwilling to try conventional treatments.

Noningestible CATs

Electro-acupuncture involves stimulation of acupoints via a needle with a pulsating electrical current. It is an intervention from traditional Chinese medicine based on the hypothesis that ADHD is caused by "effulgent gallbladder fire, Yin-Yang disharmony and noninteraction of heart and kidney" (Li et al., 2010, p. 176). Li and colleagues (2010) randomly assigned 213 4- to 6-year-olds with DSM-IV ADHD (and typical ADHD-related comorbidities) into electro-acupuncture plus behavior therapy or sham electro-acupuncture and behavior therapy. The electro-acupuncture was administered for 30 minutes a day for 6 days a week for 12 weeks using a 3- to 5-mA current, whereas the sham was identical except that the current was 0 mA, so there was no stimulation. Behavior therapy, to eliminate misbehaviors via therapist-directed rewards, punishments, and extinction, was the same for both groups and was performed 30 minutes after sham/electro-acupuncture for 40 minutes. Based on a four-point rating of ADHD symptom improvement from two blinded pediatric psychologists, Li and colleagues found that the experimental group had significantly (p <.05) more improvement than the control group immediately after treatment and at the 6-month follow-up (p <.05). Adverse effects were reported as mild and infrequent (stuck needle [local muscle spasm]: treatment group = 3.3%, sham group = 5.6%; bent needle: treatment group = 6.7%, sham group = 2.2%).

Although these are interesting preliminary data worthy of further examination, this study had several limitations, including not testing the validity of the blind by asking the psychologists, participants, parents, or experimenters which group they thought participants were assigned to; not testing the valid inertness of the sham; use of a non-standard treatment outcome measure without reported validity or reliability; and a high dropout rate (9% were treatment noncompliant and 20% dropped out at 6 months). As electro-acupuncture appears safe, seems sensible (from a traditional Chinese medicine perspective), and is easy, if not too expensive, a 12-week trial, as conducted in this study combined with behavior therapy, may be acceptable for some preschoolers with ADHD. Regarding other types of acupuncture for ADHD, a recent Cochrane review concluded that there was "no evidence base of randomized or quasi-randomized controlled trials to support [its] use" (Li, Yu, et al., 2011, p. 4).

Executive functioning (EF), also called cognitive control, is critical in goal-directed behavior and success in school (Diamond et al., 2007) and is deficient in children with ADHD (Barkley, 1997). Inhibition, working memory, and cognitive flexibility are usually considered core components of EF. EF training programs have been implemented in preschool and school-age children with ADHD. A pilot study of computerized EF remediation training in 40 school-age children showed significantly more improvement on parent-rated EF and ADHD ratings than those in the waitlist condition; however, teacher ratings were nonsignificant. Effects were maintained at the 9-week follow-up (Oord, Ponsioen, Geurts, Brink, & Prins, 2012). Two open-label trials of group-based EF training have recently been completed with preschool-age children diagnosed with ADHD; in both studies, children were taught games to improve EF skills, and parents attended a separate group to learn how to implement these activities at home (Halperin et al., 2012; Tamm, Nakonezny, & Hughes, 2012). In both studies, significant improvements in parent-rated ADHD symptoms were reported; however, results for teacher ratings of ADHD and psychometric measures of EF were mixed. Halperin and colleagues (2012) did report gains on parent-rated measures of ADHD symptoms that were maintained at the 3-month follow-up. A year-long preschool curriculum, Tools of the Mind (focused on EF-promoting activities), was compared with the school district curriculum (based on balanced literacy and included thematic units) in 18 preschool classrooms. In this randomized study, the Tools preschoolers (not selected for ADHD symptoms) significantly outperformed the preschoolers in the school district curriculum on EF tasks that taxed inhibition, working memory, and cognitive flexibility (Diamond et al., 2007). Additional research is needed to evaluate the short-term and long-term effects of EF training in preschool children with ADHD. Further studies should include randomization to a sham or alternative treatment, blinded outcome measures, and follow-up assessments. Further, it will be important to evaluate the best medium to deliver the EF training for preschoolers: group instruction with interventionists (either in clinic or at school) or using a computerized format like is most often used with school-aged children.

More specific attention and working memory trainings are most commonly delivered via computerized systematic exercises to remediate impairments in sustained and selective attention and working memory.

Attention training, via computers, has been examined by two open-label studies (Hagan, Moore, Wickham, & Maples, 2008; Tamm et al., 2010), two nonrandomized but controlled trials (Kerns, Eso, & Thompson, 1999; Semrud-Clikeman et al., 1999), and three RCTs of computerized (Rabiner, Murray, Skinner, & Malone, 2010; Shalev, Tsal, & Mevorach, 2007; Steiner, Sheldrick, Gotthelf, & Perrin, 2011) in school-age children with ADHD reported consistent improvement in psychometric measures of visual and auditory attention; however, across studies, improvements in parent- and teacher-rated ADHD symptoms and EF, academic functioning, and psychometric measures of other aspects of EF were mixed. Only one open-label study included a follow-up assessment (Tamm et al., 2010); improvements in parent-reported ADHD symptoms were maintained at 9 months after treatment.

Working memory training involves the use of systematic cognitive exercises to improve short-term retention of information necessary for more complex tasks such as reasoning, comprehension, and learning. Five RCTs comparing computerized working memory training to an alternative or sham treatment (four used low-dose working memory training and one used computerized academic training) reported significant improvements in school-age children diagnosed with ADHD on neuropsychological verbal and visual-spatial working memory tasks (Gray et al., 2012; Green et al., 2012; Johnstone, Roodenrys, Phillips, Watt, & Mantz, 2010; Klingberg, Forssberg, & Westerberg, 2002; Klingberg et al., 2005); one study reported improvements in EEG evoked response potentials (Johnstone et al., 2010); and one study reported improvement in observed child behavior during a simulated academic task (Green et al., 2012). However, results for parent- and teacher-rated ADHD symptoms, parent-rated EF, and academic performance were inconsistent. Only one study (Klingberg et al., 2005) evaluated children at follow-up; gains were maintained at 3 months after treatment. Using a similar methodology to the studies with school-aged children cited above, Nutley and colleagues (2011) randomized 112 typically developing preschool children to computerized working memory training or low-dose working memory training; significant improvements were reported for psychometric measures of nonverbal working memory, but not for verbal working memory or problem solving; neither parent nor teacher ratings of ADHD symptoms were included.

Although the data on attention and working memory training in school-age children with ADHD seem promising, currently published studies have several important limitations. First, few studies included follow-up information, and those that did primarily relied on parent ratings (Klingberg et al., 2005, is the exception). In addition, although several studies randomized participants to the study treatment or to either a sham-control treatment (usually a low-dose treatment) or an alternative treatment, none of the studies tested the validity of the blind. No convincing evidence is available regarding generalization of attention and working memory training to other cognitive skills beyond the training situation (Melby-Lervag & Hulme, 2012). Attention and working memory training is sensible and appears safe, but due to the time requirement and need for specialized equipment/technicians, it is not easy or cheap. Moreover, no information is available about applicability of the available specific attention and working memory training programs in preschoolers with ADHD. Therefore, we recommend further research to develop/modify the training programs for utility and efficacy in preschoolers with ADHD and do not currently recommend specific attention and working memory training for the younger age group.

Yoga involves modifying the body's physiology via practicing exercises such as postures and breathing techniques. It is hypothesized to work via deactivating the sympathetic nervous system while stimulating the parasympathetic system, resulting in a sense of calm, emotional balance, and increased concentration (Peck, Kehle, Bray, & Theodore, 2005). Two open-label trials and one RCT conducted in school-age children reported several significant decreases in overall ADHD symptoms ($d = 0.6$), as well as inattention ($d = 0.48$) and hyperactivity/impulsivity ($d = 0.10$) symptoms (see review by Hurt et al., 2011c). Yoga has not yet been studied in preschool children with ADHD; however, two quasi-experimental studies with preschool children at risk for developmental difficulties (Lawson, 2008; Lawson, Cox, & Blackwell, 2012) found no to minimal benefit of yoga in terms of behavior, fine motor skills, and academic performance. Differences in the results between school-age and preschool studies may be due to differences in sample (children diagnosed with ADHD vs. children at risk for developmental problems), method of delivery (DVD in preschool studies vs. yoga instructor in school-age trials), and intensity of intervention (2 to 4 total hours of yoga instruction for preschoolers over 3 to 6 weeks vs. 12 to 20 hours of total yoga instruction for school-age children over 6 to 20 weeks). Although promising, future research needs double-blind, sham-controlled RCTs with follow-up, samples of preschool children with high levels of ADHD symptoms, and greater intensity of intervention (similar to research on school-age children). Yoga appears safe, cheap, and sensible, and teachers in the preschool studies reported the yoga program was easy to use. Whether it is easy for preschool children with a high level of ADHD symptoms is not clear. Given current evidence, therefore, a short, developmentally appropriate trial may be acceptable (e.g., 10 to 15 minutes daily for 10 weeks).

Meditation, despite resulting in relaxation, is different from yoga and progressive muscle relaxation as it involves the practicing of certain techniques (e.g., being mindful of the present, repeating a mantra, listening to the breath) to train the brain to improve attention, alertness, and awareness in the present and eliminate unnecessary thoughts (Harrison, Manocha, & Rubin, 2004). Meditation is thought to relax the sympathetic nervous system, activate the parasympathetic-limbic pathways, and reduce theta while increasing beta EEG frequencies (Harrison et al., 2004). Currently, the existing four open trials and two RCTs involving school-age children with ADHD report significant improvements on overall ADHD ($d = 0.35$), inattention ($d = 0.50$), "on-task" behavior ($d = 2.15$), anxiety ($d = 0.70$), depression ($d = 0.35$), and EF ($d = 0.40$) (see review by Hurt et al., 2011c). A recent Cochrane review concluded, "As a result of the limited number of included studies, the small sample sizes and the high risk of bias, we are unable to draw any conclusions regarding the effectiveness of meditation therapy for ADHD" (Krisanaprakornkit, Ngamjarus, Witoonchart, & Piyavhatkul, 2010, p. 4). Although results are promising and there are two RCTs for meditation, additional research is needed with double-blind designs, sham or alternative treatment control groups, and follow-up studies. Meditation appears sensible, safe, and cheap, but whether it is easy for preschoolers is not known. A short, monitored, developmentally appropriate trial may be acceptable using methods described in the six studies for 5 to 10 minutes, daily, for 7 weeks.

Vestibular stimulation involves indirect physical arousal of the sensory system responsible for movement and balance located in the inner ear via stimulation of the semicircular canals or otoliths. Past research indicated vestibular processing impairments associated with ADHD (Mulligan, 1996). Two single-blind sham-controlled crossover studies of rotational vestibular stimulation, which intensively stimulates the semicircular canals, reported significant/marginally significant ($p <. 05$, ES = 0.5) decreases in ADHD symptoms (Arnold, Clark, Sachs, Jakim, & Smithies, 1985; Bhatara, Clark, Arnold, Gonnett, & Smeltzer, 1981). However, an RCT providing vestibular stimulation in all vectors through complex motion, stimulating semicircular canals only mildly and otoliths more intensely, failed to find significant differences between treatment and placebo conditions (Clark et al., 2008). Additional blinded and larger placebo-controlled RCTs with follow-up on rotational vestibular stimulation seem warranted. Although relatively safe and sensible, structured vestibular stimulation in clinical settings is expensive and difficult and therefore not recommended. However, home activities using appropriate already available play equipment/activities (e.g., swings, "Sit'N'Spin" toy, swivel chairs, carousels, spinning games) to stimulate the semicircular canals could be tried in preschoolers with ADHD. The main risks are nausea, drowsiness, and falls, which are less likely when children can regulate the intensity and duration themselves.

Massage therapy involves the manual manipulation of superficial layers of muscle and connective tissue to enhance function, relaxation, and well-being. It is thought to improve ADHD symptoms and relaxation by increasing alertness by altered brain waves, increasing vagal tone by improving parasympathetic activity, and increasing vagal control of the heart by enhancing a deficient physiologic inhibitory system (Field, Quintino, Hernandez-Reif, & Koslovsky, 1998; Khilnani, Field, Hernandez-Reif, & Schanberg, 2003). Two RCTs reported significantly ($p < .05$ to .01) less hyperactivity, daydreaming/inattention, overall ADHD symptoms, and anxiety and more on-task time and happiness in adolescent boys with ADHD (Field et al., 1998; Khilnani et al., 2003). Future research needs standardized clinical assessments to validate ADHD and control of confounds in ongoing treatments. Being sensible, seemingly safe, easy, and cheap, if parents can be taught to administer it, massage might provide a welcome addition to the bedtime ritual, improving sleep onset and the parent–child relationship.

Exercise may improve EF in children and may be particularly beneficial in children at risk of EF deficits, such as those diagnosed with ADHD (Berwid & Halperin, 2012). Three recent small pilot studies investigating the impact of exercise on ADHD symptoms of school-age children have been published. One open-label study (Smith et al., 2013) of group physical exercise (30 minutes a day, five times per week, for 5 weeks) for 17 young children (kindergarten to third grade) with ADHD symptoms found improvements in teacher-rated ADHD symptoms ($d = 0.70$), motor skills ($d = 0.96$), and psychometric measures of EF (average $d = 0.22$). Results for two non-randomized pilot studies with no-treatment controls were mixed; McKune, Pautz, and Lombard (2003) reported no significant improvement on parent-rated ADHD symptoms following a 5-week exercise program (60 minutes per day, 5 days per week) for 13 school-age children (ages 5 to 13) with ADHD. However, Verret, Guay, Berthiaume, Gardiner, and Heliveau (2012) reported significant improvement in parent-rated ADHD symptoms ($p = .01$) and on two of five measures of EF.

A pilot RCT comparing a 10-week program of "aerobically intense" physical education versus typical physical education (2 hours per week) in 5- to 6-year-old typically developing children found benefits on psychometric measures of attention and spatial memory and on parent-rated attention problems, but not hyperactive/impulsive behavior (Fisher et al., 2011). Additional research on exercise programs is needed with double-blind designs, alternative treatment control groups, and follow-up studies. Exercise appears sensible, safe, cheap, and easy; therefore, it passes the SECS criterion. Exercise programs with preschool children should adhere to the following guidelines: physical activities should follow preschoolers' "natural activity patterns," should focus on enjoyable gross motor play, should include adult facilitation to support mastery experience, and should include opportunities to use play spaces and outdoor equipment (Timmons et al., 2007).

Biofeedback (BF) and **neurofeedback** (NF) train the body and brain, respectively, via operant conditioning to change its physiologic activity to improve health and performance by providing real-time video/audio information about its electrical activity. BF is based on the theory that muscle tension and an inability to relax contribute to and augment hyperactivity (Braud, Lupin, & Braud, 1975). NF is based on the theory and empirical data indicating that ADHD is associated with abnormal electroencephalogram (EEG) brainwaves, specifically excessive theta (4 to 8 Hz) and insufficient beta (12 to 20 Hz) rhythms. Six RCTs (N = 247) of electromyograph (EMG) BF combined with relaxation training reported significant improvements, compared to controls, for overall (ES = 1.31), inattentive (ES = 0.91), and impulsive (ES = 0.93) symptoms. However, none of the studies used a double-blind format, and only one used a sham control. As 83% of the studies combined EMG-BF with relaxation (twice a week for 7 weeks), it is impossible to know which treatment component or combination caused the reported results. In a recent RCT heart-rate variability study, BF was found to significantly ($p <.05$) improve cognitive functioning (i.e., delayed word recall, immediate word recall, word recognition, and episodic secondary memory) and participant- and teacher-rated overall behaviors compared to an active control, building Legos (Lloyd, Brett, & Wesnes, 2010).

In our most recent review of NF for ADHD (Lofthouse, Arnold, & Hurt, in press), we calculated ESs for the currently available 12 RCTs and found, compared to control conditions, moderate ESs for overall ADHD problems ($d = 0.62$), inattention ($d = 0.72$), hyperactivity/impulsivity ($d = 0.70$), and all problems (ADHD or otherwise, $d = 0.57$). Four of those studies also showed neurophysiologic changes specifically associated with NF. One study also reported continued improvements on parent-rated ADHD symptoms for NF at 6 months (Gevensleben, Holl, Albrecht, et al., 2010), but that study did not identify, control, or measure potential confounds during this follow-up period (see Lofthouse, Arnold, Hersch, Hurt, & deBeus, 2012). Unfortunately, apart from one study that also had limitations, the reported benefits of NF have not been replicated in the small double-blinded studies conducted, although those studies also had some limitations. Both BF and NF appear safe and sensible, although they may not be cheap, as they require expensive equipment and a technician. Therefore, due to these drawbacks and the lack of evidence for preschoolers with ADHD, neither BF or NF is recommended for this age group.

Clinical Recommendations

1. We believe a practitioner's job is (usually) not to tell caregivers which treatment to use but to provide a well-balanced (pros and cons) summary of all treatments to help them make a well-informed decision. It is important to provide parents with a visual and user-friendly way to make this choice. We hope Tables 9.1 and 9.2 will assist practitioners with this task.

2. A simple commonsense initial guideline to consider for any treatment (Arnold et al., 2011) is that CATs that are sensible, easy, cheap, and safe (SECS) may require less evidence to justify an individual trial than CATs that are risky, unrealistic, difficult, or expensive (RUDE).

3. As many CATs target specific causes, they need to be *considered* (not necessarily used) early during the diagnostic process. Therefore, a detailed medical, psychological, developmental, family, treatment, and dietary history and physical examination are needed. When indicated, a blood count, electrolyte/mineral screen, and, in areas with high rates of subclinical lead poisoning, serum lead assessment should be considered. Preschoolers are especially prone to iron deficiency/insufficiency because of their rapid growth. Once causes amenable to specific treatments (e.g., vitamin D deficiency corrected by a vitamin D supplement) are ruled out, conventional treatments (medication and behavioral therapy) may be more confidently applied.

4. Clinicians and parents need to request the data/evidence. Many commercially advocated treatments claim to have scientific proof but provide only anecdotes, case histories, and testimonials.

5. For some individuals, a CAT may work better than an established treatment even though it is not proven by group averages. The decision to try a CAT in an individual case depends partly on data, SECS criteria and accessibility, parent preference, and response to established treatments.

6. Diverting family resources (money, time, effort) to a treatment that does not work is a risk that needs to be carefully considered for the patient and other family members.

7. Parents should be encouraged to discuss with their prescribing doctor all ingestible CATs, especially "natural" herbs, to identify any possible interactions with currently prescribed medications.

8. As with conventional treatments:
   a. Attempt one CAT at a time.
   b. Continuously monitor results and adverse effects with reliable and validated multidomain and multi-informant outcome measures of specific symptoms, psychosocial functioning, CAT-specific mechanisms of change (e.g., EEG changes for neurofeedback), and/or a simple graph (number of weeks of treatment along the x axis and effect of CAT along the y axis, 0 [not helpful] to 5 [moderately helpful] to 10 [very helpful]). If clinically significant benefit is not noted in the expected time, move on to another CAT that has supportive data and is SECS or to conventional treatment.

Table 9.1 **Summary of Ingestible CATs for Preschoolers with ADHD**

CAT	Rationale	Research Support (SC-ADHD: Schoolchildren w/ ADHD)	Sensible, Easy, Cheap, Safe (SECS)	Recommendation Trial (R) Acceptable Trial (A) Not Recommended (NR)
Sensible restriction of sugar & artificial food colorings	Sensitivity to dietary substances	Moderate for ADHD but moderate for all children	S C S; may not be E	R: 2-week trial
Breakfast containing protein & low sugar	Protein maintains cognitive performance	Poor for SC-ADHD but moderate for all children	S E C S	R: 2-week trial
RDA/RDI multivitamins	Multivitamin deficiency	Poor for SC-ADHD, but moderate for all children	S E C S	A: With medical monitoring: For picky eaters & those with stimulant-suppressed appetites
Polyunsaturated fatty acids (PUFAs)	Deficiency of PUFAs	Moderate for SC-ADHD	S E C S	A: 3- to 6-month trial for those who do not eat oily wild ocean fish at least 3x/week
Melatonin	Natural sleep hormone	Moderate for insomnia for SC-ADHD, poor for ADHD symptoms	S E C S	A: For ADHD children with sleep problems
Minerals: iron, zinc, magnesium	Mineral deficiency	Moderate for SC-ADHD	S E C; may not be safe	A: With medical monitoring only for those with documented mineral deficiency
Carnitine	Essential for PUFAs	Moderate for SC-ADHD (inattentive type)	S E C S	A: With medical monitoring but only for ADHD inattentive type
Dimethylaminoethanol (DMAE)	Neurotransmitter functioning	Moderate for SC-ADHD	S E C S	A: With medical monitoring for mild symptoms

(continued)

Table 9.1 **(Continued)**

CAT	Rationale	Research Support (SC-ADHD: Schoolchildren w/ ADHD)	Sensible, Easy, Cheap, Safe (SECS)	Recommendation Trial (R) Acceptable Trial (A) Not Recommended (NR)
Glyconutritional supplementation	Specific sugars for cell-to-cell communication	Poor for SC-ADHD	S E C S	A: With medical monitoring
Herbs	Natural medicine	Pycnogenol—moderate for SC-ADHD Gingko biloba—poor for SC-ADHD Ningdong granules—moderate for SC-ADHD St. John's wort, valerian, kava kava, chamomile—Poor	S E C; may not be safe. Not safe: valerian, kava kava, chamomile	A: With medical monitoring, Pycnogenol & Ningdong granules NR: Ginkgo biloba, St. John's wort, valerian, kava kava, chamomile
Homeopathy	Ultradiluted plant or mineral extracts thought to cause ADHD symptoms in healthy people	Moderate for SC-ADHD	E; Safe; not sure if S, not C	A: With medical monitoring
Amino acids	Deficiency of amino acid precursor for neurotransmitters	Poor	Not safe—metabolic risk	NR
Megadoses of single or multiple vitamins	Dietary deficiency or need for extra vitamins	Poor	Not sensible or safe (toxicity risk)	NR

Following not recommended for preschoolers w/ ADHD due to lack of evidence for 5- to 18-year-olds with ADHD: Antifungal treatment, thyroid treatment, immune therapy.

Table 9.2 **Summary of Noningestible CATs for Preschoolers with ADHD**

CAT	Rationale	Research Support (SC-ADHD: Schoolchildren w/ ADHD)	Sensible, Easy, Cheap, Safe* (SECS)	Recommended Trial (R) Acceptable Trial (A) Not Recommended (NR)
Massage	Relaxation to slow down	Moderate for SC-ADHD	S E C S	R: If parent can be taught massage, especially for bedtime routine
Exercise	To improve executive functioning	Moderate for SC-ADHD & for preschoolers without ADHD	S E C S	R: Physical activities that focus on enjoyable gross motor play that promotes vestibular & cerebellar activation, w/ adult facilitation to support mastery
Electro-acupuncture	Traditional Chinese medicine: ADHD caused by effulgent gallbladder fire, yin-yang disharmony & noninteraction of heart & kidney	Moderate for preschoolers w/ ADHD	S E S; may not be C	A: 12-week trial combined w/ behavior therapy as conducted in research
Executive functioning training	Trains executive functions (e.g., inhibition, working memory, cognitive flexibility)	Moderate for ADHD	S S, may not be C or E if using computerized training	A: A group-based clinic/school-based trial is acceptable for preschoolers; unclear if computerized EF training is acceptable for preschoolers
Yoga	Trains body to slow down	Moderate for SC-ADHD	S C S; may not be E	A: If child can be taught yoga, 10–15 minutes daily for 10 weeks

(continued)

Table 9.2 (Continued)

CAT	Rationale	Research Support (SC-ADHD: Schoolchildren w/ ADHD)	Sensible, Easy, Cheap, Safe* (SECS)	Recommended Trial (R) Acceptable Trial (A) Not Recommended (NR)
Meditation	Trains brain to slow down & attend	Moderate for SC-ADHD	S C S; may not be E	A: If child can be taught meditation, 5–10 minutes daily for 7 weeks
Clinical vestibular stimulation	To correct vestibular problems with movement & balance	Moderate for SC-ADHD	S S; not E or C in clinical settings	NR
Neurofeedback	Trains brain to attend & slow down	Moderate for SC-ADHD	S S; not E or C	NR
Biofeedback	Trains body to slow down	Moderate for SC-ADHD	S S; not E or C	NR
Attention memory Training	Trains attention skills	Moderate for SC-ADHD	S S not E or C	NR
Working memory training	Trains working memory skills	Moderate for SC-ADHD	S S; not E or C	NR

* Appears safe but no monitoring of potential adverse effects in research studies.

Following not recommended for preschoolers w/ ADHD due to lack of evidence for 5- to 18-year-olds with ADHD: Interactive metronome training, sensory integration therapy, mirror therapy.

Conclusion

Although research on CATs for 5- to 18-year-olds with ADHD is increasing in quantity and quality with several promising interventions, currently there are only eight published studies involving CATs for preschoolers with ADHD. As parents often ask for guidance from practitioners about alternative or adjunct treatments, the downward extension of research on CATs conducted on 5- to 18-year-olds with ADHD can be considered. Based on the SECS criteria and our clinical recommendations, the following are recommended for preschool children with ADHD:

- Sensible restriction of sugar and artificial food colorings
- Protein-containing low-sugar breakfast
- Parent-administered massage for sleep problems
- Developmentally appropriate physical exercise, including activities that promote vestibular and cerebellar activation
- RDI/RDA supplementation for picky eaters (acceptable for all)

The following CATs are acceptable for an individual trial for specific populations of preschool children with ADHD with appropriate medical monitoring:

- Polyunsaturated fatty acid (PUFA) supplementation
- Mineral supplementation for children with documented deficiencies
- Melatonin for sleep problems
- Carnitine supplementation only for children with predominantly inattentive symptoms and sluggish tempo
- DMAE for children with mild symptoms

The following CATs are acceptable for a short trial with appropriate medical monitoring for children who do not respond to traditional treatments or for whom parents do not find medication to be an acceptable option:

- Glyconutritional supplements
- Pycnogenol
- Ningdong granules (keeping in mind the risk of lead in Asian herbs)
- Homeopathy
- Group EF training
- Electro-Acupuncture
- Yoga
- Meditation

Based on available evidence, the following CATs are not recommended for preschool children with ADHD (although some may be recommended or acceptable for school-aged children with ADHD):

- Amino acid supplementation
- Megadoses of vitamins and minerals

- Herbs (aside from Pycnogenol and Ningdong granules)
- Working memory and attention training
- Biofeedback and neurofeedback

Disclosures

Nicholas Lofthouse, Ph.D., has no financial disclosures.
Elizabeth Hurt, Ph.D., has had research funding from Bristol-Meyer-Squibb.

References

Akhondzadeh, S., Mohammadi, M., & Khademi, M. (2004). Zinc sulfate as an adjunct to methylphenidate for the treatment of attention deficit hyperactivity disorder in children: A double blind and randomized trial. *BMC Psychiatry, 4*(9).

Arnold, L. E. (2004). *Contemporary diagnosis and management of ADHD* (3rd ed.). Newtown, PA: Handbooks in Health Care Co.

Arnold, L. E., Amato, A., Bozzolo, H., Hollway, J., Cook, A., Ramadan, Y.,...Manos., M. (2007). Acetyl-L-carnitine in attention-deficit/hyperactivity disorder: A multi-site, placebo-controlled pilot trial. *Journal of Child and Adolescent Psychopharmacology, 17*(6), 791–806.

Arnold, L. E., Amato, A., Gaetano, F., Bozzolo, H., Hollway, J., Cook, A.,...Zhang, D. (2005). Two carnitine pilot trials in ADHD. Poster at 12th biannual scientific meeting of International Society for Research in Child & Adolescent Psychopathology. Roosevelt Hotel, NYC, June 24, 2005.

Arnold, L. E., Bozzolo, H., Hollway, J., Cook, A.C., DiSilvestro, R. A., Bozzolo, D. R.,...Williams, C. (2005). Serum zinc correlates with parent/teacher-rated inattention in children with attention-deficit/hyperactivity disorder. *Journal of Child & Adolescent Psychopharmacology, 15*(4), 628–636.

Arnold, L. E., Christopher, J., Huestis, R. D., & Smeltzer, D. J. (1978). Megavitamins for minimal brain dysfunction: A placebo-controlled study. *JAMA, 240*(24), 2642–2643.

Arnold, L. E., Clark, D. L., Sachs, L. A., Jakim, S., & Smithies, C. (1985). Vestibular & visual rotational stimulation as treatment for attention deficit and hyperactivity. *American Journal of Occupational Therapy, 39*(2), 84–91.

Arnold, L. E., & DiSilvestro, R. A. (2005). Zinc in attention-deficit/hyperactivity disorder. *Journal of Child and Adolescent Psychopharmacology, 15*(4), 619–627.

Arnold, L. E., DiSilvestro, R. A., Bozzolo, D., Crowl, L., Fernandez, S., Ramadan, Y.,...Joseph, E. (2011). Zinc for attention-deficit/ hyperactivity disorder: Placebo-controlled double-blind pilot trial alone and combined with amphetamine. *Journal of Child and Adolescent Psychopharmacology, 21*(1), 1–19.

Arnold, L. E., Hurt, E., Mayes, T., & Lofthouse, N. (2011). Ingestible alternative & complementary treatments for attention-deficit/hyperactivity disorder. In B. Hoza & S. Evans (Eds.), *Treating attention deficit disorder*. New Jersey: Civic Research Institute.

Arnold, L. E., Lofthouse, N., & Hurt, E. (2012). Artificial food colors & attention-deficit/hyperactivity symptoms: Conclusions to dye for. *Neurotherapeutics, 9*(3), 599–609.

Bateman, B., Warner, J.O., Hutchinson, E., Dean, T., Rowlandson, P., Gant, C.,...Stevenson, J. (2004). The effects of a double blind, placebo controlled, artificial food colourings and benzoate preservative challenge on hyperactivity in a general population sample of preschool children. *Archives of Disease in Childhood, 89*, 506–511.

Baker, G. B., Bornstein, R.A., Rouget, A., Therrian, S., & van Muden, J. (1991). Phenylethylaminergic mechanisms in attention-deficit/hyperactivity disorder. *Biological Psychiatry, 29*, 15–22.

Barkley, R. A. (1997). Behavioral inhibition, sustained attention, and executive functions: constructing a unifying theory of ADHD. *Psychological Bulletin, 121*, 65–94.

Bekaroglu, M., et al. (1996). Relationships between serum free fatty acids and zinc and ADHD: A research note. *Journal of Child Psychology and Psychiatry, 37*, 225–227.

Benton, D., & Buts, J.P. (1990). Vitamin/mineral supplementation and intelligence. *Lancet, 335*, 1158–1160.

Benton, D., & Cook, R. (1991). Vitamin and mineral supplements improve the intelligence scores and concentration of six-year-old children. *Personality and Individual Differences, 12*, 1151–1158.

Benton, D., & Roberts G. (1988). Effect of vitamin and mineral supplementation on intelligence of a sample of schoolchildren. *Lancet, 331*(8578), 140–143.

Bernstein, A. L. (1990). Vitamin B6 in clinical neurology. *Annals of the New York Academy of Sciences, 585*, 250–260.

Berwid, O. G., & Halperin, J.M. (2012). Emerging support for a role of exercise in attention-deficit/hyperactivity disorder intervention planning. *Current Psychiatry Reports, 14*, 543–551.

Bhatara, V., Clark, D. L., Arnold, L. E., Gonsett, R., & Smeltzer, D. J. (1981). Hyperkinesis treated by vestibular stimulation: An exploratory study. *Biological Psychiatry, 16*(3), 269–279.

Bilici, M. Yildirim, Kandil, S., Bekaroglu, M., Yildirmis, S., Degerm, O.,…Aksu, H. (2004). Double-blind, placebo controlled study of zinc sulfate in the treatment of attention deficit hyperactivity disorder. *Progress in Neuro-Psychopharmacology & Biological Psychiatry, 28*(1), 181–190.

Bloch, M. H., & Qawasmi, A. (2011). Omega-3 fatty acid supplementation for the treatment of children with attention-deficit/hyperactivity disorder: Systematic review and meta-analysis. *Journal of the American Academy of Child and Adolescent Psychiatry, 50*, 991–1000.

Braud, L., Lupin, M., & Braud W. (1975). The use of electromyographic biofeedback in the control of hyperactivity. *Journal of Learning Disabilities, 8*, 21–26.

Brenner, A. (1982). The effects of megadoses of selected B complex vitamins on children with hyperkinesis; controlled studies with long-term follow-up. *Journal of Learning Disabilities, 15*, 258–264.

Brookes, K. J., Chen, W., Xu, X., Taylor, E., & Asherson, P. (2006). Association of fatty acid desaturase genes with attention-deficit/hyperactivity disorder. *Biological Psychiatry, 60*, 1053–1061.

Bussing, R., Zima, B. T., Gary, F. A., & Garvan, C. W. (2002). Use of complementary and alternative medicine for symptoms of attention-deficit hyperactivity disorder. *Psychiatric Services, 53*, 1096–1102.

Cala, S., Crismon, M. L., & Baumgartner, J. (2003). A survey of herbal use in children with attention-deficit/hyperactivity disorder or depression. *Pharmacotherapy, 23*(2), 222–230.

Chan, E., Rappaport, L. A., & Kemper, K. J. (2003). Complementary and alternative therapies in childhood attention and hyperactivity problems. *Journal of Developmental and Behavioral Pediatrics, 24*, 4–8.

Cohen, J. (1988). *Statistical power analysis for the behavioral sciences* (2nd ed.). Hillsdale, NJ: Lawrence Erlbaum Associates.

Clark, D. L., Arnold, L. E., Crowl, L., Bozzolo, H., Peruggia, M., Ramadan, Y.,…Cook, A. (2008). Vestibular stimulation for ADHD. *Journal of Attention Disorders, 11*, 599–611.

Coleman, M., Steinberg, G., Tippett, J., Bhagavan, H. N., Coursin, D. B., Gross, M.…DeVaeau, L. (1979). A preliminary study of the effect of pyridoxine administration in a subgroup of hyperkinetic children: a double-blind crossover comparison with methylphenidate. *Biological Psychiatry, 14*, 741–751.

Cortese, S., Konofal, E., Bernadina, B. D., Mouren, M., & Lecendreux, M. (2009). Sleep disturbances and serum ferritin levels in children with attention deficit/ hyperactivity disorder. *European Child & Adolescent Psychiatry, 18*(7), 393–399.

Crombie, I. K., Florey, C., Todman, J., Kennedy, R. A., McNeill, G., & Menzies, I. (1990). Effect of vitamin and mineral supplementation on verbal and nonverbal reasoning of schoolchildren. *Lancet, 8692*, 744–747.

Diamond, A., Barnett, W. S., Thomas, J., & Munro, S. (2007) Preschool program improves cognitive control. *Science, 318*(5855), 1387–1388.

Dykman, K. D., &, Dykman, R. A. (1998). Effect of nutritional supplements on attention-deficit/ hyperactivity disorder. *Integrative Physiological and Behavioral Science, 33*, 49–60.

Dykman, K. D., & McKinley R. (1997). Effect of glyconutritionals on the severity of ADHD. *Proceedings of the Fisher Institute for Medical Research, 1*(1)24–25.

Feingold, B. F. (1975). *Why your child is hyperactive.* New York: Random House.

Field, T. M., Quintino, O., Hernandez-Reif, M., & Koslovsky, G. (1998). Adolescents with attention-deficit hyperactivity disorder benefit from massage therapy. *Adolescence, 33*(129), 103–108.

Fisher, A., Boyle, J. M. E., Paton, J. Y., Tomporowski, P., Watson, C., McColl, J. H., & Reilly, J. J. (2011). Effects of a physical education intervention on cognitive function in young children: randomized controlled pilot study. *BMC Psychiatry, 11*, 97–105.

Flink, E. B. (1981). Magnesium deficiency. Etiology and clinical spectrum. *Acta Medica-Scandinavica—Supplementum, 647*, 125–137.

Food and Drug Agency (FDA) Food Advisory Committee, 2011. Quick Minutes: Food Advisory Committee Meeting, March 30-31, 2011. http://www.fda.gov/advisorycommittees/committeesmeetingmaterials/foodadvisorycommittee/ucm250901.htm. Accessed May 19, 2012.

Frei, H., Everts, R., von Ammon, K., Kaufmann, F., Walther, D., Hsu-Schmitz, S.,...Thurneyson, A. (2005). Homeopathic treatment of children with attention-deficit hyperactivity disorder: A randomised, double blind, placebo controlled crossover trial. *European Journal of Pediatrics, 164*, 758–767.

Frei, H., & Thurneysen, A. (2001). Treatment for hyperactive children: homeopathy and methylphenidate compared in a family setting. *British Homeopathic Journal, 90*, 183–188.

Gevensleben, H., Holl, B., Albrecht, B., Schlamp, D., Kratz, O., Studer, P., & Heinrich H. (2010). Neurofeedback training in children with ADHD: 6-Month follow-up of a randomized controlled trial. *European Child & Adolescent Psychiatry, 19*, 715–724.

Ghuman, J. K., Arnold, L. E., & Anthony, B. J. (2008). Psychopharmacological and other treatments in preschool children with attention deficit/hyperactivity disorder: Current evidence and practice. *Journal of Child & Adolescent Psychopharmacology, 18*(5), 413–447.

Gillies, D., Sinn, J. K. H., Lad, S. S., Leach, M. J., & Ross, M. J. (2012). Polyunsaturated fatty acids (PUFA) for attention deficit hyperactivity disorder (ADHD) in children and adolescents. *Cochrane Database of Systematic Reviews, 7.* Art. No.: CD007986.

Gray, S.A., Chaban, P., Marinussen, R., Goldberg, R., Gotlieb, H., Kronitz, R....Tannock, R. (2012). Effects of a computerized working memory training program on working memory, attention, and academics in adolescents with severe LD and comorbid ADHD: a randomized controlled trial. *Journal of Child Psychology and Psychiatry, 53*(12), 1277–1284.

Green, C.T., Long, D.L., Green, D., Iosif, A., Dixon, J,F., Miller, M.R....Schweitzer, J.B., (2012). Will working memory training generalize to improve off-task behavior in children with attention-deficit/hyperactivity disorder? *Neurotherapeutics.* Advance online publication. doi: 10.1007/s13311-012-0124-y.

Hagan, H., Moore, K., Wickham, G., & Maples, W. C. (2008). Effect of the EYEPORT system on visual function in ADHD children: A pilot study. *Journal of Behavioral Optometry, 19*, 37–41.

Harris, E. S., Cao, S., Littlefield, B. A., Craycroft, J. A., Scholten, R., Kaptchuk, T.,...Eissenberg, D. M. (2011). Heavy metal and pesticide content in commonly prescribed individual raw Chinese herbal medicines. *Science of the Total Environment, 409*, 4297–4305.

Harrison, L. J., Manocha, R., & Rubin, K. (2004. Sahaja yoga meditation as a family treatment program for children with attention deficit-hyperactivity disorder. *Clinical Child Psychology and Psychiatry, 9*, 479–497.

Halperin, J. M. et al. (2012). Training executive, attention, and motor skills: A proof-of-concept study in preschool children with ADHD. *Journal of Attention Disorders* [epub March 5].

Haslam, R. H. A., Dalby, J. T., & Rademaker, A. W. (1984). Effects of megavitamin therapy on children with attention deficit disorders. *Pediatrics, 74*, 103–111.

Heirs, M., & Dean, M. E. (2007). Homeopathy for attention deficit/hyperactivity disorder or hyperkinetic disorder. *Cochrane Database of Systematic Reviews,Issue 4.* Art. No.: CD005648.

Howard, A. L., Robinson, M., Smith, G. J., Ambrosini, G. L., Piek, J. P., & Oddy, W. H. (2011). ADHD is associated with a "Western" dietary pattern in adolescents. *Journal of Attention Disorders, 15*, 403–411.

Hurt, E. A., Lofthouse, N., & Arnold, L.E. (2011a). Dietary & nutritional treatments for ADHD: Current research support & recommendations for practitioners. *Current Psychiatric Reports, 13*, 323–332.

Hurt, E. A., Lofthouse, N., & Arnold, L. E. (2011b). Complimentary & alternative biomedical treatments for ADHD. *Psychiatric Annals, 41*, 32–38.

Hurt, E. A., Lofthouse, N., & Arnold, L. E. (2011c). Non-ingestible alternative & complementary treatments for attention-deficit/hyperactivity disorder. In B. Hoza & S. Evans (Eds.), *Treating attention deficit disorder*. New Jersey: Civic Research Institute.

Jacobs, J., Williams, A.L., Girard, C., Nijike, V. Y., & Katz, D. (2005). Homeopathy for attention-deficit/hyperactivity disorder: A pilot randomized-controlled trial. *Journal of Alternative and Complementary Medicine, 11*(5), 799–806.

Johnstone, S. J., Roodenrys, S., Phillips, E., Watt, A. J., & Mantz, S. (2010). A pilot study of combined working memory and inhibition training for children with ADHD. *ADHD, 2*, 31–42.

Kaplan, B. J., McNicol, J., Conte, R. A., & Moghadam, H. K. (1989). Dietary replacement in preschool-aged hyperactive boys. *Pediatrics, 83*, 7–17.

Kerns, K. A., Eso, K., & Thomson, J. (1999). Investigation of a direct intervention for improving attention in young children with ADHD. *Developmental Neuropsychology, 16*, 273–295.

Kershner, J., & Hawke, W. (1979). Megavitamins and learning disorders: a controlled double-blind experiment. *Journal of Nutrition, 159*, 819–826.

Khilnani, S., Field, T., Hernandez-Reif, M., & Schanberg, S. (2003). Massage therapy improves mood and behavior of students with attention-deficit/hyperactivity disorder. *Adolescence, 38*, 623–638.

Klingberg, T., Fernell, E., Olesen, P. L., Johnson, M., Gustafsson, P., Dahlstrom, K., Gillberg, C.G., Forssberg, H., & Westerberg, H. (2005). Computerized training of working memory in children with ADHD—A randomized, controlled trial. *Journal of the American Academy of Child and Adolescent Psychiatry, 44*, 177–186.

Klingberg, T., Forssberg, H., & Westerberg, H. (2002). Training of working memory in children with ADHD. *Journal of Clinical and Experimental Neuropsychology, 24*, 781–791.

Konofal, E., Cortese, S., Marchand, M., Mouren, M. C., Arnulf, I., & Lecendreuz, M. (2007). Impact of restless legs syndrome and iron deficiency on attention-deficit/hyperactivity disorder in children. *Sleep Medicine, 8*(7–8), 711–715.

Konofal, E., Lecendreux, M., Deron, J., Marchand, M., Cortese, S., Zaim, M., Mauren, M. C., & Arnulf, I. (2008). Effects of iron supplementation on attention deficit hyperactivity disorder in children. *Pediatric Neurology, 38*(1), 20–6.

Kozielec, T., & Starobrat-Hermelin, B. (1997). Assessment of magnesium levels in children with ADHD. *Magnesium Research, 10*, 143–148.

Kozielec, T., Starobrat-Hermelin B., & Kotkowiak, L. (1994). Deficiency of certain trace elements in children with hyperactivity. *Psychiatria Polska, 28*, 345–353.

Krisanaprakornkit, T., Ngamjarus, C., Witoonchart, C., & Piyavhatkul, N. (2010). Meditation therapies for attention-deficit/hyperactivity disorder (ADHD). *Cochrane Database of Systematic Reviews Issue 6*, Art. No.: CD006507

Lamont, J. (1997). Homeopathic treatment of attention deficit hyperactivity disorder. *British Homeopathic Journal, 86*, 196–200.

Lawson, L. M. (2008). Yoga as a school-based intervention. *ATRA Research Institute Book of Abstracts.*

Lawson, L. A. M., Cox, J., & Blackwell, A. L. (2012). Yoga as a classroom intervention for preschoolers. *Journal of Occupational Therapy, School, & Early Intervention, 5*, 126–137.

Lee, S., Burns, G. L., Snell, J., & McBurnett, K. (2013). Validity of the sluggish cognitive tempo symptom dimension in children: Sluggish cognitive tempo and ADHD-inattention as distinct symptom dimensions. *Journal of Abnormal Child Psychology* [epub Jan. 17, 2013].

Lewis, J. A., & Young, R. (1975). Deanol and methylphenidate in minimal brain dysfunction. *Clinical Pharmacology and Therapeutics., 17*(5), 534–540.

Li, J. J., Li, Z. W., Wang, S. Z., Qi, F., Zhao, L., & Li, A. (2011). Ningdong granule: a complementary and alternative therapy in the treatment of attention deficit/hyperactivity disorder.
Psychopharmacology, 216(4), 501–9.

Li, S., Yu, B., Lin, Z., Jiang, S., He, J., Kang, L.,...Wang, X. (2010). Randomized-controlled study
of treating attention deficit hyperactivity disorder of preschool children with combined
electro-acupuncture and behavior therapy. *Complementary Therapeutic Medicine, 18*, 175–183.

Li, S., Yu, B., Zhou, D., He, C., Kang, L., Wang, X., Jiang, S., & Chen, X. (2011) Acupuncture for
attention deficit hyperactivity disorder (ADHD) in children and adolescents. *Cochrane
Database of Systematic Reviews, Issue 4.* Art. No.: CD007839.

Lloyd, A., Brett, D., & Wesnes, K. (2010). Coherence training in children with attention-deficit
hyperactivity disorder: cognitive functions and behavioral changes. *Alternative Therapies in
Health and Medicine, 16*(4), 34–42.

Lofthouse, N., Arnold, L. E., Hersch, S., Hurt, E., & deBeus, R. J. (2012). A review of neurofeedback
treatment for pediatric ADHD. *Journal of Attention Disorders, 16*(5), 351–372.

Lofthouse, N., Arnold, L. E., & Hurt, E. (2012). Current status of neurofeedback for attention-deficit
hyperactivity disorder. *Current Psychiatry Reports, 14*(5), 536–542.

Lofthouse, N., Arnold, L.E., & Hurt, E. (in press). Neurofeedback for the treatment of pediatric
attention-deficit/hyperactivity disorder, autism spectrum disorders, learning disorders and
epilepsy. *Child and Adolescent Psychiatric Clinics of North America.*

Lofthouse, N., McBurnett, K., Hurt, E. A., & Arnold, L. E. (2011). Biofeedback and neurofeedback
treatments for ADHD. *Psychiatric Annals, 41*, 42–48.

McCann, D., Barrett, A., Cooper, A., Crumpler, D., Dalen, L., Grimshaw, K.,...Stevenson, J. (2007).
Food additives and hyperactive behavior in 3-year-old and 8/9-year-old children in the community: a randomised, double-blinded, placebo-controlled trial. *Lancet, 370*, 1560–1567.

McKune, A. J., Pautz, J., & Lombard, J. (2003). Behavioural response to exercise in children with
attention-deficit/hyperactivity disorder. *Sports Medicine, 15*, 17–21.

Melby-Lervåg, M., & Hulme, C. (May 21, 2012). Is working memory training effective?
A meta-analytic review. *Developmental Psychology.* Advance online publication. doi: 10.1037/
a0028228

Milte, C. M., Sinn, N., Buckley, J. D., Coates, A. M., Young, R. M., & Howe, P. R. C. (2011).
Polyunsaturated fatty acids, cognition, and literacy in children with ADHD with and without
learning difficulties. *Journal of Child Health Care, 15*, 299–311.

Milte, C. M., Sinn, N., & Howe, P. R. C. (2009). Polyunsaturated fatty acid status in attention deficit hyperactivity disorder, depression, and Alzheimer's disease: towards an omega-3 index for
mental health? *Nutrition Reviews, 67*(10), 573–590.

Mousain-Bosc, M., Roche, M., Poige, A., PradalPrat, D., Rapin, J., & Bali, J. P. (2006). Improvements
of neurobehavioral disorders in children supplemented with magnesium-vitamin B6.
Magnesium Research, 19(1), 46–52.

Mousain-Bosc, M., Roche, M., Rapin, J., & Bali, J. P. (2004). Magnesium VitB6 intake reduces central nervous system hyperexcitability in children. *Journal of the American College of Nutrition,
23*(5), 545S–548S.

Mulligan, S. (1996). An analysis of score patterns of children with attention disorders on the sensory
integration and praxis tests. *American Journal of Occupational Therapy, 50*, 647–654.National
Center for Complementary and Alternative Medicine (2011). What is Complementary and
Alternative Medicine? Publication No. D347. http://nccam.nih.gov/health/whatiscam
(Accessed November 7, 2012).

National Center for Complementary and Alternative Medicine (2011). What is Complementary
and Alternative Medicine? Publication No. D347. http://nccam.nih.gov/health/whatiscam
(Accessed November 7, 2012).

National Center for Homeopathy. What Is Homeopathy? http://www.homeopathic.org/content/
what-is-homeopathy (Accessed November 12, 2012).

Nemzer, E., Arnold, L. E., Votolato, N. A., & McConnell, H. (1986). Amino acid supplementation
as therapy for attention deficit disorder (ADD). *Journal of the American Academy of Child and
Adolescent Psychiatry, 25*(4), 509–513.

Nogovitsina, O. R., & Levitina, E. V. (2007). Neurological aspects of the clinical features, pathophysiology, and corrections of impairments in attention deficit hyperactivity disorder. *Neuroscience and Biological Psychiatry, 37*(3), 199–202.

Nutley, S.B., Soderqvist, S., Bryde, S., Thorell, L.B., Humphreys, K., & Klingberg, T. (2011). Gains in fluid intelligence after training non-verbal reasoning in 4-year-old-children: a controlled, randomized study. *Developmental Science, 14*(3), 591–601.

Oner, P., & Oner, O. (2008). Relationship of ferritin to symptom ratings children with attention deficit hyperactivity disorder: effect of comorbidity. *Journal of Child Psychiatry and Human Development, 39*(3), 323–330.

Oord, S. V., Ponsioen, A. J., Geurts, H. M., Brink, E. L., & Prins, P. J. (2012). A pilot study of the efficacy of a computerized executive functioning remediation training with game elements for children with ADHD in an outpatient setting: outcome on parent- and teacher-rated executive functioning and ADHD behavior. *Journal of Attention Disorders* [epub Aug. 9, 2012].

Peck, H. L., Kehle, T. S., Bray, M. A., & Theodore, L. A. (2005). Yoga as an intervention for children with attention problems. *School Psychology Review, 34,* 415–424.

Pelsser, L. M., Frankena, K., Toorman, J., Savelkoul, H. F., Dubois, A. E., Pereira, R. R.,… Buitelaar, J. K. (2011). Effects of a restricted elimination diet on the behaviour of children with attention-deficit hyperactivity disorder (INCA study): a randomised controlled trial. *Lancet, 377*(9764), 5–11.

Pelsser, L. M., Frankene, K., Toorman, J., Savelkoul, H. F. J., Pereira, R. R., & Buitelaar, J. K. (2009). A randomised controlled trial into the effects of food on ADHD. *European Child and Adolescent Psychiatry, 18,* 12–19.

Rabiner, D.L., Murray, D.W., Skinner, A.T., & Malone, P.S. (2010). A randomized trial of two promising computer-based interventions for students with attention difficulties. *Journal of Abnormal Child Psychology, 38,* 131–142.

Rajwan, E., Chacko, A., & Moeller, M. (2012). Nonpharmacological interventions for preschool ADHD: State of the evidence and implications for practice. *Professional Psychology: Research and Practice, 43*(5), 520–526.

Re, O. (1974). 2-Dimethylaminoethanol (deanol): a brief review of its clinical efficacy and postulated mechanism of action. *Current Therapeutic Research, Clinical and Experimental, 16*(11), 1238–1242.

Reimherr, F. W., Wender, P. H., Wood, D. R., & Ward, M. (1987). An open trial of l-tyrosine in the treatment of attention deficit disorder, residual type. *American Journal of Psychiatry, 144,* 1071–1073.

Salehi, B. (2010). *Ginkgo biloba* for attention-deficit/hyperactivity disorder in children and adolescents: A double blind, randomized controlled trial. *Progress in Neuro-Psychopharmacology and Biological Psychiatry, 34,* 76–80.

Semrud-Clikeman, M., Nielsen, K. H., Clinton, A., Sylvester, L., Parle, N., & Connor, R. T. (1999). An intervention approach for children with teacher-and parent-identified attentional difficulties. *Journal of Learning Disabilities, 32,* 581–590.

Sever, Y., Ashkenazi, A., Tyano, S., & Weizman, A. (1997). Iron treatment in children with attention deficit hyperactivity disorder: A preliminary report. *Neuropsychobiology, 35,* 178–180.

Shalev, L., Tsal, Y., & Mevorach, C. (2007). Computerized progressive attentional training (CPAT) program: Effective direct intervention for children with ADHD. *Child Neuropsychology, 13,* 382–388.

Sinha, D., & Efron, D. (2005). Complimentary and alternative medicine use in children with attention deficit hyperactivity disorder. *Journal of Pediatric Child Health, 41,* 23–26.

Shekim, W. O., Antun, F., Hanna, G. L., & McCracken, J. T. (1990). S-adenosyl-L-methionine (SAM) in adults with ADHD, RS: Preliminary results from an open trial. *Psychopharmacology Bulletin, 26,* 249–253.

Smith, A. L., Hoza, B., Linnea, K., McQuade, J. D., Tomb, M., Vaughn, A. J., Shoulberg, E. K., & Hook, H. (2013). Pilot physical activity intervention reduces severity of ADHD symptoms in young children. *Journal of Attention Disorders, 17*(1), 70–82.

Sonuga-Barke, J. E. S., Brandeis, D., Cortese, S., Daley, D., Ferrin, M.,...European ADHD Guidelines Group (2013). Nonpharmacological intervention for ADHD: systematic review and meta-analyses of randomized controlled trials of dietary and psychological treatments. *American Journal of Psychiatry, 170,* 275–289.

Starobrat-Hermelin, B., & Kozielec, T. (1997). The effects of magnesium physiological supplementation on hyperactivity in children with ADHD: Positive response to magnesium oral loading test. *Magnesium Research, 10,* 149–156.

Stein, T. P., & Sammaritano, A. M. (1984). Nitrogen metabolism in normal and hyperkinetic boys. *American Journal of Clinical Nutrition, 39,* 520–524.

Steiner, N. J., Sheldrick, R. C., Gotthelf, D., & Perrin, E. C. (2011). Computer-based attention training in the schools for children with attention deficit/hyperactivity disorder: A preliminary trial. *Clinical Pediatrics, 50*(7), 615–22.

Stevenson, J., et al. (2010). The role of histamine degradation gene polymorphisms in moderating the effects of food additives on children's ADHD symptoms. *American Journal of Psychiatry, 167,* 108–1115.

Strauss, L. C. (2002). The efficacy of a homeopathic preparation in the management of attention deficit hyperactivity disorder. *Journal of Biomedical Therapy, 18*(2), 197–201.

Stubberfield, T. G., Wray, J. A., & Parry, T. S. (1999). Utilization of alternative therapies in attention-deficit/hyperactivity disorder. *Journal of Pediatric Child Health, 35,* 450–453.

Tamm, L., Hughes, C., Ames, L., Pickering, J., Silver, C.H., Stavinoha, P...Emslie, G. (2010). Attention training for school-aged children with ADHD: Results of an open trial. *Journal of Attention Disorders, 14*(1), 86–94.

Tamm, L., Nakonexny, P., & Hughes, C.W. (2012). An open trial of a metacognitive executive functioning training for young children with ADHD. *Journal of Attention Disorders.* Advance online publication. doi: 10.1177/1087054712445782

Timmons, B., W., Naylor, P., & Pfeiffner, K. (2007). Physical activity for preschool children—how much and how? *Applied Physiology, Nutrition, and Metabolism, 32,* S122–S134.

Trebaticka, J., Kopasova, S., Hradecna, Z., et al. (2006). Treatment of ADHD with French maritime pine bark extract, Pycnogenol. *European Child and Adolescent Psychiatry, 15,* 329–335.

Tjon Pian Gi, C. V., Broeren, J. P. A., Starreveld, J. S., & Versteegh, F. G. A. (2003). Melatonin for sleeping disorders in children with attention deficit/hyperactivity disorder: a preliminary open label study. *European Journal of Pediatrics, 162,* 554–555.

Trebaticka, J., Kopasova, S., Hradecna, Z., Cinorsky, K., Skodacek, I., Suba, J.,...Durackova, Z. (2006). Treatment of ADHD with French maritime pine bark extract, Pycnogenol. *European Child and Adolescent Psychiatry, 15,* 329–335.

Uckardes, Y., Ozmert, E. N., Unal, F., & Yurdakok, K. (2009). Effects of zinc supplementation on parent and teacher behaviour rating scores in low socioeconomic level Turkish primary school children. *Acta Paediatrica, 98,* 731–736.

van der Heiiden, K. B., Smits, M. G., van Someren, J. W., Ridderinkhof, K. R., & Gunning, W. B. (2007). Effect of melatonin on sleep, behavior, and cognition in ADHD and chronic sleep-onset insomnia. *Journal of the American Academy of Child and Adolescent Psychiatry, 46*(2), 233–241.

Van Oudheusden, L. J., & Scholte, H. R. (2002). Efficacy of carnitine in the treatment of children with attention-deficit hyperactivity disorder. *Prostaglandins, Leukotrienes and Essential Fatty Acids, 67*(1), 33–38.

Verret, C., Guay, M., Berthiaume, C., Gardiner, P., & Beliveau, L. (2012). A physical activity program improves behavior and cognitive functions in children with ADHD: An exploratory study. *Journal of Attention Disorders, 16,* 71–80.

Ward, N. I. (1997). Assessment of chemical factors in relation to child hyperactivity. *Journal of Nutritional & Environmental Medicine, 7*(4), 333–342.

Ward, N. I., Soulsbury, K. A., Zettel, V. H., Colquhoun, I. D., Bunday, S., & Barnes, B. (1990). The influence of the chemical additive tartrazine on the zinc status of hyperactive children: A double-blind placebo-controlled study. *Journal of Nutritional and Environmental Medicine, 1*(1), 51–58.

Weber, W., Steop, A. V., McCarty, R. L., Weiss, N. S., Biederman, J., & McClellan, J. (2008). *Hypericum perforatum* (St. John's Wort) for attention-deficit/hyperactivity disorder in children and adolescents: A randomized controlled trial. *JAMA, 299*(22), 2633–2641.

Weiss, M. D, Wasdell, M. B., Bomben, M. M., Rea, K. J., & Freeman, R. D. (2006). Sleep hygiene and melatonin treatment for children and adolescents with ADHD and initial insomnia. *Journal of the American Academy of Child and Adolescent Psychiatry, 45*(5), 513–519.

Wender, E. H. & Salanto, M. V. (1991). Effects of sugar on aggressive and inattention behavior in children with attention deficit disorder with hyperactivity and normal children. *Pediatrics, 88,* 960–966.

Wesnes, K. A., Pincock, C., Richardson, D., Helm, G., & Hails, S. (2003). Breakfast reduces declines in attention and memory over the morning in schoolchildren. *Appetite, 41,* 329–331.

Wolraich, M. L., Wilson, D. B., & White, J. W. (1995). The effect of sugar on behavior or cognition in children. *Journal of the American Medical Association, 274,* 1617–1621.

Wood, D. R., Reimherr, F. W., & Wender, P. H. (1985a). Treatment of attention-deficit disorder with dl-phenylalanine. *Psychiatry Research, 16,* 21–26.

Wood, D. R., Reimherr, F. W., & Wender, P. H. (1985b). Amino acid precursors for the treatment of attention-deficit disorder, residual type. *Psychopharmacology Bulletin, 21,* 146–149.

10

Sleep Problems and Interventions in Preschoolers with ADHD

MARK STEIN AND MARGARET D. WEISS

Sleep Problems in Preschool-Age Children

Sleep problems are frequently reported by parents of preschool-age children and may be due to a variety of interacting factors related to the child (e.g., age, enlarged tonsils, medicines delaying sleep onset or causing sedation, inability to settle after waking, nighttime fears), the parent (e.g., overstimulating the child before bed, lack of a consistent bedtime routine, difficulty setting limits, parental sleep disturbance or psychopathology), and the environment (e.g., bed sharing, noise, light). As children enter the preschool age, naps are discontinued and the average amount of sleep decreases to approximately 10 hours a night, with marked night-to-night variability (Scott. et al., 2012).

One of the most commonly reported sleep problems in this age group is difficulty initiating or going to sleep. According to Horne (1992), "the recipe for successful sleep...is a standard, unremitting pre-sleep routine...with the bedroom being seen by all as a place for peace and sleep rather than fun and excitement."

A second common sleep problem in children with symptoms of attention-deficit/hyperactivity disorder (ADHD) that has long been recognized in the medical literature is sleep-disordered breathing (i.e., snoring, obstructive sleep apnea/hypopnea, and obstructive hypoventilation). In 1889, Dr. William Hill in the *British Medical Journal* suggested that one of the "causes of backwardness and stupidity" is the "lazy child who frequently suffers from headaches at school, breathes through the mouth instead of his nose, snores, and is restless at night."

Restless legs syndrome (RLS) is a more recently recognized sleep problem whose symptoms overlap with ADHD (Cortese et al., 2005). RLS is characterized by an uncomfortable sensation in the legs resulting in the need to kick or move the legs, typically right before going to bed. As there is increasing awareness of RLS in the general public, it is being reported more frequently. However, preschoolers will not typically complain of RLS unless specifically questioned, because they cannot distinguish the symptoms as an abnormality.

Sleep Problems and ADHD

Although there is a relative lack of research on the relationship between sleep problems and ADHD in the preschool-age population, specifically, there is now a robust and growing research literature on the relationship between sleep problems and ADHD (Scott et al., 2012; Weiss & Salpekar, 2010). A caveat, however, is that what is known about ADHD in school-age children cannot necessarily be applied to preschoolers (e.g. Charach et al., 2013). There are several possible explanations for our limited knowledge of sleep problems and ADHD in preschool-age children. First, the diagnosis of ADHD in a preschooler is clinically more difficult than in older children (Greenhill, Posner, Vaughan, & Kratockvil, 2008). Moreover, differential diagnosis is complicated by high rates of overactivity and inattention behaviors in typical preschool-age children (Lapouse & Monk, 1964) and by other conditions that can mimic or exacerbate cognitive and behavioral symptoms of ADHD, including sleep disorders such as obstructive sleep apnea (Bonuck, Freeman, & Chervin, 2012; Pearl, Weiss, & Stein, 2001). Second, the preschool period is a time of marked changes in sleep routines and expectations; thus, some degree of stress in the establishment of new sleep habits and behaviors is to be expected. Finally, as preschool children begin attending school, for the first time there is an opportunity for a non-parental figure to observe the child and compare him or her to same-age peers during social, academic, and unstructured periods. Without multiple teacher reports and/or multiple observational settings, it can be difficult to disentangle early ADHD problems from difficulties masquerading as ADHD in the context of problematic family functioning. Furthermore, beginning a half- or full-day school program also encourages the family to develop a more consistent wake-up time and sleep schedule. As demands for sustaining attention and remaining on task increase, ADHD symptoms can become more obvious and allow for easier discrimination of ADHD from developmentally appropriate levels of activity and inattention, and the identification of impairment in a setting other than the home, which is a diagnostic requirement for ADHD (American Psychiatric Association, 1994, *Diagnostic and Statistical Manual of Mental Disorders,* 4th ed.). Thus, there are multiple changes and transitions that occur during this developmental period that can improve or exacerbate sleep problems and ADHD symptoms. Moreover, this is a critical period for the establishment of both zeitgebers (routines associated with becoming sleepy) and sleeping independently.

Enlarged tonsils or adenoids, allergies, and asthma medications may interfere with breathing at night and therefore require evaluation for sleep apnea. There is a literature that notes behavioral improvement in children who displayed ADHD symptoms but responded to tonsillectomy with improved behavior and lower rates of ADHD (Chervin et al., 2006). A more recent study indicated, however, that not all cognitive and behavioral difficulties resolve after the surgical treatment (Giordani et al., 2012). Results from the Childhood Adenotonsillectomy Trial (CHAT), designed to assess neuropsychological and health outcomes in children randomized to receive early surgical treatment compared to watchful waiting, will soon be available (Redline et al., 2011) and should address many of the limitations of earlier studies that were not randomized trials.

Therefore, evaluating for sleep problems is an important differential diagnosis in all age groups, but especially in preschoolers, as being tired during the day is a common symptom of both sleep-disordered breathing and ADHD (Chervin, 2000; Weinberg & Harper, 1993). If persistent or worsening of ADHD symptoms occurs despite treatment of the sleep problem, ADHD is more likely to be the underlying disorder.

Although ADHD and sleep studies rarely focus on the preschool-age population, findings from several cross-sectional and longitudinal studies have implications for the understanding of these phenomena in preschool children. Hiscock and colleagues (2007) reported that approximately a third of preschool-age children in a large epidemiologic sample of Australian children displayed mild to moderate sleep problems based upon parent report. Snoring occurred nightly for 12% of the sample, 8% took more than 30 minutes to fall asleep each night, and 5% would wake frequently during the night. Moderate or less frequent sleep problems were more common among participants, such as falling asleep during the day (12.3%), talking in sleep (15%), and tired during the day (18%). Insomnia was highly correlated with behavior and attention problems. Children with moderate/severe sleep problems were also 12 times more likely than those with no sleep problems to receive a diagnosis of ADHD. Of the 1% of children reportedly diagnosed with ADHD, 52% had a sleep problem.

Similar rates of sleep problems and associations with behavior problems were reported in a sample of 472 children between the ages of 4 to 12 years receiving routine pediatric care (Stein, Mendelsohn, Obermeyer, Amromin, & Benca, 2001). Problems such as snoring, tiredness during the day, and excessive sleep latency were very common, occurring at least one night per week in over 20% of the sample. Although in general reports of sleep problems declined with age, previous sleep problems before age 2 years were the single best predictor of current sleep problems. Furthermore, current sleep problems were highly correlated with parent reports of both internalizing and externalizing behavior problems and inattention.

Lavigne and colleagues (1999) surveyed sleep and behavior problems in 510 2- to 5-year-old children from pediatric clinics. Less sleep was associated with both internalizing and externalizing behavior problems and with psychiatric diagnosis. Similarly, Willoughby and colleagues (2008) analyzed sleep problems in a group of 193 preschool-age children at risk for ADHD. Inattentive symptoms were related to daytime sleepiness, which was related to longer sleep duration, beyond common psychiatric comorbidities.

Thunstrom (2002) conducted a 5-year prospective study in 2,518 infants between 6 and 18 months of age and their parents, and followed children with severe sleep problems in infancy and a control group to determine if they were at increased risk of ADHD. Parents of 83% of the enrolled infants responded to a questionnaire; 27 infants with severe sleep problems and a matched control group were identified. An in-depth assessment by a multidisciplinary team was conducted when the participants were 5.5 years old; seven of the children in the sleep problem group met the criteria for the diagnosis of ADHD compared to none of the controls. The infants in the sleep problem group were characterized by psychosocial problems in the family, bedtime struggles, and extended sleep latency. Although the numbers are small, the findings from this prospective study suggest that up to a quarter of infants with severe sleep problems may be at risk for later diagnosis of ADHD in preschool years.

More recently, Scott and colleagues (2012) tracked a sample of 8,195 infants longitudinally over 11 years since birth, and 173 were eventually diagnosed with ADHD.

Shorter sleep duration and sleep disturbances appeared early in the ADHD group and predated the clinical diagnosis.

Difficulty initiating sleep was the most commonly reported sleep problem associated with ADHD across the aforementioned studies. Parents often struggle with their preschool children over bedtime, and in the past this has been largely interpreted as bedtime resistance or behavioral insomnia. The children themselves, however, often describe that they do not like to go to bed because "they cannot turn their thoughts off" and find themselves alone, restless, hyperalert, and bored. Van der Heijden demonstrated that bedtime resistance in ADHD children was often a behavioral manifestation of difficulty with circadian rhythm (Van der Heijden, Smits, & Gunning, 2006; Van der Heijden, Smits, Von Someren, & Gunning, 2005; Van der Heijden, Smits, Van Someren, Ridderinkof, & Gunning, 2007). Clearly, difficulty initiating sleep and bedtime resistance represent etiologically heterogeneous problems that have direct relevance to ADHD and its treatment with either behavioral or pharmacologic interventions (Stein, Weiss, & Hlavaty, 2012). If untreated, decreased total sleep time for the child as well as indirect effects on the family can adversely affect cognitive, behavioral, and health outcomes.

Parent-reported sleep-disordered breathing symptoms were present in 25% of 5-year-olds studied in a cross-sectional sample of 3,019 children from Massachusetts. Hyperactivity and inattention symptoms were also common, occurring in 19% and 18% of the sample, respectively. Sleep-disordered breathing was associated with a twofold increase in ADHD symptoms (Gottlieb et al., 2003).

Sleep-disordered breathing is now a well-established differential diagnosis of ADHD (Chervin, 2005; Dillon et al., 2007). What is less clear is why the preschool population, like those who are obese in late middle age, may be at particular risk of difficulty breathing at night. Some possible explanations for increased sleep-disordered breathing include the relative size of the adenoids and tonsils to the trachea in preschoolers and an excess of allergic rhinitis, colds, and asthma in this age group. Since most preschoolers are sleeping alone (unlike adults who share a bed), detection may also be less likely as parents may be unaware of apneic episodes.

Both subjective (parental report) and objective (actigraphic) approaches were employed to investigate the relationship between sleep and ADHD-like symptoms in 186 2- to 5-year-old children who had autistic disorder, developmental delay without autism, or no developmental delay (typically developing) (Goodlin-Jones, Tang, Liu, & Anders, 2009). Parent-reported ADHD composites were obtained on each child using the Child Behavior Checklist. Children who had an ADHD composite in the clinical range as rated by their parents were significantly more likely to be described as having a sleep problem. However, no significant differences in actigraphic measures were found for children who had an ADHD composite in the clinical range.

Marked differences between objective (polysomnography, actigraphy) and subjective (parent complaints) measures of sleep were common in the early stages of research on sleep and ADHD (Corkum, Moldofsky, Hogg-Johnson, Humphries, & Tannok, 1999). However, more recent studies and meta-analyses using objective sleep measures also report excessive daytime sleepiness, RLS, and periodic limb movements (Cortese, Faraone, Konofal, & Lecendreux, 2009). One potential explanation of this difference is that night-to-night variability in sleep informs parent reports. If their child has insomnia one or two nights a week that is disruptive and leads to impairments, parents will report sleep problems. On the other hand, one or two nights of polysomnography in the sleep lab will not necessarily identify this problem or the impairment it causes. Fortunately, current advances in technology allow for more ecologically valid assessment of sleep using actigraphy and in-home polysomnography (Owens, Spririto, & McGuinn, 2000).

Thus, both sleep problems and ADHD symptoms are common in preschool-age children. Although ADHD is less commonly diagnosed in preschoolers compared to older children, more than half of children with ADHD had a history of sleep problems that predate the onset of ADHD. Preschool children whose symptoms are severe enough to meet criteria for one disorder (sleep problems or ADHD) are clearly at heightened risk for the other disorder.

Clinical Presentation

Although pediatricians may receive relatively little formal training in either sleep disorders or ADHD in the preschool population, in clinical practice this is a very common reason for parents to seek help from their child's primary healthcare provider. Parents will come in with a multitude of complaints that may include refusal to go to bed, inability to settle, needing the parent present in the room, recurrent requests to leave the room, or co-sleeping with the parent. Typically, the primary healthcare provider will respond to these concerns with various parent guides, such as the Ferber "cry-it-out" method (1990). This is often where the difference between common problems with sleep entrainment and a true sleep disorder, or a sleep disorder characteristic of ADHD, becomes apparent. When the parents of such a child attempt to enforce the usual behavioral recommendations, they will often return upset and disturbed that these methods were not only ineffective but traumatic: their child screamed, vomited, and climbed out of the crib and the result was increased distress rather than improvement. In this circumstance, the primary healthcare provider should be cautious to avoid parent blaming and do a more rigorous examination of sleep patterns and other possible environmental or biologic contributing factors or refer the child to a sleep specialist.

Some problems are more specifically characteristic of the presentation of sleep difficulty in the presence of ADHD. These include the signs of sleep apnea, such as mouth breathing, snoring, being overweight, or postures during sleep indicating attempts to keep a patent airway. Excessive daytime sleepiness alongside erratic sleep patterns and night-to-night variability in sleep is also characteristic of sleep problems in children with ADHD (Cortese et al., 2009). Similarly, one of the early diagnostic criteria for ADHD, which remains a common current complaint, is restless sleep, in which the child is kicking (possible periodic limb movements) or unusually active during sleep. Enuresis occurs in up to 33% of children with ADHD and can often interfere with sleep (Stein et al., 2012). Some of these problems will come to the primary healthcare provider as a complaint by the parent. Other problems emerge in taking a good sleep history, such as asking the child about sensations of RLS or if he or she finds it hard to wind down in the evening, and/or asking the parent to observe the child while the child is sleeping. Another frequent parental complaint is about the child who cannot fall asleep easily and is in such a deep sleep in the morning that he or she cannot be wakened easily to prepare for preschool. Many parents of preschool children with a delayed sleep phase or other symptoms of a circadian rhythm sleep disorder will compensate for the problem by choosing an afternoon nursery, which entrains a sleep pattern that becomes problematic when the child starts attending a full day of school.

Assessment and Treatment Implications and Interventions

ASSESSMENT OF SLEEP PROBLEMS PRIOR TO ADHD TREATMENT

In evaluating preschool children for ADHD, a sleep history should be obtained routinely before starting treatment. Key questions include: Does the child have difficulty going to bed or falling asleep? Does the child maintain a regular sleep schedule? Does the child wake up or display unusual behaviors at night? Does the child snore? Is it hard to wake the child up in the morning? Does the child appear tired during the day? Taking a good sleep history in a complex case is time-consuming. A good place to start is with a sleep log or sleep diary in which the parent documents sleep patterns (www.sleepfoundation.org) and a simple rating scale, such as the Children's Sleep Habits Questionnaire (Owens et al., 2000) or the Pediatric Sleep Questionnaire (Chervin et al., 2007), which are available for routine use. When the parent returns the clinician can review this information in more detail and more efficiently. Nonetheless, all children should be screened for primary sleep problems. An easy acronym for routine sleep screening is BEARS (Mindell & Owens, 2003), described in detail in Table 10.1, and is appropriate to the preschool population.

MANAGEMENT OF CIRCADIAN RHYTHM ISSUES

One of the major developmental challenges of the preschool period is the "teaching of sleep hygiene." Sleep should be in a comfortable place and a sleep routine should be established. A child's sleep schedule should be as stable as possible: changing bedtime from one night to another impairs the child's ability to train his or her brain to feel fatigue and the need for sleep. Night-to-night variability in sleep can be affected by medication schedules and exacerbated by poor compliance. Other sources of sleep disturbance such as siblings keeping each other awake, use of bright light, or overstimulating video games late at night should be discouraged. Children need to "learn" to initiate sleep by themselves and to settle themselves upon waking, but this is a process that should be rewarded, described as a sign of maturity, and not presented suddenly or in a punitive manner. Further, parents need to be aware that putting a child to bed early, when the child has not built a sleep debt, is a poor way to phase-advance sleep onset. Waking a child earlier in the morning so that the child becomes tired earlier in the evening is more effective. Preschool children will also learn good sleep hygiene when they see it modeled in siblings and parents. As a result we often see sleep problems not only in one child but also in multiple members of a family. Conversely, when one child has succeeded in establishing a good sleep routine, parents will often note a beneficial impact on the rest of the family.

Table 10.1. **"BEARS" Sleep Screening Algorithm**

The BEARS instrument is divided into five major sleep domains, providing a comprehensive screen for the major sleep disorders affecting children in the 2- to 18-year-old range. Each sleep domain has a set of age-appropriate "trigger questions" for use in the clinical interview.

B = *bedtime problems*
E = *excessive daytime sleepiness*
A = *awakenings during the night*
R = *regularity and duration of sleep*
S = *snoring*

Examples of developmentally appropriate trigger questions:

	Toddler/preschool (2-5 years)
Bedtime problems	Does your child have any problems going to bed? Falling asleep?
Excessive daytime sleepiness	Does your child seem overtired or sleepy a lot during the day? Does he/she still take naps?
Awakenings during the night	Does your child wake up a lot at night?
Regularity and duration of sleep	Does your child have a regular bedtime and wake time? What are they?
Snoring	Does your child snore a lot or have difficulty breathing at night?

Source: *A Clinical Guide to Pediatric Sleep: Diagnosis and Management of Sleep Problems* by Jodi A. Mindell and Judith A. Owens; used with permission from Lippincott Williams & Wilkins.

MANAGEMENT OF STIMULANT-INDUCED SLEEP PROBLEMS

Randomized, double-blind placebo-controlled trials of stimulant medications in preschool children with ADHD have consistently found a relatively attenuated benefit-to-risk ratio compared to elementary-school–age children (Ghuman et al., 2009; Greenhill et al., 2006; Lee et al., 2012). In general, younger age is associated with more frequent side effects, including irritability, decreased appetite. and problems with sleep. It should be noted that use of a daytime stimulant in a child who is still napping may interfere both with evening insomnia and the restorative sleep of the daytime nap that the child is accustomed to. It is important for clinicians to be aware that exacerbating sleep problems in a preschool child is not just a "nuisance" side effect, and that stimulants may improve daytime behavior at the cost of mood, health, growth, and overall well-being. Therefore, sleep problems associated with stimulants should be evaluated and taken seriously. Furthermore, preexisting sleep problems should be treated and stabilized if possible before the initiation of stimulants.

There are very few data on the use of nonstimulants in preschoolers with ADHD. Both atomoxetine and alpha agonists are effective in reducing ADHD symptoms. In a study of 5- and 6-year-olds with ADHD treated with atomoxetine or placebo, 30% of the atomoxetine group displayed sedation (Kratochvil et al., 2011). These agents may contribute to daytime sleepiness, fatigue and sedation, or night wakings but generally do not increase insomnia or latency to sleep onset.

Immediate-release formulations of clonidine have been used off-label to treat sleep problems in children with ADHD. Prince and colleagues (1996) conducted a retrospective chart review of 42 children ages 4 to 12 treated with clonidine and reported that low-dose clonidine had a beneficial effect on sleep problems in 85% of the sample, most of whom were not in the preschool age range. Age, gender, comorbidity, or concurrent pharmacotherapy was not associated with response, which also did not differ by whether sleep problems were present before treatment or were medicine-induced or medicine-exacerbated. The effects on sleep of new extended-release formulations of alpha-2 agonists as yet have not been studied, although somnolence is a common side effect when used as monotherapy.

When a new sleep problem is reported during medication treatment of ADHD, the first line of intervention is to evaluate the dose, timing of medication administration, and then choice of medication to see if the sleep problems can be managed conservatively. Given the short half-life of short-acting stimulants, several trials can be done quickly with different doses, schedules, or formulations of methylphenidate or amphetamine.

If these strategies are ineffective and prolonged sleep latency persists, augmenting stimulant treatment with melatonin is often recommended. There are now several well-designed, randomized, double-blind, placebo-controlled trials using melatonin as a hypnotic at doses of 3 to 6 mg administered 30 minutes before bedtime. Melatonin may provide relief for both the insomnia associated with ADHD and worsening of the insomnia associated with stimulant treatment of ADHD. The evidence to date is that melatonin is a safe and effective treatment that can be used in children (Carr et al., 2007; Van der Heijden et al., 2007). Nonetheless, there is an absence of controlled studies evaluating medications to treat insomnia secondary to stimulants in preschoolers. Thus, we recommend consultation from a behavioral sleep medicine specialist prior to the use of a medication other than melatonin.

CLINICAL RECOMMENDATIONS

1. Screen for sleep problems with interview and rating scales as part of the differential diagnosis and evaluate further and/or treat primary sleep problems (e.g., sleep-disordered breathing).
2. Assess sleep (duration, behaviors, and variability) before and during administration of ADHD treatment.
3. Look for opportunities to improve sleep hygiene (e.g., similar bedtimes each night, limit video exposure, assess parental sleep habits and evening schedules).
4. If stimulant-induced insomnia occurs:
   4.1. Reduce the total dose.
   4.2. Change the dosing schedule.
   4.3. Change the treatment formulation so that less medication is administered later in the day.
   4.4. Change to a different stimulant (e.g., switch to methylphenidate from amphetamine or vice versa).

4.5. Consider switching to a nonstimulant (such as atomoxetine) or combining stimulant (administered during daytime) and alpha-2 agonist (administered in the evening).

4.6. Add a sleep-promoting medication (e.g., melatonin as a first-line agent, or another medication if indicated).

Summary

Inadequate and/or inconsistent sleep patterns are associated with a range of negative outcomes in preschool children, including behavior problems and ADHD. Preschool sleep issues and the prodrome of attention and sleep problems are common and intertwined complaints. Sleep problems such as difficulty initiating sleep, sleep-disordered breathing, and RLS overlap with ADHD and should be watched for, as additional interventions may be necessary. Stimulant medications adversely affect sleep, especially in younger children, and may contribute to delayed sleep onset, less total sleep, and difficulty waking up. Nonstimulants can affect alertness during the day and the quality of sleep. In preschoolers with ADHD, effective management needs to address both ADHD symptoms and sleep issues.

The research on sleep and ADHD in older children and adults shows remarkable parallels. More research is needed to see if this will also be true as we learn more about the nature of sleep issues in the preschool population. The same level of research devoted to sleep issues in later life has yet to determine the biology, the role of melatonin, and the patterns of sleep hygiene in preschool children. However, if it were in fact possible to intervene with ADHD-friendly methods of entrainment of sleep patterns in this critical phase of development, it raises the question as to whether later impairment in sleep that is characteristic of individuals with ADHD could be prevented (Kooij et al., 2010).

Disclosures

Dr. Weiss has received honoraria, speaker board fees, research funds, and consultant fees from Eli Lilly and Co, Janssen, Purdue, and Shire.

Dr. Stein receives research support from Shire and is a consultant to Novartis and Shire.

References

American Psychiatric Association. (1994). *Diagnostic and statistical manual of mental disorders,* 4th ed. Washington, DC: APA.

Bonuck, K., Freeman, K., Chervin, R. D., & Xu, L. (2012). Sleep-disordered breathing in a population-based cohort: behavioral outcomes at 4 and 7 years. *Pediatrics, 129,* e857–865.

Carr, R. Wasdell, M,. Hamilton, D., Weiss, M., Freeman, R., Tai, J. Rietveld, W. J., & Jan, J. E. (2007). Long-term effectiveness outcome of melatonin therapy in children with treatment-resistant circadian rhythm sleep disorders. *Journal of Pineal Research,* 43(4), 353–359.

Charach, A., Carson P, Fox S, Ali M., Beckett J., & Lim, C. (2013) Interventions for preschool children at high risk for ADHD: A comparative effectiveness review. *Pediatrics, 131,* e1584–e1604.

Chervin, R. D. (2000). Sleepiness, fatigue, tiredness, and lack of energy in obstructive sleep apnea. *Chest, 118,* 372–379.

Chervin, R. D. (2005). How many children with ADHD have sleep apnea or periodic leg movements on polysomnography? *Sleep, 28,* 1041–1042.

Chervin, R. D., Ruzicka, D. L., Giordani, B. J., Weatherly, R. A., Dillon, J. E., Hodges, E. K., et al. (2006). Sleep-disordered breathing, behavior, and cognition in children before and after adenotonsillectomy. *Pediatrics, 117,* e769–e778.

Chervin, R. D., Weatherly, R. A., Garetz, S. L., Ruzicka, D. L., Giordani, B. J., & Hodges, E. K. (2007) Pediatric Sleep Questionnaire: prediction of sleep apnea and outcomes. *Otolaryngology Head & Neck Surgery, 133,* 216–222.

Corkum, P., Moldofsky, H., Hogg-Johnson, S., Humphries, T., & Tannock, R. (1999). Sleep problems in children with attention-deficit/hyperactivity disorder: impact of subtype, comorbidity, and stimulant medication. *Journal of the American Academy of Child and Adolescent Psychiatry, 38,* 1285–1293.

Cortese, S., Faraone, S. V., Konofal, E., & Lecendreux, M. (2009). Sleep in children with attention-deficit/hyperactivity disorder: meta-analysis of subjective and objective studies. *Journal of the American Academy of Child and Adolescent Psychiatry, 48,* 894–908.

Cortese, S., Konofal, E., Lecendreux, M., Arnulf, I., Mouren, M. C., Darra, F., et al. (2005). Restless legs syndrome and attention-deficit/hyperactivity disorder: a review of the literature. *Sleep, 28,* 1007–1013.

Dillon, J. E., Blunden, S., Ruzicka, D. L., Giure, K. E., Champine, D., & Weatherly, R.A. et al. (2007). DSM-IV diagnoses and obstructive sleep apnea in children before and 1 year after adenotonsillectomy. *Journal of the American Academy of Child and Adolescent Psychiatry, 46,* 1425–1436.

Ferber, R. (1990). Sleep schedule-dependent causes of insomnia and sleepiness in middle childhood and adolescence. *Pediatrician, 17,* 13–20.

Ghuman, J. K., Aman, M.G., Lecavalier, L., Riddle, M. A., Gelenberg, A., & Wright, R., et al. (2009). Randomized, placebo-controlled, crossover study of methylphenidate for attention-deficit/ hyperactivity disorder symptoms in preschoolers with developmental disorders. *Journal of Child and Adolescent Psychopharmacology, 19,* 329–339.

Giordani, B., Hodges, E. K., Guire, K. E., Ruzicka, D. L., Dillon, J. E., Weatherly, R. A., et al. (2012). Changes in neuropsychological and behavioral functioning in children with and without obstructive sleep apnea following Tonsillectomy. *Journal of the International Neuropsychology Society, 18,* 212–222.

Goodlin-Jones, B., Tang, K., Liu, J., & Anders, T. F. (2009). Sleep problems, sleepiness and daytime behavior in preschool-age children. *Journal of Child Psychology and Psychiatry, 50,* 1532–1540.

Gottlieb, D., Vezina, R., Chase, C., Lesko, S., Heeren, T., Weese-Mayer, S., et al. (2003). Symptoms of sleep-disordered breathing in 5-year old children are associated with sleepiness and problem behaviors. *Pediatrics, 112,* 870–877.

Greenhill, L., Kollins, S., Abikoff, H., McCracken, J., Riddle, M., Swanson, J., et al. (2006). Efficacy and safety of immediate-release methylphenidate treatment for preschoolers with ADHD. *Journal of the American Academy of Child and Adolescent Psychiatry, 45,* 1284–1293.

Greenhill, L. L., Posner, K., Vaughan, B. S., & Kratochvil, C. J. (2008). Attention deficit hyperactivity disorder in preschool children. *Child & Adolescent Psychiatry Clinics of North America, 17,* 347–366, ix.

Hill, W. (1889). On some causes of backwardness and stupidity in children: and the relief of these symptoms in some instances by naso-pharyngeal scarifications. *British Medical Journal, 2,* 711.

Hiscock, H., Canterford, L., Ukoumunne, O. C., & Wake, M. (2007). Adverse associations of sleep problems in Australian preschoolers: national population study. *Pediatrics, 119,* 86–93.

Horne, J. (1992). Annotation: sleep and its disorders in children. *Journal of Child Psychology and Psychiatry, 33,* 437–487.

Kooij, S.J., Bejerot, S., Blackwell, A., Caci, H., Casas-Brugue, M., Carpentier, P. J., et al. (2010). European consensus statement on diagnosis and treatment of adult ADHD: The European Network Adult ADHD. *BMC Psychiatry, 10*(67), 1–24.

Kratochvil, C. J., Vaughan, B. S., Stoner, J. A., Daughton, J. M., Lubberstedt, B. D., Murray, D. W., et al. (2011). A double-blind, placebo-controlled study of atomoxetine in young children with ADHD. *Pediatrics, 127*, e862–e868.

Lapouse, R., & Monk, M. A. (1964). Behavior deviations in a representative sample of children: variation by sex, age, race, social class and family size. *American Journal of Orthopsychiatry, 34*, 436–446.

Lavigne, J. V., Arend, R., Rosenbaum, D., Smith, A., Weissbluth, M., Binns, H. J., et al. (1999). Sleep and behavior problems among preschoolers. *Journal of Developmental and Behavioral Pediatrics, 20*, 164–169.

Lee, S., Seo, W., Sung, H., Choi, T., Kim, B. K., & Lee, J. H. (2012). Effect of methylphenidate on sleep parameters in children with ADHD. *Psychiatric Investigation, 9*, 384–390.

Mindell, J., & Owens, J. (2003). *A clinical guide to pediatric sleep: Diagnosis and management of sleep problems.* Philadelphia, PA: Wolters Kluwer Health/Lippincott Williams & Wilkins.

Owens, J. A., Spirito, A., & McGuinn, M. (2000). The Children's Sleep Habits Questionnaire (CSHQ): psychometric properties of a survey instrument for school-aged children. *Sleep, 23*, 1043–1051.

Pearl, P. L., Weiss, R. E., & Stein, M. A. (2001). Medical mimics: medical and neurological conditions simulating ADHD. *Annals of the New York Academy of Science, 931*, 97–112.

Prince, J., Wilens T. E., Biederman, J., Spencer, T., & Wozniak, J (1996). Clonidine for sleep disturbances associated with attention-deficit hyperactivity disorder: a systematic chart review of 62 cases. *Journal of the American Academy of Child and Adolescent Psychiatry, 35*, 599–605.

Redline, S., Amin, R., Beebe, D., Chervin, R. D., Garetz, S. L., Giordani, B., et al. (2011). The Childhood Adenotonsillectomy Trial (CHAT): rationale, design, and challenges of a randomized controlled trial evaluating a standard surgical procedure in a pediatric population. *Sleep, 34*, 1509–1517.

Scott, N., Blair, P. S., Emond, A. M., Fleming, P. J., Humphreys, J. S., Henderson, J., et al. (2012). Sleep patterns in children with ADHD: a population-based cohort study from birth to 11 years. *Journal of Sleep Research.* [epub Oct. 12, 2012].

Stein, M., Weiss, M., & Hlavaty, L. (2012). ADHD treatments, sleep, and sleep problems: complex associations. *Neurotherapeutics, 9*, 509–517.

Stein, M. A., Mendelsohn, J., Obermeyer, W. H., Amromin, J., & Benca, R. (2001). Sleep and behavior problems in school-aged children. *Pediatrics, 107*, E60.

Thunstrom, M. (2002). Severe sleep problems in infancy associated with subsequent development of attention-deficit/hyperactivity disorder at 5.5 years of age. *Acta Paediatrica, 91*, 584–592.

Van der Heijden, K. B., Smits, M. G., & Gunning, W. B. (2006). Sleep hygiene and actigraphically evaluated sleep characteristics in children with ADHD and chronic sleep onset insomnia. *Journal of Sleep Research, 15*, 55–62.

Van der Heijden, K. B., Smits, M. G., Van Someren, E. J., & Gunning, W. B. (2005). Idiopathic chronic sleep onset insomnia in attention-deficit/hyperactivity disorder: a circadian rhythm sleep disorder. *Chronobiology International, 22*, 559–570.

Van der Heijden, K. B., Smits, M.G., Van Someren, E. J., Ridderinkhof, K. R., & Gunning, W. B. (2007). Effect of melatonin on sleep, behavior, and cognition in ADHD and chronic sleep-onset insomnia. *Journal of the American Academy of Child and Adolescent Psychiatry, 46*, 233–241.

Weinberg, W. A., & Harper, C. R. (1993). Vigilance and its disorders. *Neurologic Clinics, 11*, 59–78.

Weiss, M. D., & Salpekar, J. (2010). Sleep problems in the child with attention-deficit hyperactivity disorder: defining aetiology and appropriate treatments. *CNS Drugs, 24*, 811–828.

Willoughby, M. T., Angold, A., & Egger, H. L. (2008). Parent-reported attention-deficit/hyperactivity disorder symptomatology and sleep problems in a preschool-age pediatric clinical sample. *Journal of the American Academy of Child and Adolescent Psychiatry, 47*, 1086–1094.

Index

Tables are indicated by an italic "*t*" following the page number.